Reader's Digest Guide to
Vitamins, Minerals
and Supplements

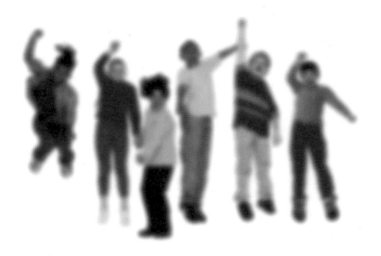

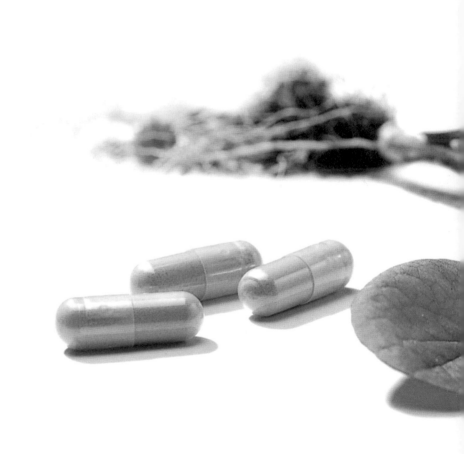

Reader's Digest Guide to
Vitamins, Minerals
and Supplements

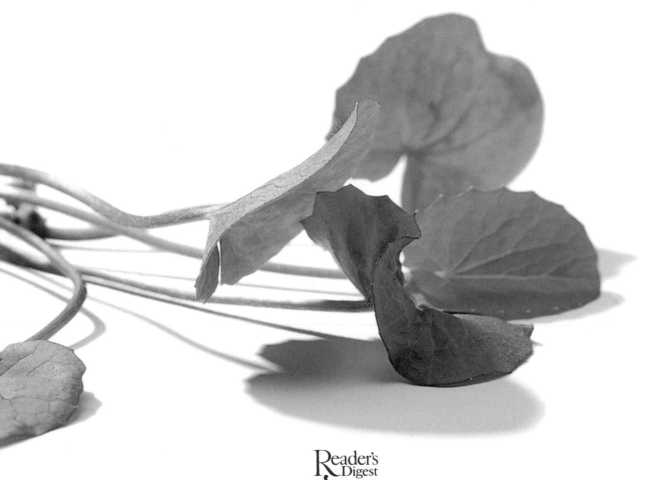

Reader's
Digest

Published by The Reader's Digest Association, Inc.
London ■ New York ■ Sydney ■ Montreal

CHIEF CONSULTANTS

DR ALAN LAKIN was Senior Lecturer on Food Chemistry at the University of Reading, where his research was centred on food proteins, before he retired in 1997. He became interested in the scientific basis of natural therapies because of their contribution to his recovery from chronic fatigue syndrome following a teaching assignment in Africa. Dr Lakin is married to Ann Walker.

DR ANN WALKER is Senior Lecturer in Human Nutrition at the University of Reading with degrees in biochemistry and food science. She is also a medical herbalist and is a member of the National Institute of Medical Herbalists and of the College of Practitioners of Phytotherapy. Her research involves clinical studies on the therapeutic applications of vitamins, minerals and herbs and their action on the human body.

DR JOHN CORMACK is a Senior Partner in a general practice in Essex. He is also Regional Press Secretary for the BMA. Both a writer and a broadcaster, he is co-author (with Dr Andrei Calin) of *Arthritis and Rheumatism – Your Questions Answered*, and was a founder member of the Media Medics team of radio broadcasters.

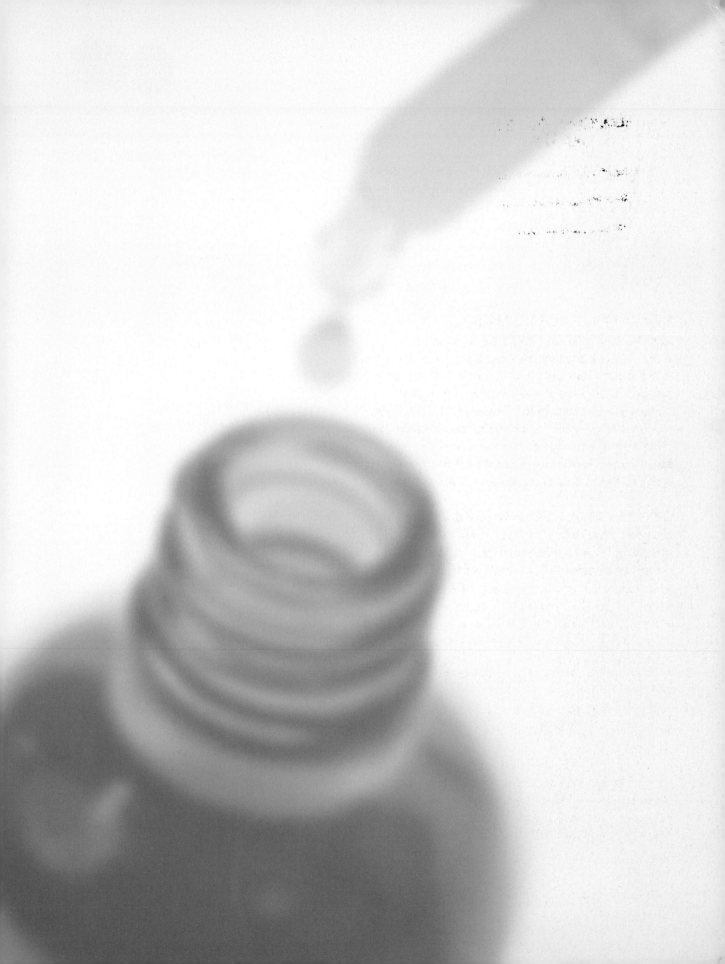

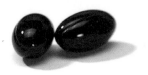

INTRODUCTION

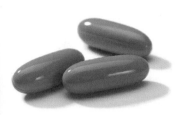

Part I SUPPLEMENTS

This colour-coded section contains:

● vitamins ● minerals ● herbs ● nutritional supplements

Part 2 PROTECTING YOUR HEALTH

A guide to the prevention and treatment of some common disorders

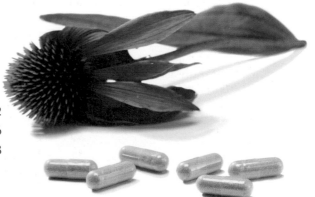

Foreword

Expectation of life at the dawn of the 21st century is higher than ever because of the reduced incidence of infectious diseases – but it could be higher still and quality of life could also be better. Unfortunately, in place of the infections to which our ancestors succumbed, chronic illnesses – including heart disease, diabetes and cancer – have now become established as the major killers. Few people realise that this epidemic of chronic disease is largely preventable through diet and lifestyle changes.

My interest in using supplements and herbs for the improvement of health stems from their successful use in treating the chronic fatigue that my husband suffered for eight years. Seeing his health steadily improve under the guidance of a herbalist inspired me to retrain in herbal medicine. Since then I have been able to observe, both in patients and from my research at the University of Reading, that a combination of good diet, nutrient supplements and herbs provides a powerful healing approach to a wide range of ailments – the rationale for this book.

Although good nutrition is the foundation of good health, many people do not reach their recommended target intakes for vitamins and minerals. This is mainly due to lack of exercise and poor food choice. Year by year, surveys show that food intakes are going down but average body weight is increasing. The explanation is lack of exercise. People reduce their food consumption to avoid becoming overweight, but this also reduces the intake of vitamins and minerals, as well as reducing calories. Lack of nutrient-rich fruit and vegetables and wholegrain cereals in the diet adds to the problem.

Poor health is often associated with low intakes of essential nutrients – the cells of the

HOW'S YOUR DIET?

If you experience symptoms of ill health such as fatigue, low mood or frequent infections, the first step towards putting things right is to consider your diet:

◻ Are you eating enough fruit and vegetables? The recommended intake of five portions a day provides potassium, vitamins and phytochemicals in quantities that no other food group provides. The antioxidant properties of these foods are particularly important, and yet most people fail to achieve even half the recommended intake.

◻ Are you eating wholegrain cereal products? These are rich sources of magnesium, trace elements and B complex vitamins. Consumption of refined cereal products may jeopardise intakes of these vital nutrients.

◻ Are you balancing your essential fatty acids (EFAs)? We require EFAs of two families: omega-6 and omega-3. Eating lots of polyunsaturated margarine (rich in omega-6 fats) and too little oily fish (rich in omega-3 fats) upsets the balance, and inflammation may result.

If the answer to any of the questions above is 'no', then changing your diet should be your first priority. The supplements described in this book are intended to augment a good diet, not to replace it. A daily 'A-Z' multivitamin and multimineral supplement is likely to be a sensible choice for people who take little exercise, for those who suffer minor illnesses and older people. In addition, higher levels of intake of some nutrients (such as vitamins C and E) will be required in order to achieve optimum health.

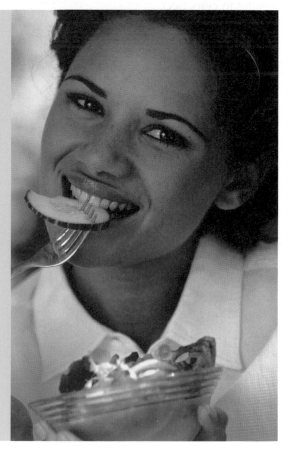

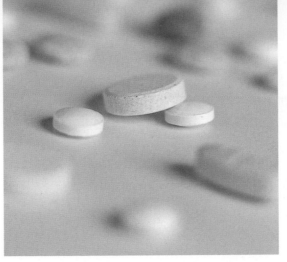

immune and nervous systems are particularly susceptible. The body's ability to maintain normal healthy functioning of cells depends on homeostasis, its self-healing capacity. An important element in homeostasis is the supply of nutrients, and each cell requires more than 40 of these, as well as protective substances, called phytochemicals, from plants.

Another important contributor to homeostasis is the elimination of toxic end-products of metabolism from a cell. Elimination requires a healthy circulation and good liver and kidney function, all of which rely on adequate intakes of vitamins, minerals and phytochemicals. Inadequate nutrition or inadequate elimination results in cells becoming stressed, so they begin to function abnormally. If this situation persists, normal homeostatic control breaks down, and eventually disease results.

Since many chronic illnesses derive from years of poor food choice, health is likely to be restored more quickly if supplements are taken at the same time as the changeover to a good diet is made. For example, the inflammation associated with asthma, eczema, psoriasis and rheumatoid arthritis is likely to respond much more quickly to supplementation with vitamins C and E and omega-3 EFAs than to dietary improvement alone – even though achieving improvement through diet is the long-term ideal. You may also find your symptoms disappear more quickly if you take a combination of supplements. This is because all cells require all nutrients at the same time.

The recommendations for the use of the vitamins and minerals described in this book are based on the results of studies with human subjects, and the levels for maximum intakes are based on *Safe upper levels for vitamins and minerals* (Expert Group on Vitamins and Minerals, 2003). These limits are safe for self-administration, although a nutritional therapist might suggest higher levels after a consultation.

Natural medicines are mild in effect and have greater therapeutic potential when taken in combination – herbs can be taken along with vitamins and minerals to help speed the healing process. Scientific research backs up the historical use of the herbs described in this book; they are rich sources of numerous phytochemicals, and, like nutrients, they have healing effects on all the body's cell, as well as on specific organs.

Since prehistory, medical herbalists throughout the world have successfully used combinations of herbs to treat their patients. This traditional knowledge cannot be conveyed in detail in a book such as this, although some information is given on pages 78-79. The use of single herbs is described instead, which should be adequate for many minor ailments, and particularly when the herb is taken with vitamins and minerals. If your illness does not respond to such self-treatment, a visit to a medical herbalist may well prove to be more effective.

My husband, Alan Lakin, and I are delighted to be associated with this book. As we have found for ourselves, natural medicine has enormous potential healing power. We hope that the wealth of information presented here will enable many more people to improve their well-being and quality of life.

Ann F Walker PhD, MNIMH, MCPP

The new age of nutritional and herbal medicines

Sneeze – and it's not unusual for someone to recommend vitamin C or echinacea. Complain about premenstrual syndrome – and the chances are that a friend will suggest that you try evening primrose oil.

A third of adults of all ages and from all walks of life in the UK now regularly use supplements as preventative therapies or to treat ailments ranging from colds and headaches to arthritis, depression and heart disease.

Food scares and poor diet

Recent scares about food safety have proved that achieving a healthy diet is much more complex than simply eating the right things.

Although there is no scientific evidence that modern farming methods have changed the nutritional value of foods, there is no doubt that subtle changes in our diet are taking place.

We are now eating varieties of fruit and vegetables that have been bred for high yields, good storage characteristics, and uniformity in appearance and texture; little consideration has been given to nutritional attributes.

These new varieties also tend to be less colourful and have less flavour than their predecessors, which suggests that they are less well endowed with phytochemicals. There are other factors too. The levels of trace elements in food crops are affected by the soil in which they are grown, and yet it is unusual for these vital minerals to be included in the fertilisers applied to intensively grown crops.

For example, government-sponsored research shows that our intake of selenium has fallen since the 1970s, mostly as a result of the growth in consumption of selenium-poor European wheat in place of selenium-rich North American wheat. In Finland, however, this problem has been addressed by adding selenium to the fertilisers applied to the land.

BAD HABITS

Despite growing awareness of the importance of healthy eating, poor dietary habits are common. National surveys consistently show that people of all ages in Britain have diets that fail to meet the recommended targets for important nutrients, and few of us eat five portions of fruit and vegetables daily.

Although it is likely that our well-being will eventually suffer because of such lapses, the implications for those currently suffering ill-health are more immediate. They may have higher requirements for certain nutrients that would aid the healing process, and the elderly could be at risk because of absorption problems. As explained on pages 15-23, many people may benefit from taking supplements.

EVEN HEALTHY GROWING CHILDREN CAN BENEFIT FROM SUPPLEMENTS

The popularity of dietary supplements

There is nothing new or unusual about dietary supplements. Vitamins in tablet form have been around for more than 50 years. Herbs have been used in cooking and in medicine for thousands of years, and, according to the World Health Organization, 80% of the world's population use herbal medicine for some aspect of primary health care. We can learn from other countries' experience of the therapeutic use of nutritional supplements. For example, cat's claw – a herb derived from the bark or roots of an Amazonian vine – may be new to us, but it has been used in South America for thousands of years to treat many diseases by enhancing the function of the immune system.

INCREASING KNOWLEDGE

Only a decade ago most dietary supplements were based on nutrients such as vitamins B and C, and minerals such as iron and calcium, that were known to be deficient in the diets of many people, and herbal remedies often had to be made up at home or bought from specialist health-food shops.

However, the advancement of nutritional knowledge has meant that many diets have been demonstrated to be lacking in several essential nutrients, including trace elements. There is also increasing evidence that insufficient attention has been paid to phytochemicals in fruit and vegetables.

This is the reason why, today, we are able to buy an enormous range of supplements that have been specially formulated to suit our individual needs. They are sold in almost all supermarkets and chemists' shops, in catalogues and over the internet, with sales rising spectacularly each year.

DOCTORS AND SUPPLEMENTS

Doctors and other practitioners of conventional medicine may be sceptical about alternative therapies, but many take dietary supplements themselves. In a survey of 181 cardiologists in the USA, nearly half were regularly taking antioxidant vitamins, including vitamin C and vitamin E, which are linked with the prevention of cancer and heart disease.

A smaller percentage of the doctors (37%) routinely recommended antioxidants to their patients. A study of 665 dieticians in Washington state found that nearly 60% of them took some kind of nutritional supplement, either daily or occasionally.

CHANGING ATTITUDES

Increasing interest in the use of supplements is reflected in the media. For example, the effects of ginkgo biloba on patients with dementia, or the fact that a common treatment for enlarged prostate in many European countries is the herb saw palmetto, are stories of interest to editors and readers alike.

The growth in knowledge about supplements has been taking place at the same time as a shift in the relationship between doctor and patient, with an increasing emphasis on patient choice. The pressure on GPs' time, coupled with the rising cost of prescription charges, has induced many patients to consider alternatives to prescription medicines. With nearly half of GPs' time taken up with minor ailments, the medical profession and the Department of Health are keen to encourage people to take more responsibility for their own well-being.

New research

Recent nutritional research has produced a flood of studies offering compelling evidence that specific foods and nutrients may help to prevent, slow down the progress of, or even reverse, serious diseases. For example, it is now well established and widely accepted that folic acid supplements taken by pregnant women can help to protect against birth defects. While maintaining that in general someone with a healthy diet does not need to take supplements, the Department of Health now recommends that women should take folic acid when trying to conceive and continue to do so during the first three months of pregnancy.

In Europe, herbs have been widely studied and scrutinised for more than 70 years, and standards have been established for their effectiveness and safety. In Germany a body of scientists and health professionals known as Commission E has been investigating the usefulness and safety of herbal remedies since 1978, gathering information from the world's scientific literature on laboratory and clinical studies. It has issued reports on more than 200 herbs that it has found to be safe and efficacious. And new clinical studies, especially from Germany, on the efficacy of herbs have persuaded many doctors and scientists to take a less dismissive view of herbal remedies.

Persistent scepticism

However, research into herbal medicine is still in its infancy, and much more work is needed to evaluate even the major health benefits that have been attributed to herbs that have been used traditionally for centuries.

Many doctors and researchers insist that studies into alternative remedies are not sufficiently rigorous: they have been small in scale, and most do not offer a long-term evaluation of benefits and side effects. Extreme claims of benefits attract criticism either because they are without merit or because they create the impression that anything 'natural' is harmless – which is not always the case. However, in more than 25 studies the herb St John's wort was found to be more effective than a placebo in treating mild to moderate depressive symptoms.

Other studies have shown that the herb works as well as standard prescription medications for treating mild depression. Moreover, when it was taken at the recommended dosage, its side effects were infrequent and mild – an appealing feature of many herbal remedies. However, St John's wort does interact with other medicines, so care should be taken before using the herb in conjunction with other medications.

Emphasis on prevention

It is now widely acknowledged that lifestyle changes – paying close attention to diet, exercise and weight, as well as limiting alcohol intake and stopping smoking – have a vital role to play in the business of staying well.

These kinds of changes can not only help to prevent or relieve common complaints, including backache and constipation, but can also reduce the risk of serious ailments such as heart disease and cancer.

Vitamins, minerals and other nutritional supplements can reinforce and enhance the benefit of these self-care measures, which are also essential to ensure not just the absence of illness but the capacity to lead a full, vital, productive life.

Integrative healing

Although medical science has found cures for many troubling health problems, including some infectious diseases that caused sickness and premature death on a grand scale in the past, it has been less successful in combating chronic illnesses such as heart disease, cancer and diabetes. And many potent modern medicines also pose the risk of powerful and distressing side effects. One complementary practitioner describes how she began treating a patient who was taking a combination of ten different medicines only to discover that each was being used to treat the side effects of the previous one.

As awareness of the limitations of conventional medicine has grown, consumers have become keener about using alternative approaches to treat ailments. Generally these methods – which include acupuncture, chiropractic medicine, homeopathy and

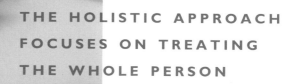

THE HOLISTIC APPROACH FOCUSES ON TREATING THE WHOLE PERSON

A RESPONSIBLE APPROACH TO TREATMENT

Whether you wish to consult a conventional doctor or a specialist practitioner, take the following guidelines into account.

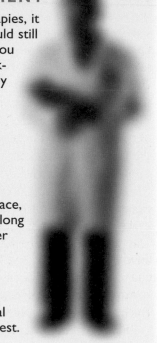

- Don't diagnose yourself. If you have symptoms that suggest an illness, the first thing you should do is to see a trained doctor who can make a skilled diagnosis – often with the aid of laboratory tests. Modern diagnostic techniques are very reliable, and any opportunity to have access to them should be welcomed. Once you have a diagnosis, you may then decide to approach a complementary therapist.
- Talk to your doctor. Be sure to report all your symptoms. Also, you should always be sure to inform your doctor about any supplements that you are already taking, because some of them might not interact well with conventional drugs that you may be asked to try (*see pages 394-7*).
- Even if your doctor is not enthusiastic about herbal or nutritional therapies, it is important that you should still discuss any supplements you are already taking or thinking about using, particularly if you have a chronic condition such as asthma, diabetes, heart disease or high blood pressure.
- Don't stop taking prescribed treatments. Some supplements may complement, or even replace, conventional drugs in the long term, but you should never discontinue or alter the dosage of any prescribed medication without first consulting your doctor.
- Accept that conventional methods are sometimes best.

aromatherapy, as well as herbal and nutritional therapies – are considered less invasive, safer and more 'holistic' than conventional treatments. The holistic approach is devoted to treating the whole person rather than suppressing symptoms.

THE HOLISTIC APPROACH
In addition to advice about which supplements to take, this book gives advice about what else you can do to alleviate particular ailments in terms of making changes to your lifestyle. The idea of 'a pill for an ill' has largely been superseded by a holistic approach. For example, the recommendations for treating fatigue may involve not only swallowing a vitamin B complex tablet but also incorporating exercise into your daily routine and eating a healthy diet.

Alternative therapies are typically less expensive than conventional treatments. Supplements, in particular, usually cost less than prescription drugs, and may be cheaper than some over-the-counter medications. Alternative therapies, such as acupuncture and chiropractic treatments, are now sometimes available on the NHS. This depends on the individual GPs and primary care organisations, but it is worth asking your doctor if he or she is prepared to make referrals.

Behind many of these alternative choices in healing is a common perspective: the body has remarkable powers of self-repair. According to this view, supplements, when used in a wise manner, can bolster the body's immune system to prevent disease. If a health problem does occur, they can also enhance and accelerate the self-healing process.

As you read the entries in this book you will see that supplements often act to enhance the body's own defences. A herb taken to help treat an infection, for example, often does not kill the bacteria, as an antibiotic would, but it strengthens the immune system so the body can marshal its own resources to kill them.

FINDING OUT ABOUT COMPLEMENTARY HEALING
The ideal of an integrative approach is that you and your doctor would work together to decide

which supplement or therapy to use for treating your particular health problem.

However, since many doctors remain sceptical about complementary healing practices, there is no single, reliable source to supply advice about these remedies. It comes down to acquainting yourself with the various types of complementary therapies, including supplements.

You and your doctor

This book aims to reflect the fact that a growing number of doctors and patients are embracing an integrative, or complementary, approach to treating health problems.

There is a move towards carefully weighing both conventional and alternative methods in order to create a strategy best suited to a patient's needs. For example, if you find it hard to cope with the side effects from a prescription drug for high blood pressure, your doctor may suggest combining supplements with relaxation techniques as an alternative solution.

Since the beginning of the 1990s, GPs have been allowed to employ complementary practitioners in their surgeries, as long as the GPs retain clinical responsibility, and to practise complementary medicine themselves. This means that around half the GPs in the UK have either practised complementary medicine or can provide access to it – so you should be able to find a doctor who is prepared to look at the whole range of options.

CONSULTING A SPECIALIST PRACTITIONER

However, even if they are open to other approaches, many GPs do not have the time to keep themselves up to date with current developments in complementary medicine. Most doctors have only a few hours of nutritional training and are taught even less, if anything, about key complementary therapies such as herbal medicine or homeopathy. A doctor who is not sufficiently knowledgeable about nutritional or herbal medicine may suggest that you work with a nutritionist or another appropriate health practitioner, especially if you have been diagnosed with a medical problem that normally responds well to these therapies.

If you find that your GP is sceptical about an integrated approach to your problem, you could consider seeking the advice of a doctor who is more receptive. You may also benefit from seeing a nutritionist, a medical herbalist or another complementary practitioner. Some of the organisations listed on pages 398-9 can help you to locate a qualified practitioner in your area.

A CAUTIONARY APPROACH

Each entry in this book provides details of the symptoms and circumstances that require you seek the advice of your GP.

It can be dangerous to seek alternative options for medical conditions that doctors excel in treating or preventing. These include medical and surgical emergencies, physical injuries, acute infections such as pneumonia, sexually transmitted diseases, kidney infections, reconstructive surgery, and prevention of serious immunisable illnesses such as polio and diphtheria.

FOOD SUPPLEMENTS

An EU Directive on food supplements came into force in the UK in August 2005. The aim is to harmonise trade in food supplements between European Union member states and to ensure that products are safe. The Directive includes a list of the vitamins and minerals that food supplements may contain and the forms in which they may be included. Fish oils and phytochemicals are not included in the list but they may be in the future. Within a few years, safe upper levels of vitamins and minerals in supplements will be set and a list of generic health claims will also be established.

Many manufacturers have reformulated their products in line with the Directive. Those using ingredients not on the permitted list can submit dossiers of evidence to the UK Food Standards Agency for inspection. Such products may remain on the market until 2009.

The best of health

Although it is a desirable goal, living constantly at the peak of good health may not be attainable with our current state of knowledge and understanding of the human body. But while we have little or no control over some factors which can make us prone to developing certain diseases, others can be influenced by individuals. Growing evidence of links between diet and health shows that, through diet, we can lessen or increase our susceptibility to many degenerative diseases.

Which factors influence health?

People studying patterns of diseases in different populations have linked certain diseases with specific characteristics or factors, including diet.

For example, the incidence of stomach cancer is far higher in Japan than in the UK, and this difference has been linked to the much greater consumption in Japan of pickled foods that are high in salt. When such links between diet and disease patterns are identified, the association is often reinforced by the results of laboratory studies and clinical trials.

A person's genetic make-up is another factor that may cause a predisposition to a certain disease. For example, people from the Indian subcontinent living in the UK are more prone to coronary heart disease than other groups in the UK, even though their diets may be similar. However, being from a particular ethnic group is an unalterable fact. Recognising which characteristics can be changed and which cannot is a useful step towards understanding how to improve our health.

FACTORS SUCH AS HEIGHT AND WHERE YOU LIVE CAN MAKE YOU PRONE TO SOME DISEASES

FACTORS AFFECTING HEALTH THAT CANNOT BE ALTERED

Height Shorter men are more likely to suffer from coronary heart disease than taller men.
Sex Women are more prone than men to osteoporosis.
Age Men in the UK have a shorter life expectancy than women.
Social class Obesity is more prevalent in lower income groups.
Race Afro-Caribbeans in the UK are more likely to suffer strokes and less likely to have coronary heart disease than other groups in the UK.
Geographical location People living in towns and cities are more likely to suffer from respiratory problems than those living in rural locations.
Birth weight Low birth weight and being born prematurely increase the risk of developing a range of diseases in later life, including type II diabetes and coronary heart disease.

FACTORS AFFECTING HEALTH THAT CAN BE ALTERED

Although it is impossible to alter factors such as height, sex, age and birth weight, there are other factors that can be influenced. By minimising those risk factors over which you have some control, you will have a greater chance of living a healthier life. For example, diet plays an important role in the development of coronary heart disease, cancer, stroke and other major diseases, so by choosing to eat healthily you can promote good health and help to protect yourself against these diseases.

There are four main factors within your control that have a crucial influence on health:
Smoking Smoking has a very bad effect on the health of both the smoker and those inhaling cigarette smoke 'second-hand'. In the UK 17% of all deaths are directly attributed to smoking, 81% of lung cancer is caused by cigarette smoking, and smoking doubles your risk of developing coronary heart disease. For the unborn baby of a mother who smokes there is a risk of being born both small and at higher

risk of developing chronic illness in later life.

HEALTH-PROMOTING STRATEGY If you smoke you should try to give it up.

Stress and work pressures

Constant pressure at home or work can have an influence on health, decreasing the effectiveness of the immune system and potentially increasing the risk of stroke and heart disease.

HEALTH-PROMOTING STRATEGY Devise ways of decreasing stress in your life.

Lack of physical activity

Regular exercise maintains the health of all organs of the body as well as improving your feeling of well-being. People who are not physically active are twice as likely to get coronary heart disease as those who exercise regularly. A recent UK survey revealed that seven out of ten men and eight out of ten women are not active enough to gain any health benefit. It is not only muscles, heart and arteries that benefit from exercise; bones are strengthened by use, and lung volume is increased.

HEALTH-PROMOTING STRATEGY Undertake about 30 minutes of moderately intense activity, such as brisk walking, on at least five days a week.

> ### GUIDE TO HEALTHY EATING
>
> ■ Enjoy your food.
>
> ■ Eat a wide variety of different foods.
>
> ■ Eat the right amount to be a healthy weight.
>
> ■ Eat plenty of foods rich in starch and fibre.
>
> ■ Do not eat too much fat.
>
> ■ Do not eat sugary foods too often.
>
> ■ Ensure a healthy intake of vitamins and minerals.
>
> ■ If you drink alcohol, keep within sensible limits.

Poor diet What you eat has a major influence on your health. Simple differences in food choice can either provide a suitable mixture of nutrients to keep your body in good health, or leave you deficient in vitamins and minerals or with the wrong balance of fat and carbohydrate. Poor diet is responsible for at least a third of all cancers and for most cases of heart disease.

HEALTH-PROMOTING STRATEGY Eat a balanced and varied diet; eat to attain and maintain the best weight for your height.

A balanced diet?

The best type of diet is one that provides all the necessary vitamins and minerals in quantities sufficient to meet your needs. Calories should be adequate but not excessive. They should be supplied by protein, fat and carbohydrate in proportions which bear the promise of good health. Although many ways of describing a balanced diet have been devised, the key messages are very similar in many countries where people eat a Western-type diet. In the UK an eight-point guide to eating healthily has been drawn up by the Food Standards Agency (*see*

THE BALANCE OF GOOD HEALTH

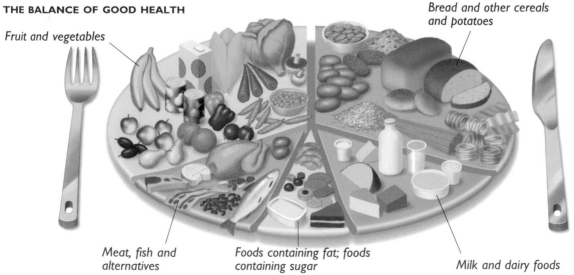

Fruit and vegetables

Bread and other cereals and potatoes

Meat, fish and alternatives

Foods containing fat; foods containing sugar

Milk and dairy foods

centre panel opposite). The most progressive approach in recent years has been in the USA, where a number of organisations, including the Department of Agriculture and the Department of Health and Human Services, have collaborated to produce a set of simple rules to achieve a healthy diet:

■ Aim for a healthy weight.
■ Become physically active each day.
■ Make grains, fruits and vegetables the foundation of your diet.
■ Eat a variety of grains daily, especially whole grain.
■ Eat a variety of fruits and vegetables daily.
■ Keep food safe to eat.
■ Choose a diet that is low in fat and cholesterol.
■ Choose drinks and foods that are low in sugars.
■ Choose and prepare food with less salt.
■ If you drink alcohol, do so in moderation.

The lists are similar, but neither indicates how much of a food should be eaten. The food models which show relative proportions of foods to be eaten are perhaps more helpful. In the USA a food guide pyramid is used, while in the UK a

WHAT THE FOOD GROUPS CONTAIN AND HOW MUCH OF EACH SHOULD BE EATEN

FOOD GROUPS	BREAD, CEREALS AND POTATOES	FRUIT AND VEGETABLES	MILK AND DAIRY FOODS	MEAT, FISH AND ALTERNATIVES	FOODS CONTAINING FAT OR SUGARS
Which foods are included	Breads and rolls, breakfast cereals; rice, oats, maize, millet, rye and other grains; pasta, noodles; potatoes, sweet potatoes, plantains, yams, green bananas	Fresh, frozen and canned fruit and vegetables; salad vegetables; beans and lentils; fruit juice; dried fruit	Milk, cheeses, fromage frais, yoghurt	Meat – beef, pork (including bacon), lamb; meat products (sausages, beef-burgers); offal (liver, kidney); chicken, turkey; fish and fish products; eggs; nuts; textured vegetable protein and other meat alternatives	Butter, margarine, low fat spreads; oils; mayonnaise and oily salad dressings; crisps, savoury snacks; biscuits, cakes and puddings; ice cream; chocolate and sweets; sugar; sweetened drinks
Advice	Eat plenty of these foods. They should form one third of the diet	Eat at least five portions a day of these foods; they should form one third of the diet	Eat or drink moderate amounts	Eat moderate amounts of all foods in this group	Use fats and oils sparingly. Don't eat fatty or sweet foods too often
Comments	Choose whole-grain varieties. These starchy foods provide energy and dietary fibre. Starchy foods are filling and can reduce desire for fatty or sweet foods	Fruit and vegetables are a major source of vitamins, minerals, dietary fibre and other metabolically active compounds	Choose lower fat products when possible. They usually contain comparable amounts of B vitamins and calcium, but may be lower in vitamins A and D	Use lean meat, removing the fat, and skin poultry. Eat fish (oily fish is best) twice a week. Beans and lentils are a rich source of B vitamins, dietary fibre and meta-bolically active plant compounds	Choose reduced fat versions when available. Don't eat many crisps, cakes, biscuits and sweets, as they contain very few vitamins or minerals

diagram named 'the Balance of Good Health' has been devised by the Food Standards Agency to illustrate the ingredients of a healthy diet (*see page 16*). The advice portrayed in the diagram applies to all people over the age of five. Under-twos need a diet that is less bulky to achieve their calorie and nutrient requirements for adequate growth and development, and so it should contain less starchy foods than that for adults. The diet of a child between the ages of two and five should increasingly resemble this model.

Key nutrients

BREAD, CEREALS AND POTATOES

This group of foods is a major source of B vitamins. Wholegrain products such as wholemeal bread – besides being rich sources of fibre – are much better sources of vitamins and minerals than refined cereals. Wholegrains also provide much of the magnesium in the diet as well as the trace elements chromium and manganese. Breakfast cereals, because they are fortified with several vitamins during manufacture, play a significant role in helping many people to achieve adequate vitamin intakes. White flour is also fortified by law in the UK, and surveys show that the added thiamin, niacin, iron and calcium markedly improves the national diet.

The humble potato, even when new, is only a moderately good source of vitamin C, but in the UK its contribution to vitamin C intake is high, because of the large quantities eaten.

FRUIT AND VEGETABLES

Eating five portions a day of a mixture of fruit and vegetables is necessary to reach dietary targets for vitamins and minerals. Fruit and vegetables that are particularly rich in vitamin C include sweet peppers, strawberries, kiwi fruit and citrus fruits. Carrots, mango and papaya are abundant sources of beta-carotene, which the body can convert to vitamin A. In addition, fruit and vegetables provide B complex vitamins, trace elements and soluble fibre. They also supply phytochemicals such as carotenoids, flavonoids and phytoestrogens.

RECOMMENDED DAILY INTAKE OF VITAMINS			
SUPPLEMENT	RNI FOR MALE 19-50	RNI FOR FEMALE 19-50	RDA
Thiamin (mg)	1.0	0.8	1.4
Riboflavin (mg)	1.3	1.1	1.6
Niacin (mg)	17	13	18
Vitamin B$_6$ (mg)	1.4	1.2	2.0
Vitamin B$_{12}$ (mcg)	1.5	1.5	1.0
Folate (mcg)	200	200	200
Vitamin C (mg)	40	40	60
Vitamin A (mcg)	700	600	800
Calcium (mg)	700	700	800
Phosphorus (mg)	550	550	800
Magnesium (mg)	300	270	300
Iron (mg)	8.7	14.8	14
Zinc (mg)	9.5	7	15
Iodine (mcg)	140	140	150
Vitamin E (mg)	no value	no value	10
Selenium (mcg)	75	60	no value
Vitamin D (mcg)	no value	no value	5
Sodium (mg)	1600	1600	no value
Potassium (mcg)	3500	3500	no value
Chloride (mg)	2500	2500	no value
Copper (mg)	1.0	1.2	no value

These antioxidant substances help to combat the body's toxic 'free radicals' – unstable molecules which circulate in the blood – and are mainly responsible for the colour, aroma and flavour of the foods in this group. To get a good mix of phytochemicals, a healthy diet should include broccoli, dark green leafy vegetables and red, orange and yellow fruit and vegetables: the brighter the colours, the better.

MEAT, FISH, EGGS, BEANS, NUTS AND MEAT ALTERNATIVES

As well as being protein-rich, this group provides some nutrients not found in abundance elsewhere in the diet. Red meat, for example, is a rich source of easily absorbed iron; although plant foods contain some iron, it is less well absorbed. Oily fish is the only dietary source of the essential omega-3 fatty acids, which reduce the risk of heart disease by thinning the blood as well as providing other health benefits.

Meat (especially red meat) and meat alternatives are also good sources of zinc. Nuts and seeds offer a wide range of nutrients, including fibre, vitamin B complex, magnesium and trace elements. They are also one of the few rich dietary sources of vitamin E, an antioxidant vital for the health of the circulatory system.

DAIRY PRODUCTS

Apart from canned fish (especially sardines), no foods contain as much calcium as milk-based foods, and it is absorbed much better from them than from other sources. This is why they are so important for achieving adequate calcium intake in the diet. As well as other vitamins, such as riboflavin, dairy products supply the fat-soluble vitamins A and D, as well as vitamin B_{12}, which is found almost exclusively in animal products. Choosing low-fat versions of dairy products helps to reduce saturated fat intakes; these contain similar or greater amounts of calcium and the B vitamins, but fewer of vitamins A and D.

FOODS CONTAINING FAT OR SUGARS

These foods tend to be low in nutritional value, supplying energy as fat or sugar but providing only small amounts of vitamins or minerals. A high intake of fat and sugar reduces the overall density of nutrients in the diet, and so decreases the chances of reaching recommended dietary targets for essential nutrients.

The UK dietary recommendations

Dietary recommendations for any nutrient are based on the daily intake thought to be adequate to satisfy safely the needs of the majority of the population. But, despite much research, values for optimum intakes of vitamins and minerals are still being debated. The Reference Nutrient Intake (RNI) measure used in the UK (*see page* 26) is calculated from studies of the physiological requirements of healthy people, but because these studies are subject to wide interpretation,

the RNI value for a nutrient can vary from country to country. European Union regulations require Recommended Daily Amounts (RDAs) to be shown on food and supplement labels. RDAs are said to apply to 'average adults' and are only very rough guides.

The table opposite shows how the RDAs differ from the UK RNIs for men and women in respect of some vitamins and minerals. Where the value is not known, no figure is given.

Food is more than nutrition

Eating can be highly pleasurable – so much so that some people just can't stop. Enjoying food is crucially important, and a congenial setting for eating enhances the enjoyment. Finding foods which both taste good and do you good can be part of the fun of eating well, whether you live alone or as part of a family.

All foods are a mixture of nutrients and other chemicals, so while a food may be rich in a particular nutrient it may also contain other valuable nutrients and health-giving factors. For instance, a wholemeal loaf of bread is not only a good source of dietary fibre but it also contains a range of B vitamins, magnesium, iron, selenium and zinc.

EAT FIVE PORTIONS A DAY OF FRUIT AND VEGETABLES

DIET AND SUPPLEMENTS

Dietary supplements should be used to augment good diet, not to replace it. They should not be used to make up deficiencies resulting from low intakes of fruit, vegetables and wholegrains. This is because these foods, as well as being rich sources of vitamins and minerals, are abundant sources of phytochemicals. In fact, the health-protective properties of fruit and vegetables may be due as much to phytochemicals as to the other nutrients they contain.

However, supplements can compensate for the great variations in the amounts of nutrients in foods and their ability to be absorbed and utilised – an attribute known as their 'bioavailability'. Interactions of a nutrient with other components in a food can reduce its bioavailability. Iron, for example, is present in many foods, but in wheat it is bound by phytates, in eggs by phosphoproteins, in tea by phenols, in spinach by oxalic acid and polyphenols,and in milk by calcium and phosphate. In each case the component that binds the iron affects the ease with which the body absorbs and utilises the mineral. Not all interactions are negative. Vitamin C, when taken with iron, can increase the latter's absorption.

Who can benefit from dietary supplements?

Intakes of vitamins and minerals vary greatly from person to person. Surveys in the UK show that, while the majority of the population reach their RNI targets, large minorities do not. Some groups are particularly prone to intakes of vitamins and minerals for a wide variety of reasons, the most outstanding being poor food choice and a sedentary lifestyle.

Certain population groups are more at risk of an inadequate intake of vitamin and minerals than others. Men, on the whole, are less at risk, because they have a higher energy expenditure and therefore eat more. Women, throughout the life cycle, are prone to nutrient deficiencies since – although their requirements for micronutrients are not very different from those of men – their average calorie intake is much lower. This is particularly so for those women who follow diets.

In addition, the recommended targets for vitamins and minerals are based on results of studies in healthy people, and may not be appropriate for sick people, whose needs may be greater. Demand for nutrients is also

A HEALTHY LIFESTYLE INCLUDES REGULAR EXERCISE AS WELL AS A BALANCED DIET

increased by stress and high toxic loads such as pesticides, pollutants and prescribed drugs.

Optimum nutrition, a concept aimed at reducing the effect of environmental toxins as well as reducing chronic disease, recommends that certain nutrients are supplied at much higher levels than the RNIs or RDAs. A diet that follows one of the healthy eating models described above provides the best possible chance of obtaining adequate nutrition, but it may still fail to provide optimum nutrition. It follows that dietary supplements are likely to be valuable health aids for many people.

FREQUENT SLIMMERS
People who often reduce their food intake while attempting to lose weight may be at risk of dietary imbalance owing to the relatively small amount of food they eat.

Although slimmers usually increase the amount of fruit and vegetables they eat – thereby maintaining a healthy intake of vitamin C, beta-carotene, folates, magnesium and potassium – other micronutrients are adversely affected. These include iron, zinc, riboflavin, iodine and calcium. Dieters who cut out all dairy products, for instance, find it hard to obtain sufficient calcium.
RECOMMENDATIONS *Avoid crash diets. A reduced-calorie diet should incorporate a mixture of foods, preferably including lean meat to provide iron, selenium and zinc, calcium-rich low-fat dairy products, starchy foods rich in vitamin B, and plenty of fruit and vegetables. A multivitamin and mineral supplement is a wise precaution for dieters, and fish oils – or flaxseed oil for vegetarians – are recommended for those who do not regularly eat oily fish.*

VEGETARIANS
A carefully planned vegetarian diet should not be deficient in micronutrients. In fact, it may well contain more micronutrients than an average non-vegetarian diet, but there are some vitamins and minerals that are more abundant

and easily absorbed in animal foods. Strict vegetarians – vegans – who do not eat any animal products are most at risk of deficiencies. The vitamins and minerals they need to monitor are vitamin B_{12}, riboflavin, calcium, vitamin D, iron, zinc and iodine. There are food sources of all of these micronutrients, but many vegans prefer to use supplements to ensure that they have an adequate supply. All vegetarians, especially women, are at increased risk of anaemia through low iron intakes, because 'haem' iron from meat is more readily available in greater quantities than the plant form of iron.

RECOMMENDATIONS *Use an appropriate multivitamin and mineral supplement formulated for vegetarians.*

FUSSY CHILDREN

Children have notoriously capricious eating habits and may suffer from nutritional inadequacy by their refusal to eat whole groups of food. The Balance of Good Health model shows the micronutrients each food group contains (*see page* 16), and if a child omits any of the four main groups there is a need to correct the imbalance with other foods rich in those vitamins or minerals, or by supplementation. If a child refuses to drink milk, say, try giving yoghurt, making milky puddings and custards, and adding low-fat cheese to foods to ensure enough calcium. A child who refuses all dairy products may need calcium supplementation. Foods for children need to be 'nutrient dense' – that is, they should contain a lot of nutritional value in a small quantity. If children's consumption of crisps, confectionery, biscuits, cakes, fizzy drinks and other foods of poor nutritional quality outweighs their consumption of the healthy elements of a diet, then multivitamin and mineral supplements are advisable.

IF A CHILD REFUSES TO EAT DAIRY PRODUCTS, THEY MAY REQUIRE SUPPLEMENTATION

CALCIUM REQUIREMENTS

The RNI for calcium of a girl of 11-14 is 800 mg. To meet this level she needs to eat a diet rich in dairy foods or take a calcium supplemement. The chart below shows how difficult it is to reach the RNI for calcium if dairy foods are restricted.

FOOD AND PORTION	AMOUNT OF CALCIUM (*mg*)
Glass of semi-skimmed milk (200ml)	248
Piece of cheddar cheese (30g)	216
Pot of low-fat fruit yoghurt (150g)	225
2 slices white bread (72g)	72
Portion broccoli (85g)	34
Small can baked beans (150g)	80
Dried apricots (56g)	52
Canned salmon without bones (100g)	93
Canned sardines with bones (100g)	460
Tablespoon sesame seeds (12g)	80
Medium orange (150g)	75

RECOMMENDATIONS *Encourage children to eat a range of different foods by involving them in the planning and making of meals, but not by forced feeding. Failing this, use a multivitamin and multimineral supplement.*

PEOPLE SUFFERING FROM STRESS

During periods of stress the need for B vitamins increases because metabolism is increased in all cells, including those of the nervous and immune systems. Having plenty of vitamin C may also help to decrease susceptibility to and duration of cold and flu viruses. If stress has led to poor eating habits, with lots of snack foods being consumed, then sodium intake is likely to increase, and consequently blood pressure too.

Eating plenty of fruit and vegetables rich in potassium – which balances out the sodium – will be beneficial.

RECOMMENDATIONS *Consider using antioxidant vitamin supplements if the diet is poor and the stress prolonged. Ensure that the supplement also contains some of the minerals involved in antioxidant systems – zinc, selenium and manganese.*

SMOKERS

Cigarette smoke stimulates the production of 'free radicals' – unstable molecules that circulate in the blood and can cause damage to cells – so vitamin C and other antioxidants are needed to mop these up.

Studies of smokers have shown that their fruit and vegetable intake is lower than that of non-smokers, even though their requirements are much higher. Taking an antioxidant supplement is advisable, but no supplement can compensate for the damage smoking causes. Studies of women who smoke in pregnancy suggest that smoking is a cause of stillbirth and low birth weight in babies.

RECOMMENDATIONS *Smokers should have a minimum of 80 mg vitamin C a day. More than 1 gram a day taken regularly may cause kidney stones.*

HEAVY DRINKERS

If alcohol replaces food in the diet, nutritional imbalances can occur. Drinking within the safe limits – between 3 and 4 units a day for men, and between 2 and 3 units a day for women – is recommended. A glass of red wine a day has been linked to a reduction in the heart disease rate – but only for men over 40 and women who have experienced the menopause.

Anything more than the recommended units of alcohol a day can increase the risk of cancers of the mouth, larynx and pharynx.

RECOMMENDATIONS *People who drink a lot of alcohol often have a low intake of fruit and vegetables, leading to dietary imbalances. Vitamin C and the B group vitamins, which are quickly depleted by high alcohol consumption, should be topped up with supplements.*

PEOPLE WHO TAKE CERTAIN PRESCRIPTION DRUGS

Taking prescription drugs, ranging from the contraceptive pill to antidepressants, may increase requirements of a range of nutrients.

RECOMMENDATIONS *If you are already taking a prescription medication, or if you are prescribed a new drug, ask your doctor about any nutritional consequences.*

Changing nutritional needs

Dietary requirements do not remain constant throughout life. For example, calcium needs fluctuate with age in accordance with growth and development, and breastfeeding makes a huge demand on calcium reserves.

PREGNANCY

In pregnancy the need for some vitamins and minerals increases. An optimum level of folic acid has been calculated which reduces the risk of having a baby with neural-tube defects. A supplement containing 400 mcg per day is recommended prior to conception up to the 12th week of pregnancy. To gain a similar amount of folic acid from diet, large quantities of specific foods would have to be eaten – such as four bowls of fortified cereal or 6.5 glasses of orange juice a day.

EXTRA FOLIC ACID PROTECTS YOUR BABY

DISEASES AND DISORDERS

Some conditions – such as ulcerative colitis and Crohn's disease in which food is not properly absorbed from the intestine – can lead to nutritional deficiencies.

Vitamin B_{12} may be particularly affected; zinc, sodium and potassium may be lost through constant diarrhoea, or iron through blood loss. Enhanced urinary losses of minerals, including zinc, occur in some conditions such as diabetes.

The balance of the fatty acid families – omega-6 (seed oils) and omega-3 (fish oils) – is very important for cell health, and many people with inflammatory diseases (eczema, arthritis, colitis, asthma) respond to supplements of omega-3 essential fatty acid. These conditions should be discussed with a medical practitioner who can advise you on treatment and diet.

How supplements can benefit you

A multivitamin and multimineral supplement is often taken as an insurance against nutritional deficiencies, but recent research provides good reasons for using a variety of supplements, including herbs, for both prevention and healing – and indicates that optimum levels may be higher than previously thought.

If you are fundamentally healthy, is there any point in taking supplements on a regular basis? If you develop a disorder or an ailment, can you expect supplements to help? What follows is a summary of the major benefits that, according to scientific researchers, most people can expect if they use the supplements covered in this book. More detailed information about the therapeutic effects of specific supplements can be found in the entries on pages 40-194.

Who needs supplements?

Conventional medical wisdom holds that healthy people who eat well enough to avoid specific nutritional deficiencies do not need to supplement their diets. The only thing they have to do is to make sure that their diets meet the RNIs – Reference Nutrient Intakes – published by the Department of Health (*see page* 26).

Even if you accept that the official standards for vitamin and mineral intakes are adequate for good health, the evidence is overwhelming that most people in the UK fail to come close to meeting those requirements.

Most of us do not eat enough fruit and vegetables, and certainly not as much as five daily servings – the quantity recommended for obtaining the minimum level of nutrients believed necessary to prevent illness.

We often make food choices that are nutritionally poor. For example, we are more likely to select chips than broccoli as a vegetable serving, and will opt for a fizzy soft drink rather than a glass of semi-skimmed milk. Eating these and other foods may not only contribute too much fat and sugar to our diet but can also result in intakes of vitamins, minerals, and disease-fighting phytochemicals that fall well short of ideal levels.

Meeting dietary targets

Government studies show that the diets of many people in the UK contain only half the recommended amounts of magnesium and folic acid. About 50% of adult women and more than 70% of adolescent girls have intakes of calcium that are below their respective RNIs of 700 mg and 800 mg.

Vitamins C and B_6, as well as iron and zinc, are other nutrients that are at notably low levels in the British diet. Even with the best nutritional planning it is hard to maintain a diet that meets the RNIs for all nutrients. Vegetarians, for example, who as a group are healthier than meat eaters (and who tend to avoid junk foods lacking in vitamins and minerals), may be deficient in some nutrients, such as iron, calcium and vitamin B_{12}.

People on a low-fat diet will find it difficult to obtain the recommended daily amounts of vitamin E from their food alone, because so many food sources for vitamin E are high in fat. Another problem is that a balanced diet may not contain some of the more specialised substances – fish oils, soya isoflavones or alpha-lipoic acid – that are now believed to promote health.

For a healthy person who is unable to eat a well-balanced diet every day, taking a supplement can fill the nutritional gaps or boost the levels of nutrients they consume from adequate to optimum.

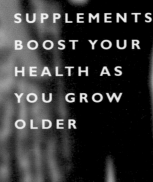

SUPPLEMENTS BOOST YOUR HEALTH AS YOU GROW OLDER

Hazards in the environment

There are various other reasons why people who maintain good eating habits might benefit from a daily supplement. Some practitioners believe that exposure to environmental pollutants – ranging from car emissions to industrial chemicals and wastes – can cause much damage inside the body at the cellular level, destroying tissues and depleting the body of nutrients.

Many supplements, particularly those that act as antioxidants, can help to control the cell and tissue damage that follows toxic exposure (*see* ANTIOXIDANTS, *pages* 46-47). Recent evidence also indicates that certain medications, excessive consumption of alcohol, smoking or persistent stress may interfere with the absorption of certain key nutrients. Even an excellent diet could not make up for such shortfalls. Specific nutritional programmes can be devised that take account of these and other lifestyle factors that affect the nutrient levels in the human body.

Prevention of disease

It used to be thought that a lack of nutrients was linked only to specific deficiency diseases such as scurvy, a condition marked by soft gums and loose teeth that is caused by having too little vitamin C. In the past three decades, however, thousands of scientific studies have indicated that particular nutrients play important roles in the prevention of a number of chronic degenerative diseases common in contemporary Western societies.

Many recent studies highlighting the disease-fighting potential of different nutrients are mentioned in this book. What most of these studies reveal is that the level of nutrients associated with the prevention of disease is often much higher than the current RNIs. The people taking part in the studies frequently had to depend on supplements to achieve these higher levels.

Some practitioners suggest that, in slowing or preventing the development of disease, nutrients (particularly the antioxidants) can also delay the wear and tear of ageing itself by

reducing the damage done to cells. This does not mean that vitamin E or coenzyme Q_{10}, for example, is a 'youth potion', but several recent studies, including work done at the US Nutritional Immunological Laboratory, have found that supplementation with single nutrients, such as vitamin E, or multivitamin and multimineral supplements seems to improve the immune response in older people.

Age-related disorders

A study of 11,178 elderly subjects by the US National Institute on Aging showed that the use of vitamin E resulted in fewer deaths than would have been expected, especially deaths from heart disease. Vitamin E users were only half as likely to die of heart disease as those who took no supplements. Antioxidant supplements have been shown to be effective in lowering the risk of cataracts and macular degeneration, two age-related conditions in which vision slowly deteriorates.

Nutritional supplements that serve as high-potency antioxidants against ageing disorders include selenium, carotenoids, flavonoids, certain amino acids and coenzyme Q_{10}. Clinical research suggests that the herb ginkgo biloba may improve many age-related symptoms, especially those involving reduced blood flow, such as dizziness, impotence and short-term memory loss.

Substances found in echinacea and other herbs are reported to strengthen the immune system, and phytoestrogens such as soya isoflavones may help to delay or prevent some of the effects of the menopause as well as to prevent cancer and heart disease. (A fuller discussion of ageing appears on pages 198-9.)

Treating ailments

Many practitioners of complementary medicine recommend supplements for a wide range of health problems affecting virtually every system

ANTIOXIDANTS PROVIDE POTENT DEFENCE AGAINST MANY AILMENTS

in the body. Traditional doctors would be more likely to prescribe drugs for such conditions, although they might treat some disorders with supplements; for example, iron is sometimes prescribed for some types of anaemia, vitamin A (in the drug isotretinoin, or Accutane) for severe acne, and high doses of the B vitamin niacin for reducing high cholesterol levels.

In this book certain vitamins and minerals are suggested for the treatment of specific ailments – but the use of nutritional supplements as remedies, especially for serious conditions, is controversial. Doctors practising conventional medicine are often sceptical of their efficacy, and believe that it is sometimes dangerous to rely on them. However, drawing on published data and their clinical observations, nutritionally orientated doctors and practitioners think the use of these supplements is justified – and that to wait years for unequivocal proof to appear would be wasting valuable time.

Until there is clearer and more consistent evidence available you should be careful about depending on nutritional supplements alone to treat an ailment or injury.

A tradition of herbal medicine

For thousands of years various cultures have employed herbs for soothing, relieving or even curing many common health problems – a fact not ignored by medical science. After all, the pharmaceutical industry grew out of the tradition of using herbs as medicine.

Recent studies suggest that many of the claims made for herbs are valid, and the pharmacological actions of the herbs covered in this book are often well documented by clinical studies as well as historical practice. A number of herbal remedies, including St John's wort, ginkgo biloba and saw palmetto, are now accepted and prescribed as medications for treating disorders such as allergies, depression, impotence and heart disease. But even herbs and other supplements with proven therapeutic effects should be used judiciously for treating an ailment. Guidelines for using these remedies safely and effectively are given on pages 35-36.

TOO MANY BENEFITS TO BE TRUE?

When you see a supplement label that lists a variety of functions and benefits for a single herb or substance, you may wonder if this owes more to marketing 'hype' than to fact. But some supplements do have multiple effects that are well documented, and misleading claims are unlikely because manufacturers of dietary supplements are obliged to observe statutory regulations to conform to the requirements of the Advertising Standards Authority; many belong to the Health Food Manufacturers' Association, which advises its members on label claims.

Consider a herb such as green tea, whose benefits may include helping to control several cancers, protecting against heart disease, inhibiting bacterial action, combating tooth decay and boosting the immune system. Given that various active components have been identified in green tea, it is not very surprising that it can offer all these benefits.

Many common medications were initially developed for one purpose. As more people take the drugs and their effects are studied, new uses come to light. Imagine a drug that can cure headaches, relieve arthritis, help to prevent heart disease, ease the pain of athletic injuries and reduce the risk of colon cancer. It is aspirin, of course – and its precursor came from a herbal source: the bark of the white willow tree.

What supplements will not do

Despite the benefits of supplements, it is important to be aware of their limitations – and some of the questionable claims made for them.
■ As the word itself suggests, a 'supplement' is not meant to replace the nutrients available from foods. Supplements can never compensate for a poor diet: they cannot counteract a high intake of saturated fat (linked to an increased risk of heart disease), nor can they replace every nutrient found in food groups that do not form part of your diet. Also, although scientists have isolated and extracted a number of disease-fighting phytochemical compounds from fruit,

vegetables and other foods, there may be many others that are undiscovered – and that you can get only from food sources. And some of the known compounds may work only when used in combination with others in various foods, rather than as single ingredients in a supplement form.

■ Supplements cannot compensate for habits known to contribute to ill health, such as smoking or lack of exercise. Optimum health requires a wholesome lifestyle (*see pages* 14-21) – particularly if, as people get older, they are intent on ageing well.

■ Although some of the benefits ascribed to supplements are unproved but plausible, other claims are far-fetched, particularly those made for some weight-loss preparations. It is questionable whether any such preparation can help you to shed pounds without making the right food choices and taking regular exercise at the same time. Products that claim to 'burn fat' won't burn enough on their own for significant weight loss.

■ Similarly, claims about supplements that are alleged to boost mental or physical performance are difficult to prove – and in a healthy person any 'enhancement' will be at best a limited one. Although a particular supplement may improve mental function in someone experiencing mild to severe episodes of memory loss, it may have a negligible effect on most adults' memories or their ability to concentrate. A supplement that has been shown to counteract fatigue will not transform the average jogger into an endurance athlete. Nor is there any convincing evidence that 'aphrodisiac' supplements are effective in enhancing sexual performance.

■ No supplements are known to have the capacity to cure serious diseases such as cancer, heart disease, diabetes and HIV/AIDS. However, the right supplement may help to improve a chronic condition and to relieve symptoms such as pain and inflammation. But you should always consult your doctor before taking supplements as a treatment for any condition.

RNIs: WHAT DO THE NUMBERS MEAN?

■ In 1991 the Department of Health published *Dietary Reference Values for Food Energy and Nutrients for the United Kingdom.* Dietary Reference Value (DRV) is a generic term for daily dietary recommendations.

■ The most important of these is the Reference Nutrient Intake (RNI) – the amount of a nutrient that should be taken daily in order to meet the requirements of the majority of a specified population group. For example, the RNI for iron for a woman in the age group 19-50 is 14.8 mg, but for a man in the same group it is only 8.7 mg.

■ RNI values are derived from studies of the physiological requirements of healthy people. For example, the RNI for a vitamin may be based on the amount needed to maintain its correct blood level in a test group of people.

■ These studies are subject to wide interpretation, so the RNI value (or its equivalent) for a nutrient can vary from country to country. RNI values in the UK tend to be modest compared with other countries, especially the USA.

■ The RNI is not the amount of a nutrient recommended for optimum nutrition. This is especially the case with regard to intakes of the vitamins and minerals thought necessary to prevent degenerative diseases, such as cancer or heart disease. Despite much research, values for optimal intakes of vitamins and minerals are still being debated.

■ Some guidelines for optimal intakes have been produced by authoritative scientists, but none have yet been adopted by the government.

■ However, in the case of fat as an energy source in the diet, optimum levels for health have been agreed. The 1991 report recommends that no more than 33% of total energy should come from fat, and no more than 10% from saturated fatty acids.

■ When there is not enough information on the physiological requirements for a particular nutrient for an RNI to be set, a Safe Intake (SI) is recommended. This is based on the intake level that is believed to be consistent with maintaining good health. Nutrients for which SIs, rather than RNIs, have been set are biotin, chromium, manganese, molybdenum, pantothenic acid, vitamin E and vitamin K.

Basic types of supplement

If you visit a health-food shop, or stroll down the dietary supplement aisle in a supermarket or any large pharmacy, you cannot fail to be struck by the huge variety of products on the market.

Taking into account different brands and combinations of supplements, there are literally thousands of choices available. You are not likely to encounter as many as this in one location, but even a far more limited selection in your local chemist's shop can be confusing.

Manufacturers are constantly trying to distinguish their own brands from others, and so they devise different dosages, new combinations and creatively worded claims for their products. At the same time, scientists have found new and better ways of extracting nutritional components from plants and synthesising nutrients in a laboratory, resulting in many new and purer products.

Making informed decisions

In order to find your way through the jungle it is helpful to be familiar with the natures and properties of specific supplements – more than 70 of which are examined in detail in Part 1 of this book (*pages* 38-195). It is also essential to understand the terms used on supplement labels – advice on how to read a label is given on pages 33-34. But, to avoid feeling over-whelmed by all the choices facing you, it is useful first of all to learn about the basic types of supplement that are available and the key functions they perform in helping to keep you healthy.

The characteristics of vitamins, minerals, herbs and other supplements, including phytochemicals, are described below and on the next page. Some substances, such as amino acids, have been known to scientists for many years but only recently marketed as dietary supplements.

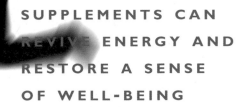

SUPPLEMENTS CAN REVIVE ENERGY AND RESTORE A SENSE OF WELL-BEING

Vitamins

- A vitamin is an organic substance that is essential for regulating both the metabolic functions within the body's cells and the processes that release energy from food.
- Evidence is growing that certain vitamins are anti-oxidants. These are substances that protect tissues from cell damage and may possibly help to prevent a number of degenerative diseases.
- There are 13 known vitamins, which can be categorised as either fat-soluble (A, D, E and K) or water-soluble (the eight B vitamins and C).

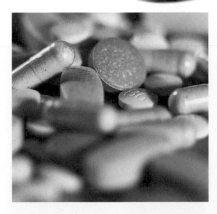

- The distinction between fat-soluble and water-soluble vitamins is important because the body stores fat-soluble vitamins for relatively long periods, such as months or even years; on the other hand, water-soluble vitamins, except vitamin B_{12}, remain in the body for a short time and therefore need to be replenished more frequently.
- With a few exceptions, notably vitamins D and K, the body does not have the capacity to manufacture vitamins – so, to maintain good health, they must be ingested through food or in nutritional supplements.

Minerals

- Minerals are present in the body in small amounts: in total they add up to only 4% of body weight.
- These inorganic substances are essential for a wide range of vital processes, from basic bone formation to the normal functioning of the heart and digestive system.
- A number of minerals have been linked to the prevention of cancer, osteoporosis and other chronic illnesses.
- Humans must replenish their mineral supplies through food or with supplements.
- Of more than 60 different minerals in the body, only 22 are considered essential.
- Of these, seven – including calcium, chloride, magnesium, phosphorus, potassium, sodium and sulphur – are usually called macrominerals, or major minerals.
- The other 15 minerals are called trace minerals, or microminerals, because the amount needed each day for good health is tiny (usually measured in micrograms, or millionths of a gram).

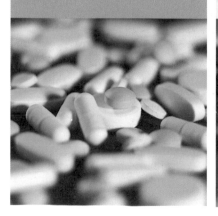

Herbs

- Herbal supplements are prepared from plants, often using the leaves, stems, roots and/or bark, as well as the buds and flowers.
- Many plant parts can be either used in their natural forms, or refined into tablets, capsules, powders, tinctures and other formulations.
- A herbal supplement may contain all the compounds found in a plant, or just one or two of the isolated compounds that have been successfully extracted.
- Many herbs have several active compounds that interact with one another to produce a therapeutic effect.
- In some herbs the active agents simply have not been identified, so it is necessary to use the entire herb to obtain all its benefits.
- Of the hundreds of remedies that feature in the current rebirth of interest in herbal medicines, the majority are being used to treat chronic or mild health problems.
- Herbs are also used to attain or maintain good health – for example, to enhance the immune system, to help to keep cholesterol levels low or to protect against fatigue.

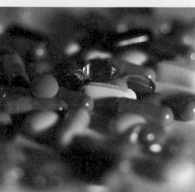

Other supplements

- These nutrients include a diverse group of products. Some, such as fish oils, are food substances believed by scientists to possess disease-fighting potential.
- Flavonoids, soya isoflavones, and carotenoids are phyto-chemicals – compounds found in fruit and vegetables that work to lower the risk of disease and may alleviate the symptoms of some ailments.
- Other nutritional supplements, such as coenzyme Q_{10}, are substances present in the body that can be re-created synthetically in a laboratory.
- Among similar examples is acidophilus, a 'friendly' bacterium in the body that, taken as a supplement, may aid in the treatment of some digestive disorders.
- Amino acids are the building blocks for proteins that may play a role in strengthening the immune system and in other health-promoting activities and are now available as supplements.

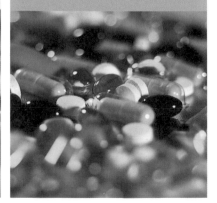

Buying supplements: preparations and forms

The number of different forms and strengths of supplements available theoretically allows you to find the kind that is best for you, but the wide choice and the varying label claims can make shopping for supplements confusing.

Some 'special' formulas – including those described as 'timed-release' or 'chelated' – may provide little additional benefit and are often not worth the extra expense.

Common forms

Tablets and capsules are frequently the most convenient forms of supplement to use, but other forms may be more appropriate in some cases.

TABLETS AND CAPSULES

Both tablets and capsules are easy to use and store, and they generally have a longer life than some other supplement forms.

As well as their vitamin or nutrient content, tablets are also likely to contain more, usually inert, additives known as excipients. These compounds bind, preserve or give bulk to the supplement, and some can help tablets to break down more quickly in the stomach. Increasingly, supplements are available in capsule-shaped, easy-to-swallow tablets called 'caplets'.

Essential fatty acids, such as those found in fish oils and evening primrose oil, and sometimes the fat-soluble vitamins A, D and E are available as 'softgel' capsules. Other vitamins and minerals are processed into powders or liquids and then encapsulated.

Capsules tend to have fewer additives than tablets, and there is evidence that they dissolve more readily, although this does not necessarily mean that they are absorbed better by the body.

POWDERS

People who find pills hard to swallow may choose to use powders, which can be mixed into juice or water or stirred into food. Ground seeds such as psyllium often come in this form.

Powdered vitamin C can be mixed with water for use as a skin compress. Dosages of powders can be easily adjusted, and because single nutrient powders have fewer additives than tablets or capsules they are useful for individuals who are allergic to certain substances. Powders are often cheaper than tablets or capsules.

LIQUIDS

Liquid formulas for oral use are easy to swallow and can be flavoured; many children's formulas are in liquid form. Some supplements, such as vitamin E, also come in this form for applying topically to the skin.

CHEWABLE TABLETS

Such supplements are usually flavoured, and are particularly useful for people who have trouble swallowing pills. They do not need to be taken with water.

Deglycyrrhised liquorice (DGL) is activated by saliva, so the tablets should be chewed rather than simply swallowed. Vitamin C is often found in chewable form. These tablets are often high in sugar or artificial sweeteners.

LOZENGES

Some supplements can be bought in the form of lozenges that dissolve slowly in the mouth. Zinc lozenges, for example, help in the treatment of colds and flu.

SUBLINGUAL LIQUIDS AND TABLETS

A few supplements in liquid or tablet form are formulated to dissolve sublingually (under the tongue), providing quick absorption into the bloodstream without interference from stomach acids and digestive enzymes.

TIMED-RELEASE FORMULAS

These consist of tiny capsules contained within a standard-size capsule. The microcapsules gradually break down, releasing the vitamin into the bloodstream over a period of about 2 to 10 hours. Vitamin C is often sold in this form because it cannot be stored in the body. Timed-release formulas may allow a more natural and even absorption of a vitamin into the bloodstream, but there are no reliable studies showing that they are more efficiently utilised by the body than conventional capsules or tablets.

CHELATED MINERALS

Minerals in supplements are chelated, or bonded, to another substance; this may be an inorganic mineral, an organic substance or an amino acid. The substance to which a mineral is chelated dictates how well it is absorbed. Inorganic chelates, such as oxides, sulphates, phosphates, chlorides and carbonates, tend to be cheaper than organic chelates but less well absorbed. Organic chelates, including ascorbates, citrates, succinates and malates, are better absorbed.

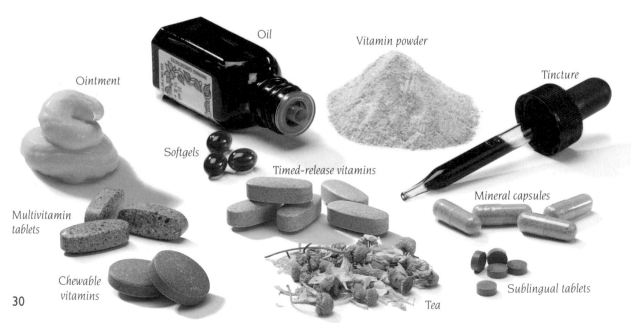

Ointment

Oil

Vitamin powder

Tincture

Softgels

Timed-release vitamins

Mineral capsules

Multivitamin tablets

Chewable vitamins

Tea

Sublingual tablets

Herbal remedies

You can buy whole herbs and make up your own formulas, but the tablets, capsules and other prepackaged forms described below, including forms for external use, are readily available in supermarkets, chemists' and health-food shops.

For a discussion of the preparations that combine one herb with another, and herbs with other nutritional supplements, *see pages* 78-79.

TABLETS AND CAPSULES
Tablets and capsules are prepared using either a whole herb or an extract containing a high concentration of the herb's active components. Either form allows you to avoid the often bitter taste of the herb. The constituents are ground into a powder that can be pressed into tablets or encapsulated.

Some herbs are available in 'enteric'-coated capsules. These pass through the stomach into the small intestine before dissolving. This minimises potential gastrointestinal discomfort and also enhances the absorption of some herbs into the bloodstream.

TINCTURES
These concentrated liquids are made by soaking the whole or part of a herb in water and alcohol. The alcohol acts to extract and concentrate the herb's active components. In certain cases some or all of the alcohol is then removed. Non-alcoholic concentrations can also be made using glycerine.

Tinctures are typically taken in small doses several times a day. The dose is measured in drops with a pipette and usually diluted in water or juice.

TEAS, INFUSIONS AND DECOCTIONS
Less concentrated than tinctures, teas and infusions are brewed from the fresh or dried flowers, leaves or roots of a herb. They can be

purchased in bulk or as tea bags. Although tea is normally made with boiling water, the herbal teas recommended in this book are prepared as infusions, using hot water that is just on the verge of boiling – this preserves the beneficial oils that can be dissipated by the steam of boiling water. To make a decoction the tougher parts of a herb, such as the stem or bark, are generally simmered for at least half an hour.

These liquid remedies should be used as soon as possible after being brewed because they start to lose their potency within a few hours of exposure to air. If stored in tightly sealed glass jars in the refrigerator they will retain some strength for up to three days.

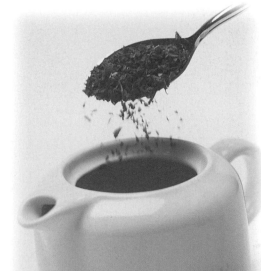

ESSENTIAL OILS
Oils extracted from herbs can be distilled to form potent concentrations for external use in massage or on particular areas of the skin. These 'essential' oils are usually placed in a neutral 'carrier' oil, such as almond oil, before use on the skin. (Milder 'infused' oils can be prepared at home.) Essential

herbal oils should never be ingested, with one exception – a few drops of peppermint oil on the tongue may be recommended for bad breath, and capsules of the same oil can be beneficial in the treatment of digestive problems.

GELS, OINTMENTS AND CREAMS

Gels and ointments made from the fats or oils of aromatic herbs are applied to the skin to soothe rashes, heal bruises or wounds, and serve other therapeutic purposes. Creams are usually light oil-and-water mixtures that are partly absorbed by the skin, allowing it to breathe while also keeping in moisture. Creams can be used for moisturising dry skin, for cleansing, and for relieving rashes, insect bites or sunburn.

Standardised extracts

To obtain a concentrated extract, a herb is soaked in alcohol or water (which is allowed to evaporate) and then put into a heavy press. Extracts are the most effective form of herbs, which makes them particularly useful for people with absorption difficulties or severe disorders.

When herbs are recommended in this book for the treatment of ailments, it is usually suggested that 'standardised extracts' should be chosen. Herbalists and manufacturers use this term to guarantee the potency of the active ingredients of a product.

The quality of a herb is dependent on many factors, including the sunlight, water, tempera-ture and soil quality to which it was exposed when growing as well as storage conditions and extraction and manufacturing procedures. A change in any of these conditions can affect potency. The standardisation of an extract ensures that the product you are buying is not affected by these variations.

To achieve standardisation the active components of a whole herb – such as the allicin in garlic or the ginsenosides in ginseng – are

extracted, concentrated and made into a form of supplement, such as a tablet, capsule or tincture. By this method a precise amount of the active ingredient can be supplied in each dose.

Sometimes, instead of standardised extracts, manufacturers process the whole, or crude, herb. In this case the whole herb is simply air or freeze-dried, made into a powder then converted into capsule, tablet, tincture or other form ready for packaging. Herbalists continue to debate the comparative merits of standardised extracts and crude herbs. Crude herbs may contain unidentified active ingredients, and only by ingesting the whole thing can all its benefits be obtained. In many cases you would have to use a much greater amount of a whole herb to gain an effect similar to that of a standardised product, but although stan-dardised products are more consistent from batch to batch, this does not mean that they are more effective.

Buying supplements: how to read a label

Understanding the key terms that may be found on supplement labels can help you to make a better informed decision about which supplement is right for you.

Manufacturers are required by law not to be misleading about their products. However, because there is no standardisation of information with regard to supplements, you are likely to see differences in the wording and details that appear on packaging.

Health-improving claims

Most nutritional supplements for sale in the UK are classed as foods, which restricts what can be said about them. A limited number of health maintenance claims are allowed, but suggesting that such a product has the property to treat, prevent or cure any condition is prohibited.

Certain products with a licence granted by the Medicines and Healthcare products Regulatory Agency (MHRA) can cite health-improving claims. This is why you may read on an echinacea bottle 'a traditional herbal remedy for the symptomatic relief of colds and influenza', but packaging for vitamin C could usually only go as far as to say that the product is 'important for a healthy immune system'. If a vitamin C product is licensed for the relief of colds, however, then the label could make that claim. There are licensed vitamin supplements on the market – look for a PL (Product Licence) number on the packaging.

What the terms mean

QUANTITY The amount in the container, in terms either of the number of capsules or tablets or volume or weight.

'HIGH POTENCY' This term could be used to compare strengths between different products in a manufacturer's range, but is potentially misleading without other information. It is better to check nutrient quantities and compare them with other products than to set store by this term.

DIRECTIONS FOR USE Instructions on the amount of the supplement to take, as recommended by the manufacturer. This normally includes advice about when and how to take the product – with or between meals or with a glass of water, for

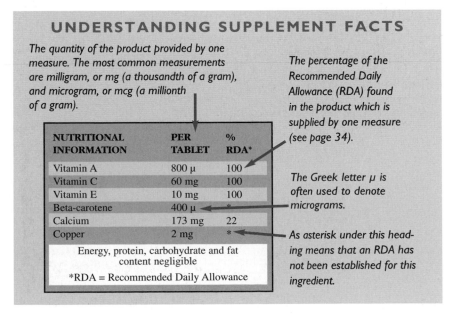

UNDERSTANDING SUPPLEMENT FACTS

The quantity of the product provided by one measure. The most common measurements are milligram, or mg (a thousandth of a gram), and microgram, or mcg (a millionth of a gram).

The percentage of the Recommended Daily Allowance (RDA) found in the product which is supplied by one measure (see page 34).

NUTRITIONAL INFORMATION	PER TABLET	% RDA*
Vitamin A	800 µ	100
Vitamin C	60 mg	100
Vitamin E	10 mg	100
Beta-carotene	400 µ	*
Calcium	173 mg	22
Copper	2 mg	*
Energy, protein, carbohydrate and fat content negligible		
*RDA = Recommended Daily Allowance		

The Greek letter µ is often used to denote micrograms.

As asterisk under this heading means that an RDA has not been established for this ingredient.

example. If a product is classed as a food it should not refer to a 'dose' or 'dosage', which suggests a medical use.

INGREDIENTS A list of everything in the supplement, arranged in decreasing order according to weight, is required by law. Ingredients include binders, fillers, coatings, preservatives, colouring agents and other substances, including inert ones.

CAUTION A statement warning that, for example, pregnant women or those with an allergy to niacin should not use a product, or to advise that a doctor should be consulted if a user is under medical supervision. Cautions about the dangers of exceeding the stated measure of vitamin A and iron are required by law.

CHILD WARNING A precautionary statement that all supplements should be kept in a place where children cannot reach them. Some supplements can be toxic to children in large amounts.

STORAGE ADVICE This is advice on how best to store the product. When this information appears on a bottle or packet it is found next to the 'best before' date or a reference to it. Most supplements should be kept in a cool, dry place, which means they should not be stored in a refrigerator or in a damp place where moisture could cause damage to them. There are, however, some products that should be refrigerated after opening. If this is the case, the label on the product will tell you.

'BEST BEFORE' DATE A date up to which the supplement can be expected to retain its full potency, if properly stored. In effect, it is a pledge from the manufacturer that the product will remain 'fresh' up to that point.

NAME AND PLACE OF BUSINESS The name and address of the manufacturer, packager or distributor. This is the address you can write to for more product information. There may also be a telephone number on the label.

UNDERSTANDING 'BP'
■ You may see the letters 'BP' on the packaging of certain supplements. This is the stamp of the British Pharmacopoeia, a commission that is appointed by the government and works closely with the Medical Controls Agency.
■ A BP specification for a particular preparation, sometimes known as a monograph, provides an indication that the product contains the right amount of the right active ingredient of the right quality.
■ 'BP' on the label indicates that the quality of the ingredients has been checked, even though their potency has not necessarily been assessed. For products that are intended for medicinal use it applies whether or not the letters 'BP' appear on the label.
■ Products that are not sold for medicinal purposes, such as certain vitamins, do not have to comply with the BP, but are permitted to carry the designation if they are of the required quality.

WHY DO LABELS USE THE TERM RDA?

■ As required by European Union regulations, labels on foods and dietary supplements give their contents of nutrients as Recommended Daily Amounts (RDAs).
■ RDAs approximate to the average quantities of key nutrients that people should obtain from their diets, and are said to apply to 'average adults'.
■ Since they are based on the requirements of men, RDAs are only a very rough guide to healthy eating for other groups of people – they take no account of differences in individual nutritional requirements according to age, gender, occupation and other factors. For example, an RDA does not differentiate between a man of 18 and a woman of 45, who have very different dietary needs.
■ The EU RDA is therefore a simple approximation that is used for labels only.
■ For all other purposes, including the provision of nutritional advice, the DRVs, including the RNIs, are used (see page 26).

Using supplements safely and effectively

Responsible manufacturers print instructions about proper use on their supplement labels, but you may encounter many brands that do not include instructions.

The entries in this book provide detailed information about the benefits, uses, side effects and forms of supplements, as well as the doses that are considered safe and effective. Set out below are some general guidelines about the safe and effective use of supplements, and on pages 392-5 you will find a section listing interactions between supplements and commonly prescribed medications.

The proper balance

Some nutrients may interact with one another, which can affect their absorption or utilisation by the body. For example, fat-soluble vitamins (A, D, E and K) require some dietary fat to facilitate absorption so they should be taken with food.

Iron taken with meals is best absorbed with small amounts of meat and foods containing vitamin C. Calcium absorption is improved by taking supplements with meals, and the effect of calcium on building healthy bones is enhanced when it is taken with magnesium.

Other nutrients, when taken in combination, likewise enhance one another's benefits. For example, vitamin C helps to regenerate vitamin E after it has been modified by neutralising reactive free radicals – so, because these antioxidant nutrients work together, they are best taken at the same time.

The proper amounts

Dietary supplements are generally safe when consumed in the appropriate dosages. But more is not necessarily better – and sometimes it can be worse. For example, the mineral selenium is recommended for many disorders, from cataracts to cancer prevention, but taking doses even slightly higher than those recommended can cause loss of hair and other toxic reactions. When using supplements it is advisable to avoid high doses, particularly the extremely high ones known as 'megadoses'. Whatever the circumstances, follow dosage recommendations closely. In addition, notify your doctor at once if your condition worsens or if any serious adverse reactions develop.

VITAMINS AND MINERALS

Most vitamins can be taken in significantly higher doses than their RNIs (*see page* 26) without incurring adverse reactions. However, some fat-soluble vitamins, which are stored in the body rather than excreted, may be toxic at high doses. In particular, taking an excessive amount of vitamin A or vitamin D is dangerous. Although very high doses of some other vitamins – such as vitamin C – are not toxic, certain individuals may experience side effects. Reducing the dosage will usually remedy the situation.

Some minerals taken in large doses or over time can block the absorption of other minerals; zinc, for instance, can impede the absorption of copper. Also, large amounts of certain minerals are linked to disease – several studies have shown that too much iron in men, for example, increases their risk of heart disease.

For these reasons, even researchers who believe that the RNIs for many vitamins are too low think that the levels for minerals are generally adequate for optimum health.

HERBS

Surveys by toxicologists conclude that serious side effects or toxic reactions associated with herbal medicines are rare; nevertheless, some once-popular medicinal herbs, such as foxglove and chaparral, are now recognised as toxic.

Occasionally some people have serious allergic reactions to a herb; these may include a rash or difficulty in breathing. Furthermore, because no uniform quality control for herbal preparations exists, the chemical composition of a herbal remedy can vary greatly from batch to batch. It may also contain potentially toxic contaminants and other ingredients that could influence the herb's effectiveness or cause side effects.

Products that contain standardised extracts are more likely to provide a proper dose of a particular supplement than those that do not, but whenever you buy a supplement – whether it is a standardised extract or a whole herb in tablet, tincture or another form – you are always dependent on the manufacturer's integrity.

PEOPLE WHO SHOULD BE WARY OF HERBS

Using some herbs for medicinal purposes can be dangerous for people with certain conditions or for those on particular medications (*see pages* 392-5). Garlic, for example, may intensify the effects of anticoagulant drugs, while liquorice – which aids digestive problems and enhances the immune system – can raise blood pressure. Even so, apart from the few contra-indications that have been identified, the tonic herbs which are described in this book have no adverse effects and can be safely taken over the long term.

The issue of quality control

How do you know what a product contains? Manufacturers are required by law to list all the active ingredients on each label, but monitoring of the contents of supplements can be sporadic, so no one is sure about the degree of compliance.

Established manufacturers of supplements have reputations to protect, and so they try to ensure that their products contain what is stated on the labels. But herbal supplements can sometimes be problematic.

For example, in a survey sponsored by the Good Housekeeping Institute of America, the levels of an active ingredient in St John's wort were found to vary considerably between brands. A study published in the leading British medical journal *The Lancet* reported that some supplements that purported to be ginseng contained varying amounts of active ginsenosides, and others none at all. However, it was later pointed out that the latter (although called 'ginseng') were actually different species and could not be expected to contain ginsenosides.

SAFETY GUIDELINES

Supplements, especially herbs, can have potent primary effects and side effects, so keep these points in mind when using them:

■ Shop carefully. There is no independent guarantee of purity or potency, so it is up to you to select brands with a reputation for quality.

■ Do not exceed the recommended dosages. Overdosing with a supplement can have serious consequences. In the case of herbs and nutritional supplements, start with the lowest dose when a dosage range is given.

■ Monitor your reactions. At the first sign of a problem, stop using the supplement. You should also stop taking the herb if it does not seem to be working (but give it time – you may need to take a herb for a month or more before noticing an effect).

■ Take a break. If you are treating a particular condition with supplements, it is advisable to take them for specified periods, then stop temporarily to see if the condition has improved. If the problem returns you may need to take the supplement over a long period as a 'maintenance' medication.

■ Avoid risks. If you have symptoms that indicate a serious problem, do not self-treat it with supplements but arrange to see your doctor immediately.

■ Very young or elderly people, and pregnant or breastfeeding women, should also consult their doctors before using supplements.

■ Always ask your doctor or pharmacist about possible interactions with any drugs you are taking (*see pages* 392-5).

Practitioners

If you are suffering from a particular ailment, consult your GP for at least an initial diagnosis. In general, practitioners of complementary medicine have less training in making diagnoses, and most would recommend that you see a conventionally trained doctor, particularly for more serious ailments. The two approaches can usually work alongside each other. Your GP may be able to recommend an alternative practitioner, or friends and family may be able to make personal recommendations.

Because anyone can legally call themselves a herbalist, even after completing a course as short as week, you should obtain a register of accredited practitioners in your area. The Complementary Medical Association and the Institute for Complementary Medicine can provide details of registered of naturopaths, herbalists and nutritionists as well as other complementary medicine practitioners (*see pages* 396-7). Registered practitioners have usually completed an accredited course, are insured and have accepted their organisation's code of ethics.

Practitioners should be willing to talk to you on the telephone, explaining their approach and answering your questions. Be wary of anyone who suggests a long, and probably expensive, course of treatment, and of any practitioner who is very dismissive of other approaches. During the initial consultation you should be asked for a full medical history and also for details of any drugs or supplements you are taking – to ensure that any possible adverse interaction between them is avoided. The number and frequency of follow-up visits will depend on the ailment and the practitioner.

MEDICAL HERBALISTS

Although medical herbalists learn the same diagnostic skills as ordinary doctors, they take a holistic approach to healing and use herbs rather than drugs. A member of the National Institute of Medical Herbalists has had four years of training.

NATUROPATHS

Naturopaths have the same training in diagnostic skills as ordinary doctors. Their approach is based on principles which involve non-suppression of symptoms and non-interference with the body's natural defence systems. Treatment may include nutritional advice, hydrotherapy and relaxation techniques.

The letters ND after a name mean that a naturopath has acquired a national diploma after a four-year degree course. The letters MRN indicate a practitioner who is a member of the General Council and Register of Naturopaths, the largest in the UK, which recognises only full-time degree courses.

NUTRITIONISTS

These practitioners specialise in the study of nutrition. The letters RNUT denote a registered nutritionist, while RPHNUT indicates a registered public health nutritionist who has studied 'population' nutrition – for example, in regard to elderly people or some other segment of the population. To be registered with the Nutrition Society a nutritionist must complete a three-year degree course and three years' practical experience.

PHARMACISTS

These are often the most accessible kind of health professional. Although their role is to manage and check the safety and accuracy of prescription drugs, they can also advise patients on how to manage their medicines for optimum treatment. This usually means conventional medicine, but some pharmacists are also knowledgeable about supplements. Any trained pharmacist has completed a four-year degree course and should be registered with the Royal Pharmaceutical Society of Great Britain.

Part I

Supplements

In this section of the book you will find detailed profiles of more than 70 popular supplements, arranged alphabetically from aloe vera to zinc. Each entry is colour-coded according to basic supplement type (for a general explanation of these basic types see pages 27-28). Look for:

- ○ Vitamins
- ● Minerals
- ● Herbs
- ● Nutritional Supplements

Each profile describes what the supplement is, the forms in which it comes and the way it works to promote good health and to prevent or relieve specific ailments. How much you need, the amount you should take at any one time and other guidelines for using the supplement are explained, along with possible side effects. Key food sources of vitamins and minerals are also indicated.

This section also includes special features on antioxidants, combination supplements, functional and fortified foods, and phytochemicals.

To learn more about a particular disorder, refer to Part 2 of this book, Protecting Your Health (pages 194-391). If you have any serious medical or psychiatric condition – or one that may not have been properly diagnosed – always consult your doctor before treating it with any supplement.

ABOUT THE RECOMMENDATIONS

Specific dosage suggestions are listed in each of the profiles that follow. These are the total daily amount of a supplement that you need to treat a disorder or condition. In practical terms you may have to adjust these numbers to take account of the additional amounts of these same nutrients that you may be getting in any daily multivitamin or individual supplements that you are taking for other health reasons.

For example, we suggest taking 250 mg vitamin E daily for the promotion of a healthy prostate gland. If you are already taking a daily multivitamin tablet that supplies 250 mg vitamin E, you do not need any additional supplement of that vitamin. If you also have angina (which calls for 500 mg vitamin E),

you will have to take only 250 mg more each day to meet that requirement as well. The dosages are meant to be accurate, but each person is different. Always read the label on a supplement packet, and do not exceed recommended dosages, even though you may be treating several ailments. If you have a serious medical condition, consult your doctor about using supplements.

A final word: We have tried to include widely available dosages in the pages that follow but the strengths of individual supplement products vary greatly. If the information on a bottle or packet confuses you there are many qualified people, including health professionals and pharmicists, who can help you to choose the appropriate dose.

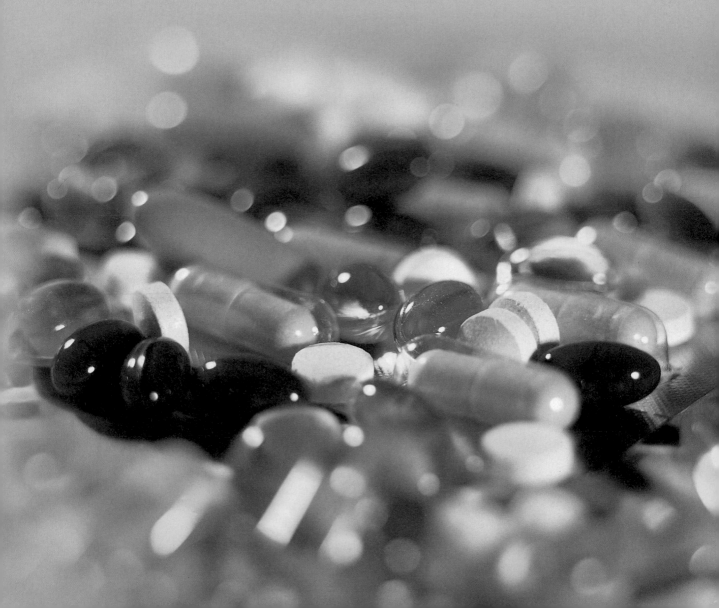

Aloe vera

Aloe vera
A. barbadensis
A. vulgaris

Long before the reign of Cleopatra, the ancient Egyptians discovered the power of the aloe vera plant. The cool, soothing gel from its leaf has been used ever since to treat burns and minor wounds, and is the basis of aloe vera juice, which is effective in calming digestive complaints.

Common uses

Applied topically

- Heals minor burns (including sunburn), cuts and abrasions, insect bites and stings, small skin ulcers and frostbite.

- Relieves the itching of shingles (herpes zoster).

- May help to clear up warts.

Taken internally

- Soothes ulcers, indigestion and other digestive complaints.

Forms

- Capsule
- Cream/ointment
- Fresh herb/gel
- Liquid
- Softgel

What it is

A succulent of the lily family, aloe vera has fleshy leaves that provide a gel widely used as a topical treatment for skin problems – a practice dating back to at least 1500 BC, when Egyptian healers described it in their treatises. The plant is native to the Cape of Good Hope and grows wild in much of Africa and Madagascar. Commercial growers cultivate it in the Caribbean, the Mediterranean, Japan and the USA.

What it does

Scientists are not sure how aloe vera works, but they have identified many of its active ingredients. Rich in anti-inflammatory substances, the gel contains a gummy material called acemannan that acts as an emollient, as well as bradykininase, a compound that reduces pain and swelling, and components which sooth itching. Aloe vera also dilates the tiny blood vessels known as capillaries, allowing more blood to reach the site of an injury and thereby speeding up the process of healing. Some studies show that it destroys, or at least inhibits the spread of, a number of bacteria, viruses and fungi.

CAUTION!

- Aloe vera should not be confused with the bitter yellow aloe latex, a laxative which can cause severe cramps and diarrhoea. Pregnant or breast-feeding women, in particular, should avoid aloe latex.

REMINDER: If you have a medical condition, consult your doctor before taking supplements.

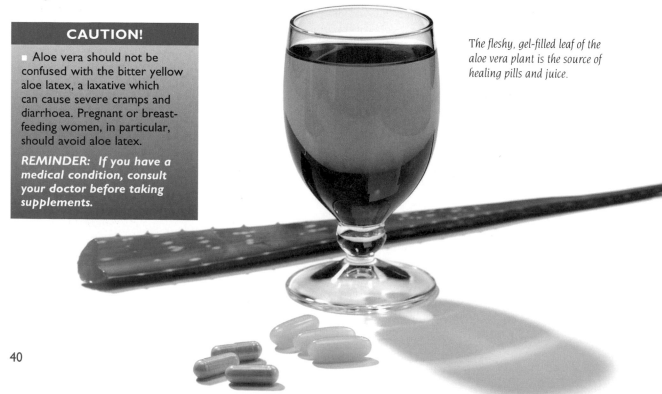

The fleshy, gel-filled leaf of the aloe vera plant is the source of healing pills and juice.

⊗ **Major benefits:** Aloe vera gel is particularly effective when applied to damaged skin. It aids in the healing of minor burns, sunburn, mouth ulcers and minor skin wounds, as well as relieving pain and reducing itching in people suffering from shingles. The gel also provides a hygienic moisturising barrier, so that wounds do not dry out. Its capillary-dilating properties increase blood circulation, speeding the regeneration of skin and alleviating mild cases of frostbite. The gel's antiviral effects may also promote the healing of warts.

Though effective against minor cuts and abrasions, aloe vera may not be a good choice for more serious, infected wounds. In a study of 21 women in a Los Angeles hospital whose caesarean-section wounds had become infected, applying aloe vera gel actually increased the length of time it took for the wounds to heal – from 53 to 83 days.

⊗ **Additional benefits:** Aloe vera gel is used to make a juice that may be taken internally to combat inflammatory digestive disorders, including ulcers and indigestion. However, research into its effectiveness in this form has been very limited. In Japan, purified aloe vera compounds have been found to inhibit stomach secretions and lesions. In one study, aloe vera juice cured 17 out of 18 patients with peptic ulcers, but there was no comparison group taking a placebo. A commercial laboratory in the USA is conducting trials with an aloe-derived compound as a treatment for people with ulcerative colitis, a common type of inflammatory bowel disease.

Other studies are exploring aloe vera's effectiveness as a possible antiviral and immune-boosting agent for people suffering from AIDS; as a treatment for victims of leukaemia and other types of cancer; and as a therapy for diabetics.

How to take it

⊘ **Dosage:** *For external use:* Liberally apply aloe vera gel or cream to the injured skin as needed or desired. *For internal use:* Take a half to three-quarters of a cup of aloe vera juice three times a day; or take one or two capsules as directed on the label.

⊙ **Guidelines for use:** Topically, aloe vera gel can be applied repeatedly, especially in the case of burns. Simply rub it on the affected area, let it dry and reapply when needed. Fresh gel from a live leaf is the most potent – and economical – form of the herb. If you have an aloe vera plant, cut off several inches from a leaf, then slice the cutting lengthwise. Spread the gel found in the centre onto the affected area. For internal use, take aloe vera juice between meals. Aloe latex, a yellow extract from the inner leaf of the plant, is a powerful laxative that should be used only sparingly on the advice of a doctor.

Possible side effects

Topical aloe vera is very safe. On rare occasions a mild itching or rash may develop; if this happens to you, simply discontinue use. Aloe vera juice may – as the result of poor processing – contain small amounts of the laxative ingredient found in aloe latex. If you experience cramping, diarrhoea or loose stools after taking the juice, stop taking it immediately and replace it with a new supply. Never take aloe vera juice if you are pregnant or breastfeeding.

Alpha-lipoic acid

Supplements of alpha-lipoic acid have been shown to alleviate the effects of nerve damage in people with diabetes. They may also protect the liver and brain cells, prevent cataracts and serve as a powerful general antioxidant.

Common uses

- *Relieves numbness, tingling and other symptoms of nerve damage in people with diabetes.*

- *Protects the liver in hepatitis sufferers, and in cases of alcohol abuse, or exposure to poisons or toxic chemicals.*

- *Inhibits the development of cataracts.*

- *May help to preserve memory in people with Alzheimer's disease.*

- *Acts as a high-potency antioxidant and, possibly, an immunity booster; may alleviate a wide range of disorders, including psoriasis, chronic fatigue syndrome and AIDS.*

Forms

- Capsule
- Tablet

What it is

It had been known since the 1950s that alpha-lipoic acid (also called thioctic acid or, simply, lipoic acid) worked with enzymes throughout the body to speed up the processes involved in energy production. More recently, in the late 1980s, it was discovered that this vitamin-like substance also had the capacity to act as a powerful antioxidant, neutralising naturally occurring, highly reactive molecules called free radicals that can damage cells. Although the body manufactures alpha-lipoic acid in minute amounts, it is mainly present in foods such as spinach, meats (especially liver) and brewer's yeast. It is difficult to obtain therapeutic amounts of alpha-lipoic acid through diet alone, however, and some people find that they need to take supplements in order to benefit fully from its healing properties.

What it does

Alpha-lipoic acid affects nearly every cell in the body. It helps all the B vitamins – including thiamin, riboflavin, pantothenic acid and niacin – to convert carbohydrates, protein and fats found in foods into energy that the body can store for later use. Alpha-lipoic acid is a cell-protecting antioxidant that may stimulate the body to recycle other antioxidants, such as vitamins C and E, thereby boosting their potency. Owing to its unique chemical properties, alpha-lipoic acid is easily absorbed by most tissues in the body, including the brain, nerves and liver, which makes it valuable for treating a wide range of ailments.

✪ **MAJOR BENEFITS:** One of alpha-lipoic acid's primary uses is to treat nerve damage, including the effects of diabetic neuropathy, a long-term complication of diabetes that causes pain and loss of feeling in the limbs. The nervous condition may be partly the result of free-radical damage to nerve cells caused by runaway levels of glucose in the blood. Alpha-lipoic acid may play a role in countering nerve damage through its antioxidant action. In addition, it can help people with diabetes to respond to insulin,

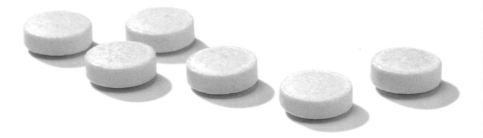

the hormone that regulates glucose levels. In a study of 74 people with type II diabetes who were given 600 mg or more of alpha-lipoic acid daily, all benefited from lowered glucose levels. Studies in animals also show that alpha-lipoic acid increases blood flow to the nerves and enhances the conduction of nerve impulses. These effects may make alpha-lipoic acid suitable for the treatment of numbness, tingling and other symptoms of nerve damage from any cause, not only diabetes.

Alpha-lipoic acid also benefits the liver, protecting it against damage from free radicals and helping it to eliminate toxins from the body. It is sometimes used to treat hepatitis, cirrhosis and other liver ailments, as well as in cases of poisoning by lead or other heavy metals or by industrial chemicals such as carbon tetrachloride.

✚ **ADDITIONAL BENEFITS:** Alpha-lipoic acid may have other potential medicinal uses, but more research is needed. Some compelling studies in animals show that it can prevent cataracts from forming. Other animal experiments suggest that it may improve memory (making it beneficial in cases of Alzheimer's disease, for example) and protect brain cells against damage caused by an insufficient supply of blood to the brain – the result of surgery or stroke, for instance.

Some evidence indicates that alpha-lipoic acid's antioxidant properties make it effective in the suppression of viral reproduction. In one study, alpha-lipoic acid supplements were shown to boost the immune system and liver function in a majority of patients infected with AIDS. It may also help in the fight against cancer, especially the forms of the disease thought to be related to free-radical damage. There is evidence, too, that alpha-lipoic acid may help to slow the development of atherosclerosis, for which people with diabetes are at higher risk. Other studies are investigating the effectiveness of alpha-lipoic acid in Alzheimer's disease and Parkinson's disease. Finally, as part of a general high-potency antioxidant formula, alpha-lipoic acid may prove effective against disorders ranging from chronic fatigue syndrome to psoriasis, which may be aggravated, in part, by free-radical damage.

How to take it

⊘ **DOSAGE:** *To treat specific disorders*: Alpha-lipoic acid is usually taken in doses of 100 to 200 mg three times a day. *For general antioxidant support*: Lower doses of 50 to 150 mg a day may be used.

◈ **GUIDELINES FOR USE:** Supplements of alpha-lipoic acid can be taken with or without food.

Possible side effects

There have been no reports of serious side effects in people taking alpha-lipoic acid. Occasionally the supplement may produce a mild upset stomach, and in rare cases allergic skin rashes have occurred. If side effects appear, lower the dose or stop using the supplement.

RECENT FINDINGS

In a study of people suffering from diabetic nerve damage, 328 patients were given 100 mg, 600 mg or 1200 mg of alpha-lipoic acid a day over a three-week period. Patients receiving 600 mg reported the most significant reduction in pain and numbness compared with the other groups.

Alpha-lipoic acid may also benefit the 25% of diabetes sufferers at risk of sudden death from nerve-related heart damage. After four months of taking 800 mg of alpha-lipoic acid a day, these patients showed a notable improvement in heart function.

A study of ageing mice indicated that alpha-lipoic acid improved long-term memory, possibly by preventing damage to brain cells by free radicals.

DID YOU KNOW?

Doctors have used an injectable form of alpha-lipoic acid to save the lives of people who became ill after eating poisonous amanita mushrooms picked in the wild.

Amino acids

The proteins in food and in the human body are combinations of chemical units called amino acids. A diet deficient in even one amino acid can have a damaging effect on health. Supplements may be needed to help the body to work more efficiently and to treat disease.

Common uses

- Treatment of heart disease.
- Lowering of blood pressure.
- Boosting immune function.
- Relieving some nervous disorders.

Forms

- Capsule
- Liquid
- Powder
- Tablet

CAUTION!

- Pregnant or breastfeeding women, diabetics or anyone with high blood pressure or a liver or kidney disease should be particularly wary about using amino acid supplements.

REMINDER: If you have a medical condition, consult your doctor before taking supplements.

What they are

Every cell in the body needs and uses amino acids. When you eat a meal, your digestive system breaks down the protein from foods into separate amino acids, which are then recombined to create the specific types of protein required by the body. (Each cell is programmed to produce exactly the right combination for its needs.) There are two types of amino acid: non-essential and essential. The body can manufacture non-essential amino acids but must obtain essential amino acids from foods. Non-essential amino acids include alanine, arginine, asparagine, aspartic acid, cysteine, glutamic acid, glutamine, glycine, proline, serine, taurine and tyrosine. Essential amino acids include histidine, isoleucine, leucine, lysine, methionine, phenylalanine, threonine, tryptophan and valine.

What they do

Amino acids are needed to maintain and repair muscles, tendons, skin, ligaments, organs, glands, nails and hair. They also assist in the production of hormones (such as insulin), neurotransmitters (message-carrying chemicals within the brain), various body fluids, and enzymes that trigger bodily functions.

Though the major cause of an amino acid deficiency is poor diet (particularly a diet low in protein), amino acids may also be affected by infection, trauma, stress, medication, age and chemical imbalances within the body. Nutritionally aware doctors may suggest a blood test to determine whether a patient has a deficiency. Amino acid supplements can compensate for deficiencies and can also be taken therapeutically to alleviate a number of health problems.

✪ **MAJOR BENEFITS:** Various amino acids, and their by-products, are very effective in the treatment of heart disease. Highly concentrated in the cells of the heart muscle, carnitine – a substance similar to an amino acid that the body produces from lysine – strengthens the heart, aids the

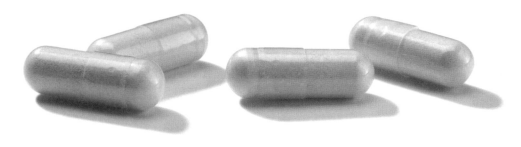

recovery of people who have suffered heart failure and can improve the chances of surviving a heart attack. As it is also involved in fat metabolism, carnitine may help to lower high levels of triglycerides (blood fats related to cholesterol). Arginine, a non-essential amino acid, reduces the risk of heart attack and stroke by widening blood vessels and lowering blood pressure; it can also ease the symptoms and pains of angina. Taurine treats heart failure and lowers high blood pressure by balancing the blood's sodium-to-potassium ratio and by regulating excessive activity of the central nervous system.

N-acetylcysteine (NAC), a by-product of cysteine that is more easily absorbed than cysteine, stimulates the body's production of antioxidants and may itself be an antioxidant. As such it aids in the repair of cell damage and boosts the immune system. NAC also thins the mucus of chronic bronchitis and has been used to protect the liver in overdoses of acetaminophen (Tylenol). It may also relieve disorders involving damage to brain or nerve cells, such as multiple sclerosis.

✤ **ADDITIONAL BENEFITS:** Concentrated in the cells of the digestive tract, glutamine soothes irritable bowel syndrome and diverticular disorders and helps to heal ulcers. By enhancing the production of certain brain chemicals, taurine may be a boon to people with epilepsy. It is also a key element in bile and may prevent gallstones. People with diabetes can benefit from taurine because it facilitates the body's use of insulin.

Carnitine feeds the muscles by making it possible for them to burn fat for energy. Lysine is one of the most effective treatments for cold sores and is also useful for shingles and mouth ulcers. (Arginine, on the other hand, can trigger outbreaks of cold sores or genital herpes.)

How to take them

▨ **DOSAGE:** For the recommended dose of a particular amino acid supplement, refer to the appropriate ailment in the section Protecting Your Health. If you use an individual amino acid for longer than a month, take it with a mixed amino acid complex – a supplement that contains a variety of amino acids – to ensure that you are receiving adequate, balanced amounts of all the amino acids.

◉ **GUIDELINES FOR USE:** Amino acid supplements are more effective when they do not have to compete with the amino acids present in high-protein foods. For this reason, take the supplements at least 1½ hours before or after meals – the best times are probably first thing in the morning or at bedtime.

Individual amino acid supplements should not be used for longer than three months except under the supervision of a doctor familiar with their use. Take mixed amino acid supplements on an empty stomach and at a different time of day from when you take the individual supplement.

Possible side effects

As long as they are taken in the recommended amounts, amino acid supplements have no side effects. High doses of certain amino acids, however, may be toxic and induce nausea, vomiting or diarrhoea.

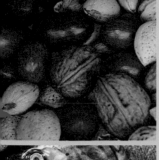
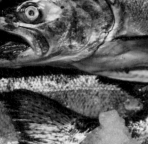
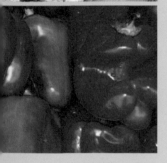

Antioxidants

Antioxidants are substances in food used by the body as protection against free radicals, molecules produced during normal metabolism which can wreak havoc if they proliferate in an uncontrolled way as a result of illness, ageing or overexposure to toxins or the sun.

HOW FREE RADICALS CAUSE DAMAGE

Free radicals are highly unstable and quickly react with nearby molecules, setting off a process called oxidation which can have harmful effects on the body.

■ If free radicals oxidise DNA (the body's genetic code) in the nucleus of a cell, the reaction can cause cell mutations, which may initiate cancer.

■ The oxidation of cholesterol particles in the blood can trigger the build up of fatty deposits in the arteries, which may lead to heart disease or stroke.

■ Free radicals have also been associated with cataracts, immune deficiency, arthritis and premature ageing, and their role in these conditions is still the subject of extensive research.

THE ROLE OF ANTIOXIDANTS

The body produces its own antioxidants, which neutralise the effects of free radicals, but vitamins, minerals and compounds known as phytochemicals in plant foods provide a valuable extra supply, so additional dietary sources are essential for the main-tenance of good health. The table opposite lists the antioxidant vitamins and min-erals as well as their food

sources, and gives the officially recommended daily intakes, or RNIs (*see page 26*). In some cases the RNI is adequate for the maintenance of good health; in others the suggested opti-mum intake is higher. Even more doses may be recom-mended during illness or when diet has been inadequate.

■ A well-balanced multivitamin and multimineral formulation will supply enough mineral antioxidants, but extra supplies of vitamins C and E are required for optimum nutrition.

■ Other supplements can help to ease symptoms of certain ill-nesses. For example, coenzyme Q_{10} may be particularly helpful for heart disease sufferers, and alpha-lipoic acid for those with diabetic neuropathy or AIDS.

■ Antioxidant phytochemicals can be taken as supplements.

■ Studies suggest that green tea extract, grapeseed extract and flavonoid preparations such as rutin can reduce the risk of cancer and heart disease.

■ Some phytochemicals seem to favour specific types of tissue. Extracts of bilberry are rich in anthocyanosides (flavonoid pigments), which improve the health of the retina of the eye.

■ Antioxidants in ginkgo extracts are effective in enhancing cerebral circulation and correcting memory loss.

ANTIOXIDANT VITAMINS AND MINERALS

VITAMINS	ANTIOXIDANT EFFECTS	FOOD SOURCES	RECOMMENDED DAILY INTAKE (RNI)	SUGGESTED OPTIMUM DAILY INTAKE
Vitamin A, as retinol or as carotenoids	Diets high in carotenoids (some of which the body can convert into vitamin A) are linked with a reduced risk of some cancers; preliminary findings suggest that two carotenoids, lutein and zeaxanthin, may protect against age-related macular degeneration, a common cause of blindness in adults.	**Retinol**: animal foods such as liver, oily fish, eggs, milk, cheese and butter. **Carotenoids**: brightly coloured plant foods such as carrots, broccoli, dark green leafy vegetables, sweet red peppers, pumpkins, mangoes, canteloupe melons and dried apricots.	700 mcg for men; 600 mcg for women. Caretonoids: no RNI.	Supple-mentation not advised. Mixed caretonoids: 15 mg (see page 64)
Vitamin C	Scavenges for free radicals and regenerates the antioxidant potential of vitamin E after it has reacted with free radicals.	Citrus fruit, kiwi fruit, soft fruit such as blackcurrants and strawberries; potatoes, green and red peppers, tomatoes, bean sprouts and green leafy vegetables.	40 mg (80 mg for smokers)	200 mg (see page 180)
Vitamin E	Helps to prevent oxidation by free radicals of polyunsaturated fatty acids in cell membranes; the more polyunsaturated fats you eat, the more vitamin E you need to protect them from oxidation.	Vegetable oils such as sunflower and nut oils, margarine, almonds, hazelnuts, sunflower seeds, tuna, salmon, avocados.	No RNI; safe intake 10 mg, depending on intake of poly-unsaturated fat	100 mg (see page 184)
MINERALS				
Copper	Present in many enzymes that protect against free radical damage; required for healthy bone growth, for connective tissue formation, and to aid iron absorption from food.	Shellfish, liver, nuts, mushrooms and whole-grain cereals.	1.2 mg	RNI is adequate (see page 80)
Manganese	Present in enzymes that protect against free radical damage.	Nuts, brown rice, whole-grain bread, pulses and cereals; levels of manganese in plant foods depend on the amounts contained in the soil in which they are grown.	No RNI; safe intake 1.4 mg	
Selenium	Present in the enzyme that protects DNA against free radical damage; deficiency increases the risk of prostate cancer.	Brazil nuts, meat and offal, seafood and seaweed; avocados, whole grains and sunflower seeds also contain selenium, although levels depend on the amounts in the soil in which they were grown.	75 mcg for men; 60 mcg for women	RNI is adequate (see page 164)
Zinc	Present in enzymes that protect against free radical damage.	Shellfish (particularly oysters), lean meat, poultry, eggs and dairy products, pumpkin seeds, sunflower seeds, nuts and whole grains.	9.5 mg for men; 7 mg for women	RNI is adequate (see page 192)

Artichoke

Cynara scolymus

Artichoke's benefits were first documented by a pupil of Aristotle in the 4th century BC. The plant extract has long been popular in Germany for its positive dietary effects. It can bolster the actions of the gall bladder and liver, aid digestion and help to control cholesterol levels.

Common uses

- *Promotes healthy functioning of the gall bladder and liver.*
- *Improves digestion.*
- *Maintains and lowers levels of cholesterol.*
- *May help to control blood sugar levels, which is particularly important for diabetics.*

Forms

- Capsule
- Juice

CAUTION!

- If you are suffering from obstructive gall bladder disease, consult your doctor before taking artichoke extract because it increases bile secretion.

- A very small minority of people are allergic to artichoke and artichoke extract.

REMINDER: If you have a medical condition, consult your doctor before taking supplements.

What it is

Artichoke is a member of the botanical family that includes milk thistle, daisy and sunflower. Growing up to 2 metres in height, it is crowned with a large purple and green flower head. The young, unopened flower heads are cooked and the fleshy bases of the bracts, together with the receptacle, or 'heart', are eaten as a delicacy.

Also known as globe artichoke, the plant should not be confused with Jerusalem artichoke, the edible root vegetable. However, the globe artichoke is thought to have evolved from the cardoon that is grown in Mediterranean countries, and which has very similar medicinal qualities to the artichoke. The leaves of the globe artichoke contain several substances that have beneficial health effects when consumed at the recommended levels. They include cynarin (the key, active component) and various flavonoids, particularly luteolin.

What it does

Although artichoke leaf extract has been popular in Germany for some time, its benefits have only recently been recognised in the UK. Laboratory studies in Germany have shown it to be useful in the protection and regeneration of the liver following intoxication.

Scientific research dating back to 1933 shows that artichoke stimulates the production of bile from the liver, which then passes into the duodenum. This effect accounts for the successful use of the

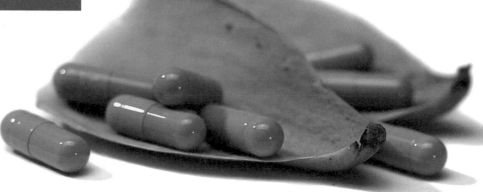

Artichoke supplements are made from the plant's leaves, and the edible bracts around the flower head (shown here) can help to control blood sugar levels.

herb in the treatment of people with impaired digestion of fat. Work undertaken as early as the 1930s showed that artichoke leaf extract was able to reduce blood cholesterol levels in patients with raised values. These findings have been confirmed by recent research, and one study has found that, while levels of LDL ('bad') cholesterol were lowered, there was a slight increase in levels of HDL ('good') cholesterol. It would seem that these cholesterol-lowering properties of artichoke extract are due to its content of luteolin, which inhibits the synthesis of cholesterol by the liver.

✪ **MAJOR BENEFITS:** Cynarin and the flavonoids of artichoke, including luteolin, are powerful antioxidants that can help to prevent cell damage in the liver, protect the body from damage by the unstable oxygen molecules known as free radicals, and hence help to fight disease. Several clinical studies have shown the extract to alleviate digestive disorders, such as abdominal pain, nausea and flatulence.

Artichoke contains inulin, a polysaccharide that slows down the rate at which the body digests food. This property means that, when eaten as a vegetable, artichoke may help to control blood sugar levels after meals, which makes it particularly useful for diabetics. People with high cholesterol levels may also benefit from the extract, which can reduce the synthesis of cholesterol in the liver.

✪ **ADDITIONAL BENEFITS:** Artichoke leaf has been traditionally used for its cleansing and detoxifying action in the treatment of gout, arthritis and rheumatism. Also, its diuretic action may help to alleviate urinary tract problems. Research is under way into other possible benefits, including its value for people suffering from irritable bowel syndrome. A recent study found significant reduction in the severity of symptoms in this condition.

How to take it

⬟ **DOSAGE:** *For improved digestion, liver function and cholesterol levels:* Take two 320 mg capsules daily. *For improved digestion at times of high fat intake:* Take up to six 320 mg capsules daily either at the same time or at different times during the day.

⬟ **GUIDELINES FOR USE:** Take capsules with or immediately after a meal and swallow them whole with cold liquid. If you suffer from gall bladder obstruction problems, consult your doctor before using artichoke. Anyone with an allergy to plants in the daisy family may experience an allergic reaction and should discontinue use at once.

Possible side effects

Many studies have confirmed that artichoke leaf extract is very well tolerated by most people, even after continuous long-term use. When taken as a food, artichoke presents minimal risks, but in a small minority of people it may cause side effects such as flatulence and mild gastrointestinal problems.

BUYING GUIDE

■ Buy standardised leaf extract to ensure that you obtain a concentrated dose of cynarin. Tablets made from the dried and powdered leaf (rarely available) provide a much less potent form.

RECENT FINDINGS

A 1998 study of people with digestive problems showed that 85% experienced an improvement in their health from taking artichoke leaf extract. After the patients had taken five capsules a day for an average of 23 weeks their symptoms – which included nausea, flatulence, bloating, abdominal pain and fat intolerance – were all dramatically reduced.

A recent Germany study involving 553 people aged 20-87 found that artichoke extract had a beneficial effect on blood cholesterol levels. After six weeks of treatment the subjects found that their blood cholesterol levels had dropped by an average of 11.5%.

DID YOU KNOW?

The ancient Greeks introduced globe artichoke into Europe from North Africa. It has long been popular in France, where it is served in salads or as an appetiser.

Astragalus

For more than 2000 years astragalus has played an integral part in the traditional medicine of China, where it is used to balance the life force, or *qi*. The Chinese name for the herb is *huang qi*, meaning 'yellow leader', reflecting its therapeutic importance.

Astragalus membranaceus

Common uses

- *Enhances immunity.*
- *Helps to fight respiratory infections.*
- *Bolsters the immune system in people undergoing cancer treatment.*

Forms

- Capsule
- Dried herb/tea
- Tablet
- Tincture

CAUTION!

■ Pregnant or breastfeeding women should seek medical advice before using this herb.

REMINDER: *If you have a medical condition, consult your doctor before taking supplements.*

What it is

Astragalus contains a variety of compounds that are known to stimulate the body's immune system, and in China this native plant has long been used both to prevent and to treat disease. Botanically, astragalus is related to liquorice and the pea. Although its sweet-smelling, pale yellow blossoms and delicate structure give the plant a frail appearance, it is actually a very hardy species. Medicinally, the most important part of the astragalus plant is its root, which is loaded with health-promoting substances including polysaccharides, a class of carbohydrate, that appear to be responsible for its immune-boosting effects. Astragalus is harvested when it is four to seven years old; after they have been sliced for use, its yellowish roots resemble the broad flat sticks that are used to hold ice-lollies.

What it does

A tonic in the true sense of the word, astragalus has the capacity to enhance overall health by improving resistance to disease, increasing stamina and vitality, and promoting general well-being. It also acts as an antioxidant, helping the human body to correct or prevent cell damage caused by free radicals. It may also have antiviral and antibiotic properties. Supplements derived from the herb can be safely used in combination with conventional medicines.

♥ **PREVENTION:** Astragalus is particularly effective in fighting off colds, flu, bronchitis and sinus infections because it inhibits viruses from establishing themselves in the respiratory system. Like echinacea, astragalus can destroy harmful bacteria as soon as the symptoms of respiratory infection start to appear. If an illness does develop, astragalus can shorten its duration and reduce its severity. People who frequently suffer from respiratory illnesses should consider using

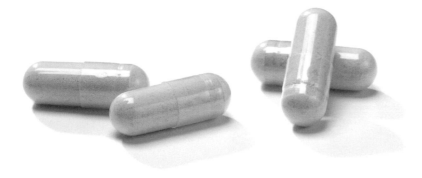

astragalus on a regular basis to prevent recurrences. It also helps to minimise the detrimental effects on health caused by excessive stress.

✳ **ADDITIONAL BENEFITS:** Astragalus is widely used in China to rebuild the immune systems of cancer patients who have received radiotherapy or chemotherapy – a practice that is also gaining popularity in the West. The herb increases the body's production of T-cells, macrophages, natural killer cells, interferon and other immune cells. Astragalus may also protect bone marrow from the immunosuppressive effects of chemotherapy, radiotherapy, toxins and viruses. The herb, which stimulates the immune response, is a possible treatment for people infected with HIV, the virus that causes AIDS.

In addition, astragalus widens blood vessels and increases blood flow, which makes it useful in controlling excessive perspiration (such as night sweats) and lowering blood pressure. Research has also shown that astragalus can have beneficial effects on the heart and it can enhance the motility of sperm.

How to take it

🗐 **DOSAGE:** For *strengthening the immune system*: Take 200 mg of astragalus extract once or twice a day for three weeks, then alternate, in three-week stints, with echinacea, cat's claw and pau d'arco. For *acute bronchitis*: Take 200 mg four times a day until the symptoms ease. Choose a product that contains a standardised extract of astragalus with 0.5% glucosides and 70% polysaccharides.

◔ **GUIDELINES FOR USE:** Astragalus can be taken at any time during the day, with or without meals.

Possible side effects

Remarkably, even after thousands of years of use in China, there are few (if any) negative reports associated with the medicinal use of astragalus.

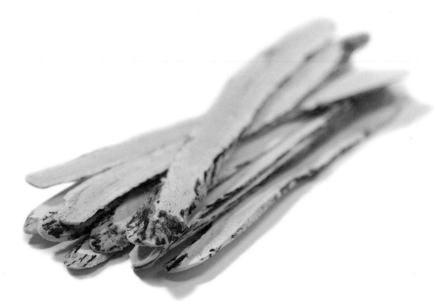

Bee products

Although many intriguing claims have been made for the healing powers of bee products, there is little evidence to support most of them. But bee pollen, royal jelly and propolis are popular nutritional supplements, and continue to be the subject of scientific studies.

Common uses

- *May relieve symptoms of hay fever.*
- *Propolis helps to heal skin abrasions.*

Forms

- Capsule
- Cream
- Dried and fresh pollen
- Liquid
- Lozenge
- Powder
- Softgel
- Tablet

What they are

There are three types of bee products available in health-food shops: bee pollen, propolis and royal jelly. Bee pollen, which comes from flowers, is distinct from the airborne pollen produced by grasses that often causes hay fever. After bees have gathered pollen, they compress it into pellets, which can be collected from their hives. (A second type of pollen, also sold as bee pollen, is collected directly from plants.) Bee pollen contains protein, B vitamins, carbohydrates and various enzymes. Propolis – also called bee glue – is a sticky resin that bees collect from the buds of pine trees and use to repair cracks in their hives. Royal jelly is a milky-white substance produced by the salivary glands of worker bees as a food source for the queen bee. The specialised nutritional content of royal jelly may account for the fertility, large size and longevity of the queen.

What they do

Bee products, especially bee pollen, have been touted as virtual cure-alls. Proponents assert that, among other things, these products slow ageing, improve athletic performance, boost immunity, contribute to weight loss, fight bacteria and alleviate the symptoms of allergies and hay fever. Although bee pollen shows some promise in treating allergies, and propolis may be effective as a salve for cuts and bruises, the scant research that has been conducted into bee products does not support the extravagant claims made for them.

✪ **MAJOR BENEFITS:**

Bee pollen may help to prevent the sneezing, runny nose, watery eyes and other symptoms suffered by people susceptible to seasonal allergies triggered by flower pollen. Some scientists believe that ingesting small amounts of pollen can desensitise an individual to its allergenic compounds, much as allergy inoculations do. The theory is that, when

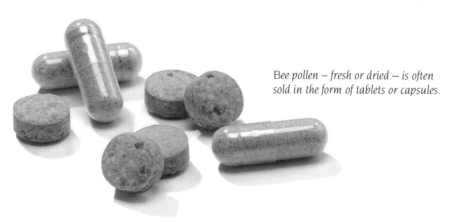

Bee pollen – fresh or dried – is often sold in the form of tablets or capsules.

exposed to even a tiny amount of pollen, the human immune system produces antibodies whose task is to provide protection against the extreme reaction that causes classic allergy symptoms. Tests of this theory continue, but meanwhile bee pollen poses no apparent danger to most people. Some advocates maintain that, for best results, sufferers need to use bee pollen from a local source, in order to desensitise them to the flower pollens in their own particular environment.

✤ **ADDITIONAL BENEFITS:** Propolis may have a role as a skin softener or a wound healer. Although it contains antibacterial compounds, research has shown that these are not as effective as standard antibiotics or over-the-counter antibiotic ointments in fighting infection.

The fact that royal jelly enhances the growth, fertility and longevity of queen bees has led many people to think that it will do the same for humans. There is no evidence to support this view, but royal jelly has long been highly regarded in traditional Chinese medicine for its efficacy in restoring strength after illness.

How to take them

✐ **DOSAGE:** The amount of bee pollen needed to relieve allergy symptoms varies from person to person. In general, start with a few granules a day and increase the dose gradually until you reach 1 to 3 rounded teaspoons a day.

◉ **GUIDELINES FOR USE:** Before the hay-fever season begins, take very small amounts of bee pollen each day – a few granules or a portion of a tablet. If you do not suffer any adverse reaction, increase the dosage slowly until you experience relief from allergy symptoms. Bee-pollen supplements should be consumed with plenty of water; you can also mix dried or fresh pollen with juice or sprinkle it over food.

Possible side effects

Some individuals have allergic reactions to bee pollen, which can include asthma, eczema and a runny nose. Start by taking a small amount so that you can determine if you are susceptible. If you develop a rash, an itchy throat, skin flushing, wheezing or headaches, stop using it immediately.

CASE HISTORY
A killer drink

Aware from childhood that he was allergic to bee stings, Martin H. did all he could to avoid the buzzing, venom-carrying insects. He could not have foreseen that his life would be put in danger by a health-food drink.

An insurance broker in the City of London, Martin was in the habit of missing lunch and stopping off at his favourite health-food bar on the way home for a quick pick-me-up.

On the fateful day he took the advice of an enthusiastic waiter and ordered the Kitchen Sink Smoothie, a new yoghurt drink. He did not know that, in addition to the advertised ginseng and spirulina, it contained a generous scoop of some 'energising' bee product.

The last thing Martin remembers about the incident was 'putting the glass to my lips'. When he awoke he found himself in an intensive care unit recovering from anaphylactic shock. His advice to other allergy sufferers is: 'Don't try a new health food unless you're quite sure what's in it.'

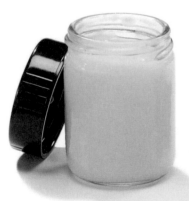
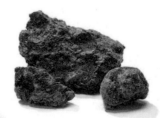
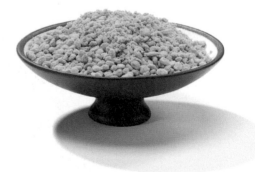

The three types of bee product on the market are royal jelly (left), the sticky resin called propolis (centre) and bee pollen (right).

Bilberry

Vaccinium myrtillus

During the Second World War, RAF pilots noted the curious fact that their night vision improved after eating bilberry jam. Their anecdotal reports stimulated scientific research into bilberry, which is now used to treat a wide range of visual disorders and other complaints.

Common uses

- *Maintains healthy vision as well as improving night vision and poor visual adaptation to bright light.*
- *Treats a wide array of eye disorders, including diabetic retinopathy, cataracts and macular degeneration.*
- *Relieves varicose veins and haemorrhoids, especially in pregnant women.*

Forms

- Capsule
- Dried herb/tea
- Softgel
- Tablet
- Tincture

What it is

Although the fruit of the bilberry bush has been eaten with pleasure since prehistoric times, its first recorded medicinal use was in the 16th century. Historically, dried berry or leaf preparations were recommended for the treatment of a variety of conditions, including scurvy (caused by vitamin C deficiency), urinary tract infections and kidney stones.

Bilberry is a short, shrubby perennial that grows in the forests and on the moors of northern Europe. Bushes of the sweet blue-black berries are also found in western Asia and the Rocky Mountains of North America. The health-promoting components of the ripe fruit consist primarily of flavonoid compounds known as anthocyanosides, and the modern medicinal form of bilberry is an extract containing a highly concentrated amount of these compounds.

What it does

Many of the medicinal qualities of bilberry derive from anthocyanosides, the plant's main constituents, which are potent antioxidants. These compounds help to counteract cell damage caused by the unstable oxygen molecules known as free radicals.

MAJOR BENEFITS: Bilberry extract is the leading herbal remedy for maintaining healthy vision and managing various eye disorders. In particular, bilberry helps the retina, the light-sensitive portion of the eye, to adapt properly to dark and light. It has been widely used to treat night blindness as well as poor vision resulting from daytime glare. With its ability to strengthen the tiny blood vessels called capillaries – and, in

Bilberries, available in capsule form, provide a popular herbal remedy for a variety of eye disorders.

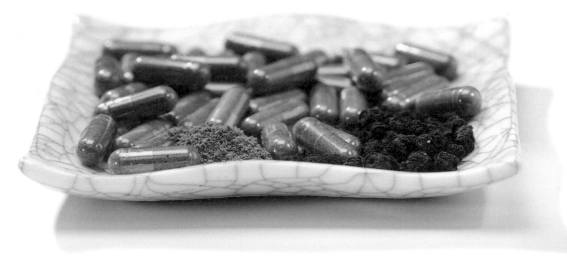

54

turn, facilitate the delivery of oxygen-rich blood to the eyes – bilberry may also play a significant role in preventing and treating degenerative diseases of the retina (retinopathy). In one study, 31 patients were treated with bilberry extract daily for four weeks. Use of the extract fortified the capillaries and reduced haemorrhaging in the eyes, especially in cases of diabetic retinopathy.

Bilberry is used to treat two leading causes of sight loss in older people: macular degeneration, a progressive disorder affecting the central part of the retina, and cataract, the loss of transparency in the lens of the eye. A study of 50 patients with age-related cataracts found that bilberry extract combined with vitamin E supplements inhibited cataract formation in almost all participants. Bilberry is known to strengthen collagen – the abundant protein that forms the 'backbone' of healthy connective tissue – which may make it valuable in the prevention and treatment of glaucoma, a disease caused by excessive pressure within the eye.

✳ **ADDITIONAL BENEFITS:** As the anthocyanosides in bilberry improve the blood flow in capillaries as well as in larger blood vessels, bilberry in standardised extract form may be efficacious for people with poor circulation in their extremities. It is helpful in treating varicose veins and in easing the pain and burning of haemorrhoids, particularly during pregnancy when both these conditions can be very troublesome. People who bruise easily may also benefit from bilberry's effect on capillaries.

Although more research is needed, there are indications that the plant may have other medicinal uses. One study demonstrated that long-term use of bilberry extract improved the vision of normally short-sighted people – but how it produced this effect is unknown. Preliminary results from tests on women showed that bilberry helps to relieve menstrual cramps because anthocyanosides relax smooth muscle, including the uterus. Animal studies suggest that bilberry anthocyanosides may fight stomach ulcers and may also reduce levels of triglycerides (a type of fat) in the blood.

How to take it

⌀ **DOSAGE:** Normal doses range from 40 to 160 mg of bilberry extract two or three times a day. The lower dose is generally recommended for long-term use, including prevention of macular degeneration; higher doses – up to 320 mg a day – may be needed by people with diabetes.
◑ **GUIDELINES FOR USE:** Bilberry can be taken with or without food. No adverse effects have been noted in pregnant or breastfeeding women who use the herb. In addition, there are no known adverse interactions with prescription or over-the-counter drugs.

Possible side effects

In therapeutic doses, bilberry appears to be very safe and has no known side effects, even when taken over a long period of time.

Biotin and pantothenic acid

These two B vitamins play a vital role in sustaining efficient metabolic function. Deficiencies are rare, but supplements can help in treating various disorders and may be useful for people whose diets include a lot of processed foods.

Common uses

Biotin

- *Promotes healthy nails and hair.*
- *Helps the body to use carbohydrates, fats and protein.*
- *May improve blood-sugar control in people with diabetes.*

Pantothenic acid

- *Promotes a healthy central nervous system.*
- *Helps the body to use carbohydrates, fats and protein.*
- *May alleviate chronic fatigue syndrome, migraines, indigestion and the symptoms of some allergies.*

Forms

- Capsule
- Liquid
- Softgel
- Tablet

CAUTION!

REMINDER: *If you have a medical condition, consult your doctor before taking supplements.*

What they are

Biotin and pantothenic acid are vitamins contained in many foods, so deficiencies are virtually non-existent. Biotin is also produced by intestinal bacteria, though the vitamin may be hard for the body to use in this form. Multivitamins and B-complex vitamins usually include biotin and pantothenic acid (also called vitamin B_5), and both are available as individual supplements. The main form of biotin is D-biotin. Pantothenic acid comes in two forms, pantethine and calcium pantothenate; the latter is suitable for most purposes and is less expensive than pantethine.

What they do

Both biotin and pantothenic acid are involved in the production of various enzymes and in the breaking down of carbohydrates, fats and protein from foods so that they can be used by the body. Biotin plays a special role in helping the body to use glucose, its basic fuel, as well as promoting healthy nails and hair. The body needs pantothenic acid to maintain proper communication between the brain and the nervous system and to produce certain stress hormones.

⊛ **MAJOR BENEFITS:** Biotin supplements improve the quality of weak and brittle fingernails and help to slow down hair loss caused by a biotin deficiency. Pantothenic acid is used to manufacture stress hormones, and during long periods of emotional upset, depression or anxiety – which are generally accompanied by an overproduction of stress hormones – the body's need for the vitamin appears to increase. The stress caused by migraines or chronic fatigue syndrome, or by the challenge of giving up smoking, may be alleviated by pantothenic acid supplements. In combination with the B vitamins choline and thiamin, pantothenic acid can be an effective remedy for indigestion; it also relieves the nasal congestion caused by certain allergic reactions, such as hay fever.

⊛ **ADDITIONAL BENEFITS:** Biotin in very high doses may benefit diabetics, increasing the body's response to insulin so that levels of blood sugar (glucose) stay low. It may protect against the nerve damage that can occur in diabetes. Diabetics should seek medical advice.

Biotin (left) and pantothenic acid (right) are important B vitamins.

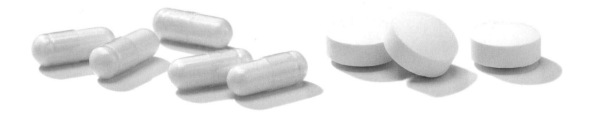

How much you need

There is no RDA for biotin or pantothenic acid, but 30 to 100 mcg of biotin and 4 to 7 mg of pantothenic acid a day appear to be enough to maintain healthy bodily functions. For the treatment of specific diseases or disorders, higher doses may be needed.

⊖ **IF YOU GET TOO LITTLE:** Deficiencies of biotin or pantothenic acid are virtually unknown in adults. Long-term use of antibiotics or anti-seizure medications, however, can lead to less-than-optimal levels of biotin.

⊕ **IF YOU GET TOO MUCH:** Although no serious adverse effects from high doses of biotin or pantothenic acid have been recorded, the daily recommended upper safe levels of, respectively, 900 mcg and 200 mg should not be exceeded.

How to take them

⬚ **DOSAGE:** *For hair and nails:* Take up to 900 mcg of biotin a day. *During periods of stress:* Take 100 mg of pantothenic acid a day as part of a vitamin B complex. *For migraines:* Take 100 mg of pantothenic acid twice a day. *For chronic fatigue syndrome:* Take 100 mg of pantothenic acid twice a day. *For chronic indigestion:* Take 100 mg of pantothenic acid twice a day along with 50 mg of thiamin first thing in the morning and 500 mg of choline three times a day. *For allergies:* Take 100 mg of pantothenic acid twice a day. *For diabetes:* Consult your doctor about taking high doses of biotin to relieve or even to prevent diabetic neuropathy.

◉ **GUIDELINES FOR USE:** A multivitamin or a B-complex supplement will provide enough biotin and pantothenic acid for most people. Individual supplements are necessary only to treat specific disorders. In most cases, individual supplements should be taken with meals.

Other sources

Biotin is found in liver, soy products, nuts, oatmeal, rice, barley, legumes, cauliflower and whole wheat. Offal, fish, poultry, whole grains, yoghurt and legumes are the best sources of pantothenic acid.

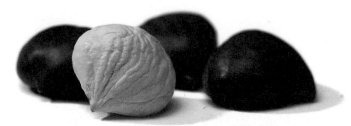

Nuts such as sweet chestnuts are a useful natural source of biotin.

Black cohosh

Cimicifuga racemosa

The gnarled black root of the black cohosh plant was identified more than a century ago as the source of one of the most useful natural medicines for women. The name 'cohosh', derived from a Native American word for 'rough', refers to the twisted appearance of the root.

Common uses

- *Reduces menopausal symptoms, particularly hot flushes.*
- *Eases menstrual pain and associated conditions, such as PMS.*
- *Works as an anti-inflammatory; relieves muscle pain.*
- *Helps to clear mucous membranes and to relieve coughs.*

Forms

- Capsule
- Dried herb/tea
- Tablet
- Tincture

What it is

Long used to treat 'women's problems', the black cohosh plant grows up to 2½ metres high and is distinguished by its tall stalks of fluffy white flowers. Native to North America, this member of the buttercup family is also known as bugbane, squawroot or rattle root. However, its most common nickname, black snakeroot, describes its gnarled black root, the part of the plant that is used medicinally. Contained in the root is a complex mixture of natural chemicals, some as powerful as the most modern pharmaceuticals.

What it does

Traditionally, black cohosh has been prescribed to treat menstrual problems, pain after childbirth, nervous disorders and joint pain. Today the herb is recommended primarily for relief of the hot flushes that some women experience during the menopause.

☆ **MAJOR BENEFITS:** Black cohosh is an increasingly popular remedy for hot flushes, excessive sweating, vaginal dryness and other menopausal symptoms. Scientific study has shown that it can reduce levels of LH (luteinising hormone), which is produced by the brain's pituitary gland. The rise in LH that occurs during the menopause is thought to be one cause of hot flushes.

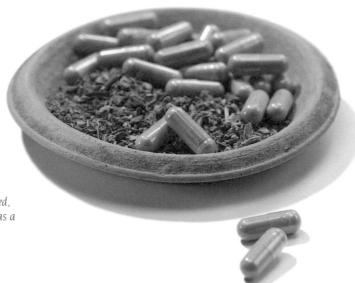

The root of black cohosh is dried, ground to a powder and sold as a supplement in capsule form.

In addition, black cohosh contains phytoestrogens, plant compounds that have an effect similar to that of oestrogen produced by the body. Phytoestrogens bind themselves to hormone receptors in the breasts, uterus and elsewhere in the body, easing menopausal symptoms without increasing the risk of breast cancer, a possible side effect of hormone replacement therapy. Some phytoestrogens may even help to prevent breast cancer by inhibiting the body's own oestrogen from locking onto breast cells.

❉ **ADDITIONAL BENEFITS:** Black cohosh's antispasmodic properties mean that it has the power to alleviate menstrual cramps by increasing blood flow to the uterus and reducing the intensity of uterine contractions. This action also makes it useful during labour and after childbirth. Black cohosh 'evens out' hormone levels, offering possible benefits to women suffering from premenstrual syndrome (PMS), but chasteberry is probably more effective in relieving this condition.

Although these capabilities are less frequently noted, black cohosh has demonstrated some mildly sedative and anti-inflammatory effects, which may be particularly valuable in treating muscle aches as well as nerve-related pain caused by, for example, sciatica or neuralgia. It can help to clear mucus from the body and has been recommended for coughs. The herb has also been shown to be an effective treatment for tinnitus (ringing in the ears).

How to take it

❑ **DOSAGE:** Look for capsules or tablets containing extracts that have been standardised to contain 2.5% of triterpenes, the active components in black cohosh. *For menopausal or* PMS *symptoms*: Take 40 mg of black cohosh extract twice a day. For PMS, begin treatment a week to 10 days before the start of your period. *For menstrual cramps*: Take 40 mg three or four times a day as needed.

◉ **GUIDELINES FOR USE:** Black cohosh can be taken at any time of day, but to reduce the chance of stomach upset you may prefer to take it with meals. Allow four to eight weeks to see its benefits. Many researchers recommend a six-month limit on taking black cohosh, though recent studies show that longer use seems to be safe and free of significant side effects.

Possible side effects

Though it has virtually no toxic effects, black cohosh may cause stomach upsets in certain people. One study suggested that it may induce slight weight gain and dizziness in some women. It may also lower blood pressure. A very high dose can cause nausea, vomiting, reduced pulse rate, heavy perspiration and headaches.

FACTS & TIPS

■ Compresses soaked in black cohosh tea can be used to soothe sore muscles and aching joints. Boil the dried root in water for 20 to 30 minutes. Let the liquid cool a bit (it should still be hot, but not hot enough to burn your skin). Then apply the warm compress to the affected area and leave it there for about 20 minutes.

■ Recent research suggests that black cohosh helps to relieve the menopausal symptoms of hot flushes and night sweats by acting on the receptors in the brain used to control body temperature, and not by influencing oestrogen.

Bromelain

A digestive enzyme with anti-inflammatory properties, bromelain is derived from the pineapple plant. It has been used since the 1950s for a wide variety of therapeutic purposes, relieving conditions from sports injuries to heart disease.

Common uses

- *Reduces pain and swelling caused by minor injuries.*
- *Aids healing of wounds and post-operative recovery.*
- *Reduces mucous congestion in bronchitis and sinusitis.*
- *Improves the effectiveness of some antibiotics.*
- *Helps in the digestion of protein.*

Form

- Tablet

CAUTION!

- Do not take bromelain supplements if you have an allergy to pineapple.

- Because bromelain acts as a blood thinner, it should be avoided by anyone taking anti-coagulant drugs; little is known about how they interact.

REMINDER: If you have a medical condition, consult your doctor before taking supplements.

What it is

Bromelain is a protein-digesting, milk-clotting enzyme found in fresh pineapple. The commercial supplement is usually obtained only from the pineapple stem, which is different from the enzyme in the fruit. It is produced mainly in Japan, Taiwan and Hawaii.

What it does

Bromelain is a powerful anti-inflammatory agent which can reduce pain and swelling and promote tissue repair. Its effectiveness is thought to spring from its interaction with hormone-like substances known as prostaglandins. Bromelain can inhibit the action of prostaglandins that cause pain and inflammation while promoting the formation of different, anti-inflammatory prostaglandins. It also stimulates the breakdown of fibrin, an insoluble protein that can be associated with fluid retention. Bromelain is unusual as a protein-digesting enzyme in that it bypasses the digestive tract to be absorbed intact.

MAJOR BENEFITS: Bromelain's anti-inflammatory action makes it useful in the treatment of the pain and swelling associated with sprains and muscle injuries as well as in the healing of wounds and burns. In one study involving 700 firemen with burns, those who took bromelain found that their injuries healed in half the time that they took to heal in those who were not given the enzyme.

Other evidence shows that bromelain helps to reduce the bruising and pain that can follow minor operations, especially in women who have had surgery after childbirth. When combined with another

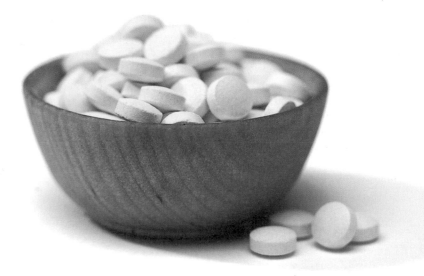

proteolytic enzyme called trypsin, bromelain may be effective against urinary tract infections. In a preliminary study 78% of sufferers said that their symptoms were eased by taking the enzyme combination. Taken together with papain, bromelain may also ease period pain by reducing spasms in the uterus.

✚ **ADDITIONAL BENEFITS:** By counteracting excessive stickiness of blood platelets the enzyme helps to combat cardiovascular disease, reducing the threat of thrombosis and the pain of angina, and relaxing arterial constriction. Angina sufferers who took between 1000 mg and 1400 mg of bromelain reported a disappearance of all their symptoms within a period of 4 to 90 days. (The length of time it took for the improvements to become evident was related to the severity of the patients' original symptoms.)

As a protein-digesting enzyme, bromelain may have an anticancer effect, but more evidence is needed. Also, it may boost the effectiveness of chemotherapy and possibly inhibit the growth of cancer cells. When taken orally, the enzyme has been shown to bring about the synthesis of anticancer compounds.

Bromelain appears to reduce the thickness of mucus, which may be helpful in the treatment of asthma or chronic bronchitis. It has also been shown to be effective in alleviating sinusitis. Other studies show that the enzyme can aid the absorption of antibiotics such as amoxicillin and penicillin, as well as assisting the absorption of curcumin, the active ingredient in turmeric. There is some evidence to suggest that, when used with papain, a proteolytic enzyme found in unripe papaya, bromelain may relieve painful menstrual periods.

As an anti-inflammatory, bromelain may be useful for relieving rheumatoid arthritis. In a preliminary study 73% of patients given a supplement for periods of between three weeks and 13 months reported good to excellent results. Since bromelain can reduce the swelling and bruising that may follow an operation, while leaving the blood-clotting process unaffected, it may sometimes be given to patients who are about to undergo liposuction.

How to take it

☑ **DOSAGE:** A typical recommended dose of bromelain is between 250 mg and 500 mg three times a day.

◉ **GUIDELINES FOR USE:** Bromelain should generally be taken on an empty stomach, but when used as a digestive aid it should be taken with food, especially to assist in the digestion of fatty or high-protein meals. For the relief of swelling or inflammation continue to take the supplement until symptoms subside.

Possible side effects

Even when bromelain is taken in very large doses, side effects are extremely rare. Some people with particular sensitivity may experience allergic reactions and skin irritation. There has been a preliminary report of increased heart rate associated with the use of the enzyme.

RECENT FINDINGS

Research in Germany has highlighted a combination therapy that may drastically reduce the risk of a second heart attack. Patients who take potassium, magnesium and bromelain capsules with every meal have been shown to reduce their risk by 95%. The magnesium and potassium combination is thought to strengthen the heart, while bromelain both prevents the clustering of blood platelets and dissolves fibrin, a protein that can contribute to blood clots.

DID YOU KNOW?

'Raw' bromelain has such a powerful action that people who work in pineapple plantations and canning factories have to wear protective clothing to prevent damage to their skin.

Calcium

Renowned for its importance in combating osteoporosis, calcium is now thought to have a role in lowering blood pressure and preventing colon cancer. But modern diets are often severely lacking in calcium; many adults get only half the daily recommended quantities of the mineral.

Common uses

- *Maintains healthy bones and teeth.*
- *Helps to prevent progressive bone loss and osteoporosis.*
- *Aids heart and muscle contraction, nerve impulses and blood clotting.*
- *May help to lower blood pressure in people with hypertension.*
- *Eases indigestion.*

Forms

- Capsule
- Liquid
- Powder
- Softgel
- Tablet

CAUTION!

- **People with thyroid or kidney disease should seek medical advice before taking calcium.**

- **Calcium may interact with some drugs, notably the tetracycline antibiotics.**

REMINDER: If you have a medical condition, consult your doctor before taking supplements.

What it is

An essential constituent of bones and teeth, calcium is also required for bodily functions such as blood clotting and muscle contraction. Eating enough calcium-rich foods may be difficult, but supplements can prevent the development of a deficiency. The most common forms are calcium carbonate, calcium citrate, calcium citrate malate, calcium gluconate, calcium phosphate and calcium lactate. The amount of elemental – or pure – calcium in a supplement varies from compound to compound. Calcium carbonate (used in antacids to relieve indigestion) provides 40% elemental calcium, while calcium gluconate supplies 9%: the lower the calcium content, the more pills needed to meet recommended amounts.

What it does

Most of the body's calcium is stored in the bones and teeth, where it provides structure and strength. The small amount circulating in the bloodstream helps to move nutrients across cell membranes and plays a role in producing the hormones and enzymes that regulate digestion and metabolism. Calcium is also needed for normal communication between nerve cells and for blood clotting, wound healing and muscle contraction. To have enough of the mineral available in the blood to perform vital functions, the body will steal it from the bones. Over time, too many calcium 'withdrawals' leave bones porous and fragile. Only an adequate daily calcium intake will maintain healthy levels in the blood – and provide enough extra for the bones to absorb as a reserve.

PREVENTION: Getting enough calcium throughout life is a central factor in preventing osteoporosis, the bone-thinning disease that leads to a higher risk of hip and vertebra fractures, spinal deformities and loss of height. The body is best equipped to absorb calcium and build up bone mass before the age of 35, but several studies have shown that even people aged over 65 can maintain bone density and reduce the risk of fractures by taking calcium supplements and eating calcium-rich foods.

ADDITIONAL BENEFITS: By limiting the irritating effects of bile acids in the colon, calcium may reduce the incidence of colon cancer. Research

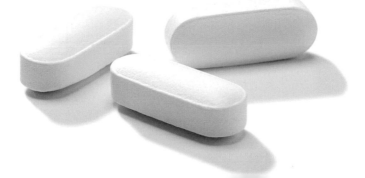

indicates that diets including plenty of calcium – as well as fruit and vegetables – may be as effective as some prescription drugs in lowering blood pressure. But people with hypertension should not substitute calcium supplements for regular medication except on a doctor's advice. Calcium may also be useful for treating the symptoms of premenstrual syndrome and period pain. A trial of 497 women with PMS found that 100 mg of calcium daily for three months reduced symptoms significantly more than a placebo.

How much you need

In the UK the current recommended daily target of calcium, for both men and women, is 700 mg, with no extra amount recommended for pregnant women. But the equivalent recommendation in the USA is 1000 mg for men and women aged from 19 to 50 and 1200 mg for those from 50 to 70.

⊟ **IF YOU GET TOO LITTLE:** A prolonged calcium deficiency can lead to bone abnormalities, such as osteoporosis. Low levels of calcium in the blood can cause muscle spasms.

⊞ **IF YOU GET TOO MUCH:** A daily calcium intake of 1500 mg from supplements appears to be safe. However, taking calcium supplements may impair the body's ability to absorb zinc, iron and magnesium. Very high doses of calcium from supplements could lead to kidney stones. If calcium carbonate supplements cause flatulence or constipation they can be replaced by calcium citrate.

How to take it

◨ **DOSAGE:** Ensure that you get the recommended amount of 700 mg of elemental calcium a day from foods, supplements or both. When taking calcium, it may be advisable to take magnesium supplements as well, in a ratio of 1 to 2. So if you take 500 mg of supplemental calcium, take 250 mg of magnesium with it.

◉ **GUIDELINES FOR USE:** To enhance efficient absorption, split up your supplement dose so that you do not consume more than 600 mg of calcium at any one time. Always take the supplements with food. Those containing calcium citrate or malate are more easily absorbed by the body than those containing calcium carbonate.

Other sources

The most plentiful sources of calcium are dairy products, such as milk, yoghurt and cheese. Low-fat or fat-free varieties contain slightly more calcium than the full-fat types. Orange juice fortified with calcium malate, tinned salmon and sardines (eaten with the soft bones), broccoli and almonds are good non-dairy sources.

A 100 *gram serving of boiled broccoli provides only one twentieth of an adult's daily calcium needs.*

Carotenoids

The pigments that give some vegetables and fruits their rich red, orange and yellow colours are called carotenoids. These natural antioxidants are also potent disease fighters. A popular way of enjoying the benefits of carotenoids is by taking a combination supplement.

Common uses

- May *lower the risk of certain types of cancers*, including prostate and lung cancer.
- May *provide protection against heart disease*.
- *Slow the development of macular degeneration*.
- *Enhance immunity*.

Forms

- Capsule
- Softgel
- Tablet

CAUTION!

- High doses of carotenoids should be avoided in pregnancy.

REMINDER: *If you have a medical condition, consult your doctor before taking supplements.*

What they are

Although more than 600 carotenoid pigments have been identified in foods, it appears that only six of them are used in significant ways by the blood or tissues of the body. Apart from beta-carotene, which is probably the best-known carotenoid, these are alpha-carotene, cryptoxanthin, lycopene, lutein and zeaxanthin.

Carotenoids are found in a wide variety of fruits and vegetables, but the foods that represent the most concentrated sources may not be part of your daily diet. Alpha-carotene is found in carrots and pumpkin; lycopene is abundant in red fruits, such as watermelon, red grapefruit, guava and, in particular, cooked tomatoes. Lutein and zeaxanthin are plentiful in dark green vegetables, pumpkin and red peppers; and cryptoxanthin is present in mangoes, oranges and peaches. To prevent certain diseases it may be advisable to choose supplements that provide a mixture of the six key carotenoids.

What they do

The primary benefit of carotenoids lies in their antioxidant effect – protecting the cells of the body from damage by unstable oxygen molecules called free radicals. Although carotenoids are similar to one another, each acts on a specific type of bodily tissue. In addition, alpha-carotene and cryptoxanthin can be converted into vitamin A in the body, but not to the same extent as beta-carotene.

PREVENTION: Carotenoids may guard against certain types of cancer, apparently by limiting the abnormal growth of cells. Lycopene, for instance, appears to inhibit the development of prostate cancer. Researchers at Harvard University found that men who ate ten or more servings a week of tomato-based foods – tomatoes are the richest dietary source of lycopene – cut their risk of prostate cancer by nearly 45%. Lycopene may also be effective against cancers of the stomach and digestive tract. Studies show that high intakes of alpha-carotene, lutein and zeaxanthin decrease the risk of lung cancer, and that cryptoxanthin and alpha-carotene lower the risk of cervical cancer. Carotenoids may also fight heart disease. In a survey of 1300 elderly people, those who

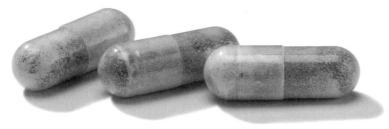

Though capsules of individual carotenoids such as lycopene (left) are available, it is even more beneficial to take a mixed carotenoid supplement.

consumed the greatest amount of carotenoid-rich foods were shown to have half the risk of developing heart disease, and a 75% lower chance of heart attack, than those who ate the least amount of these foods. This was true even after taking account of other risk factors for heart disease, such as smoking and high cholesterol levels. Scientists believe that all carotenoids, particularly alpha-carotene and lycopene, block the formation of LDL ('bad') cholesterol, which can lead to heart attacks and other cardiovascular problems.

✪ **ADDITIONAL BENEFITS:** Lutein and zeaxanthin are important for eye health, *see page* 136. Other carotenoids may also help protect the eye, reducing the risk of diseases such as cataracts. Studies have identified protective effects for lycopene against oxidative damage in the human lens and reduced incidence of cataract in test animals. A survey of 372 older people also found that the risk of cortical cataract was lowest in the people with the highest blood concentrations of lycopene.

A recent study found that increasing lycopene intake from tomato paste to 16mg/day over a 10-week period offered significant protection against sunburn following UV radiation, although the protective effects appear to develop slowly. Lycopene should not be used as a substitute for protective sunscreens.

How to take them

✐ **DOSAGE:** If you do not eat a wide variety of carotenoid-rich foods, choose a supplement that contains a mixture of carotenoids – alpha-carotene, beta-carotene, cryptoxanthin, lycopene, lutein and zeaxanthin.

◉ **GUIDELINES FOR USE:** Take carotenoid supplements with foods that contain a little fat, which allows the body to absorb them more effectively. If you divide in half the total daily amount of supplements you plan to take, and take each half at a different time, your body may be able to absorb more of them.

Possible side effects

Large doses of carotenoids, consumed in food or in the form of supplements, can turn your skin orange, especially the palms of your hands and the soles of your feet. This effect is harmless and will gradually go away if you reduce your intake. Although there are no other known side effects associated with large amounts of mixed carotenoids, taking high doses of particular carotenoids may interfere with the workings of the other carotenoids. Beta-carotene supplements, on their own, do not appear to reduce the risk of any disease, and may increase risk in smokers and those at high risk of lung cancer.

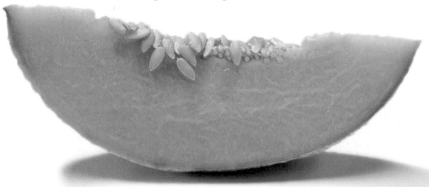

Cantaloupe melon is a good source of beta-carotene.

Cat's claw

First used in European medicine as recently as the 1980s, cat's claw has long been popular among South American Indians as a treatment for wounds, stomach disorders, arthritis, cancer and other ailments. It is a herb derived from the bark or roots of an Amazonian vine.

Uncaria tomentosa
U. guianensis

Common uses

- *May enhance immunity, which makes it useful for sinusitis and other infections.*
- *Supports cancer treatment.*
- *May help to relieve chronic pain.*
- *Reduces pain and inflammation from gout or arthritis.*

Forms

- Capsule
- Dried herb/tea
- Softgel
- Tablet
- Tincture

CAUTION!

- **Do not take cat's claw if you are pregnant, considering pregnancy or breastfeeding. Its safety is not established in these situations, and it may bring on a spontaneous miscarriage.**

REMINDER: If you have a medical condition, consult your doctor before taking supplements.

What it is

In the Amazon basin, one woody tropical vine twining up trees in the rain forest has two curved thorns that resemble the claws of a cat at the base of its leaves. The herb derived from the inner bark or the roots of this plant is known as cat's claw or, in Spanish, *uña de gato*. Although there are dozens of related species, two specific ones, *Uncaria tomentosa* and U. *guianensis*, are harvested in the wild (primarily in Peru and Brazil) for medicinal purposes. Large pieces of their bark are a common sight in South American farmers' markets.

What it does

Modern scientific studies have identified several active ingredients in cat's claw that enhance the activity of the immune system and inhibit inflammation. Their presence may help to explain why this herb has traditionally been used to fight cancer, arthritis, dysentery, ulcers and other infectious and inflammatory conditions. However, there is a lack of clinical evidence to confirm these uses.

✪ **MAJOR BENEFITS:** Doctors in Germany and Austria prescribe cat's claw to stimulate the immune response in cancer patients who may be weakened by chemotherapy, radiotherapy or other conventional treatments. Several compounds in the herb – some of which have been studied for decades – may account for its cancer-fighting and immunity-boosting effects. In the 1970s researchers reported that the inner bark and root contained compounds called procyanidolic oligomers (PCOs), which inhibit the growth of tumours in animals, and in the 1980s German scientists identified other compounds in cat's claw that enhance the immune system, in part by stimulating immune cells called phagocytes that engulf and devour viruses, bacteria and other disease-causing

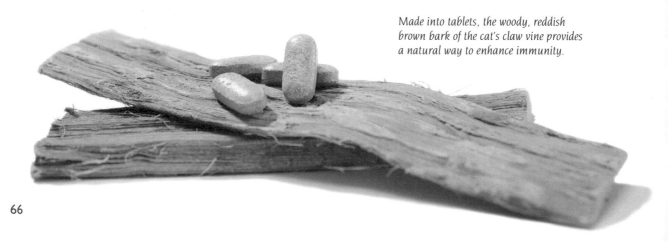

Made into tablets, the woody, reddish brown bark of the cat's claw vine provides a natural way to enhance immunity.

microorganisms. Then in 1993 an Italian study detected another class of compound, quinovic acid glycosides, which have multiple benefits; they act as antioxidants, ridding the body of cell-damaging molecules called free radicals and also kill viruses, reduce inflammation and inhibit the transformation of normal cells into cancerous ones.

In addition to its potential for impeding the growth of tumours, cat's claw may also combat stubborn infections such as sinusitis.

✷ **ADDITIONAL BENEFITS:** Traditionally cat's claw has been relied on to treat pain. Its anti-inflammatory properties apparently make it effective in relieving joint pain caused by arthritis or gout. Additional research is needed, however, to define the precise role that the herb plays in treating arthritis and other inflammatory complaints.

Preliminary reports found that, when used in conjunction with conventional AIDS drugs, cat's claw may benefit people infected with HIV, because it seems to boost the immune response. Some researchers caution against taking the herb for chronic conditions affecting the immune system, including tuberculosis, multiple sclerosis and rheumatoid arthritis, because they believe it may overstimulate the immune system and make symptoms worse. There are doctors, however, who recommend it for autoimmune disorders, including rheumatoid arthritis and lupus. Further studies are required.

How to take it

⌀ **DOSAGE:** Take 250 mg of a standardised extract in tablet form twice a day. Alternatively, take 1 to 2 ml (20 to 40 drops) of the tincture twice a day. The crude herb (the ground root or inner bark of cat's claw in a non-concentrated form) is available in the form of 500 or 1000 mg capsules; these should be taken twice daily (up to 2000 mg a day). Cat's claw tea is sold in health-food shops; use 1 or 2 teaspoons of dried herb per cup of very hot water, following the instructions on the packet. You can drink up to three cups a day.

◉ **GUIDELINES FOR USE:** You can combine or rotate cat's claw with other herbs that stimulate the immune system, such as echinacea, goldenseal, reishi and maitake mushrooms, astragalus and pau d'arco.

Pregnant or breastfeeding women should avoid cat's claw. In Peru it has been valued for a long time as a contraceptive; in animals it stimulates uterine contractions. This effect suggests that the herb could induce miscarriages. It should not be used as a contraceptive.

Possible side effects

Although few studies have been conducted into the safety of cat's claw, there have been no reports that it is toxic at recommended doses. Taking higher doses, however, may cause diarrhoea.

Cayenne and chilli

Hot peppers renowned for the fiery taste they bring to Indian, Mexican and other cuisines, cayenne and chilli are also used medicinally to stimulate digestion and to relieve pain. Their healing properties come from oily compounds called capsaicinoids.

Capsicum genus

Common uses

Topical ointment
- Alleviates arthritis pain.

- Reduces nerve pain associated with shingles (post-herpetic neuralgia), diabetes, surgery or trigeminal neuralgia (tic douloureux).

Capsule, tablet and tincture
- Relieve indigestion.

Forms
- Capsule
- Fresh or dried herb
- Ointment/paste
- Tablet
- Tincture/liquid

CAUTION!

■ Never apply chilli ointment to raw or open skin. Avoid eyes and contact lenses: the burning can be intense.

REMINDER: If you have a medical condition, consult your doctor before taking supplements.

What they are

Derived from several varieties of capsicum, cayenne and chilli are cousins of the red and green peppers used in salads and stir-fry dishes, but they are not related to black table pepper. The main active ingredients in the peppers – and what gives them their hotness – are capsaicinoids, particularly capsaicin (pronounced cap-SAY-i-sin), oily irritants that are also the principal ingredients of pepper sprays used in self-defence. Capsaicin is usually described on medicinal labels as 'capsicum'.

What they do

When applied to the skin, capsicum is an effective painkiller. It causes the depletion of a component in nerve cells called substance P, which transmits pain impulses to the brain. When taken as a supplement or in food, capsicum appears to have a highly beneficial effect on the digestive system, and it is sometimes used to counteract poor circulation.

✷ **MAJOR BENEFITS:** Regular application to the skin of an ointment, or paste, containing capsicum can be very effective in relieving arthritis pain. It can also relieve lingering pain in people recovering from shingles, postoperative pain, and pain from nerve damage caused by diabetes.

Preliminary studies indicate that chilli ointment has other medicinal uses. It may reduce the itching of psoriasis (the itching sensation follows the same nerve pathways as pain). The ointment has also shown promise in relieving the aches and pains of fibromyalgia and the coldness in the extremities caused by Raynaud's disease.

✷ **ADDITIONAL BENEFITS:** Fresh peppers, tinctures, tablets and capsules are said to stimulate digestion and to relieve flatulence and ulcers by increasing blood circulation in the stomach and bowel and by promoting the secretion of digestive juices. Liquid products containing tinctures of capsicum can ease symptoms of colds and flu. Claims that capsicum may reduce heart disease risk – by lowering blood cholesterol and triglyceride levels – or help to prevent cancer lack the support of clinical evidence.

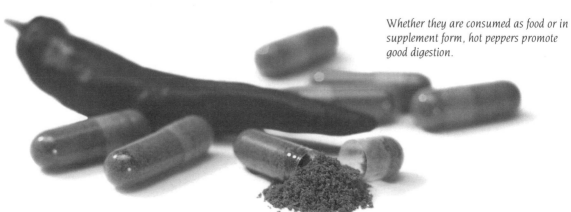

Whether they are consumed as food or in supplement form, hot peppers promote good digestion.

How to take them

⊘ **DOSAGE:** *For external use*: Chilli ointment containing 0.025% to 0.075% capsaicin is most effective with regular, daily use; apply it thinly over the affected areas at least three or four times a day for pain, rubbing it in well. The pain may take several weeks to subside. *Cayenne for internal use*: Follow the instructions on the packet or on the jar of tablets.

◉ **GUIDELINES FOR USE:** *For external use*: Sensitivity to chilli varies from person to person, so test the ointment first on a small, particularly painful area. If it proves effective – which may take a week or more – and causes no lasting discomfort, you can enlarge the coverage area. To avoid getting chilli in the eyes, wash your hands afterwards with warm, soapy water, or wear rubber gloves during application and then discard them; you can also cover the area with a loose bandage. (If you are using chilli ointment to relieve pain in the fingers or hands, wait 30 minutes before washing it off to allow the ointment to penetrate the skin. In the meantime, avoid touching contact lenses and sensitive areas, such as eyes and nose.) Store chilli ointment away from light and extremes of heat or cold, and keep it out of reach of children.

For internal use: Cayenne supplements can be taken with or without food. No adverse effects have been reported in pregnant or breastfeeding women, but discontinue use if a breastfeeding baby becomes irritable.

Possible side effects

Chilli ointment often causes a mildly unpleasant burning sensation that lasts half an hour or so in the first few days of application, but this effect usually disappears after several days of regular use. Using too much ointment or inhaling it may trigger coughing, sneezing, tears or an irritated throat. Chilli can also cause intense pain and burning – though no lasting damage – if it gets in your eyes (or other moist mucous membranes). If this happens, flush the affected area with water or milk. To remove chilli from the skin, wash with warm, soapy water. Vinegar may also work, but do not use it in or near your eyes.

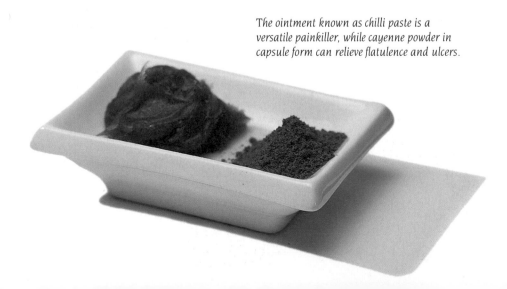

The ointment known as chilli paste is a versatile painkiller, while cayenne powder in capsule form can relieve flatulence and ulcers.

Chamomile

Sometimes called the most soothing plant on earth, chamomile has traditionally been enjoyed as a tea to relax the nerves and ease digestive complaints. The herb is found in concentrated form in pills and tinctures, and in skin formulas designed to treat sores and rashes.

Matricaria recutita

Common uses

- *Promotes general relaxation and relieves anxiety.*
- *Alleviates insomnia.*
- *Heals mouth sores and treats gum disease.*
- *Soothes skin rashes and burns, including sunburn.*
- *Relieves red and irritated eyes.*
- *Eases menstrual cramps.*
- *Treats bowel inflammation, digestive upset and indigestion.*

Forms

- Capsule
- Cream/ointment
- Dried herb/tea
- Oil
- Tincture

CAUTION!

REMINDER: If you have a medical condition, consult your doctor before taking supplements.

What it is

The more popular of the two chamomile herbs (and the one discussed in this book) is German – sometimes called Hungarian – chamomile. It comes from the dried daisy-like flowers of the *Matricaria recutita* plant (its older botanical names are *Matricaria chamomilla* and *Chamomilla recutita*). The other type of chamomile is Roman or English chamomile (*Chamaemelum nobile* or *Anthemis nobilis*), which has properties similar to those of the German species.

The herb has long been used to prepare a gently soothing tea. Its pleasing apple-like aroma and flavour (the name chamomile is derived from the Greek *kamai melon*, meaning 'ground apple') make the ritual of brewing and sipping the tea a relaxing experience in itself.

Concentrated chamomile extracts are added to creams and lotions or packaged as capsules or tinctures. The healing properties of the herb are related in part to its volatile oils, which contain a compound called apigenin as well as other therapeutic substances.

What it does

Chamomile is a great soother. Its anti-inflammatory, antispasmodic and infection-fighting effects can benefit the whole body. When taken internally it calms digestive upsets, relieves cramps and relaxes the nerves. It also works externally on the skin and the mucous membranes of the mouth and eyes, relieving rashes, sores and inflammation.

MAJOR BENEFITS: When Peter Rabbit's mother put him to bed to recover from an adventure, she gave him a spoonful of chamomile tea. Scientists have since confirmed the wisdom of Beatrix Potter's character; studies in animals have shown that chamomile contains substances that act on the same parts of the brain and nervous system as those affected by anti-anxiety drugs, promoting relaxation and reducing stress.

Chamomile appears to have a mildly sedative effect, but more importantly it also calms the body, making it easier for the person taking it to fall asleep naturally. In addition the herb has a relaxing, anti-inflammatory effect on the smooth muscles lining the digestive tract. It helps to relieve a wide range of gastrointestinal complaints, including indigestion, diverticular disorders and inflammatory bowel disease. Its muscle-relaxing action may alleviate menstrual cramps.

ADDITIONAL BENEFITS: Used externally, chamomile helps to soothe skin inflammation. It contains bacteria-fighting compounds that may also speed the healing of infections. A dressing soaked in chamomile tea is often beneficial when applied to mild burns. For sunburn, chamomile oil can be added to a cool bath or mixed with almond oil and rubbed on sunburnt areas. The oil should always be diluted before application, and should never be taken internally. Chamomile creams can also relieve sunburn and skin rashes such as eczema. Alternatively, the herb is used to treat inflammation or infection of the eyes or mouth. Eyewashes made from the cooled tea may relieve the redness or irritation of conjunctivitis and other eye inflammations; prepare a fresh batch of tea daily and store it in a sterile container. Used daily as a gargle or mouthwash, the tea can help to heal mouth sores and prevent gum disease. Inhaled chamomile vapours may also help colds. A study of 60 patients with colds found a better reduction in symptoms with a steam inhalation using chamomile extract, than one using alcohol.

How to take it

☑ **DOSAGE:** *To make a cup of chamomile tea:* Pour a cup of very hot (not boiling) water over 2 teaspoons of dried flowers. Steep for five minutes and strain. Drink up to three cups a day or a cup at bedtime. If you are using the tea on the skin or eyes, it should be cooled thoroughly, poured into a sterile container and kept covered until needed. *For the skin:* Add a few drops of chamomile oil to 3 teaspoons of almond oil (or another neutral oil), or buy a ready-made cream. Capsules and tinctures are also available; follow instructions on the packet. A single capsule, or up to 1 teaspoon of tincture, often has the therapeutic effects of a cup of tea.

◉ **GUIDELINES FOR USE:** Chamomile is gentle and can be used over long periods. It can be combined safely with prescription and over-the-counter drugs as well as with other herbs and nutritional supplements. At recommended doses, the herb seems to be safe for children and pregnant and breastfeeding women.

Possible side effects

Whether the herb is used internally or externally, side effects are virtually unknown. Those taking doses higher than recommended of the herb have reported a few instances of nausea and vomiting. Although some concerns have been raised about possible allergic reactions which cause bronchial tightness or skin rashes, these appear to be extremely rare.

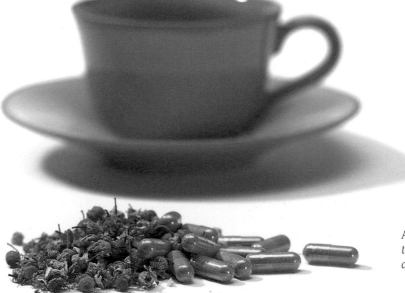

A single capsule can produce the same relaxing effect as a cup of chamomile tea.

71

Chasteberry

Vitex agnus-castus

The physicians of ancient Greece, including Hippocrates, recommended chasteberry for the treatment of a variety of conditions. It is now one of the herbs most often prescribed to relieve the symptoms of premenstrual syndrome (PMS) and other menstrual problems.

Common uses

- *Alleviates symptoms of premenstrual syndrome (PMS).*
- *Regulates menstruation.*
- *Promotes fertility.*
- *Eases menopausal hot flushes.*

Forms

- Capsule
- Dried herb/tea
- Tablet
- Tincture

CAUTION!

■ Chasteberry affects hormone production, so it should not be used by women taking hormonal medications, including contraceptive pills and oestrogen, or by those who are pregnant.

REMINDER: If you have a medical condition, consult your doctor before taking supplements.

What it is

Also called vitex, chaste tree berry, or monk's pepper, chasteberry is the fruit of the chaste tree. Actually a small shrub with violet flower spikes and long, slender leaves, the chaste tree is native to the Mediterranean region but grows in subtropical climates throughout the world. Its red berries are harvested in the autumn and then dried. They resemble peppercorns in shape, and the taste they impart to a therapeutic cup of tea is distinctively peppery.

What it does

The use of chasteberry for 'female complaints' dates back to Hippocrates in the fourth century BC. Although the herb does not contain hormones, or hormone-like substances, it prompts the pituitary gland (located at the base of the brain) to send a signal to the ovaries to increase production of the female hormone progesterone. Chasteberry also inhibits the excessive production of prolactin, a hormone that primarily regulates breast-milk production but has other less understood actions as well.

☆ **MAJOR BENEFITS:** Some scientists believe that women who routinely suffer from PMS produce too little progesterone in the last two weeks of their menstrual cycle. This deficiency causes an imbalance in the body's natural oestrogen-progesterone ratio. Chasteberry restores hormonal equilibrium, relieving such PMS-related complaints as irritability, bloating and depression. Studies in Germany indicate that the herb offers at least some relief for PMS symptoms in about 90% of women – and in a third of them the symptoms disappear. Chasteberry's prolactin-lowering action helps to reduce the breast pain and tenderness that some women experience before menstruation even if they have no other premenstrual symptoms.

The easiest way to enjoy the benefits of chasteberry is to take it in tablet or capsule form.

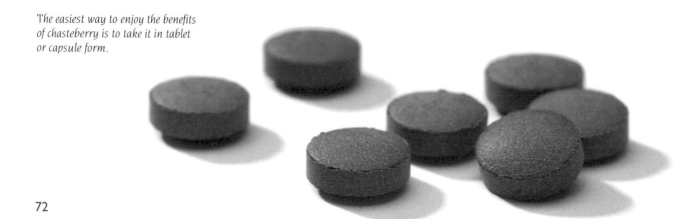

✱ **ADDITIONAL BENEFITS:** Because high levels of prolactin and low levels of progesterone in the body can inhibit monthly ovulation, chasteberry may be useful to those who are having trouble becoming pregnant. The herb works best in women with mild or moderately low progesterone levels. When too much prolactin causes menstruation to stop (a condition called amenorrhoea) the herb can help restore a normal monthly cycle.

Menopausal hot flushes are also the result of hormonal changes controlled by the pituitary gland, so women who are experiencing the menopause may want to try chasteberry. Used either alone or in combination with other herbs such as dong quai or black cohosh, it can alleviate the periodic flushing and sweating that occur.

Chasteberry is sometimes also recommended in the treatment of menstrual-related acne.

How to take it

▢ **DOSAGE:** Whether you are using chasteberry to treat PMS, breast tenderness, infertility, amenorrhoea or other menstrual disorders, the dose is the same. In tincture form, add a ½ teaspoon twice a day to a glass of water. The equivalent dose for the powdered extract in tablet or capsule form is 225 mg, standardised. For menopausal hot flushes take the same dose (½ teaspoon/225 mg) twice a day.

◉ **GUIDELINES FOR USE:** Take chasteberry on an empty stomach to increase absorption; your first dose should always be taken in the morning. Even after just 10 days a woman with PMS symptoms will probably notice at least some improvement during her next menstrual cycle. However, it may take three months of use to benefit from the full effect of this herb. Six months of treatment with chasteberry may be necessary to correct infertility or amenorrhoea.

Possible side effects

Most people will not notice any adverse side effects from taking chasteberry, but studies have shown that stomach irritation, headache or an itchy rash can occur in a small percentage of women. Discontinue using it if you develop any sign of a rash. In addition, some women may experience an increased menstrual flow after taking this herb.

FACTS & TIPS

■ As with other herbs, the action of chasteberry is the result of the combined effects of several active components; the berry's biological action cannot be reproduced when the components are used individually.

■ Women who are having trouble breastfeeding may want to try chasteberry, because it can increase milk production. Take 225 mg of chasteberry extract, in tablet or capsule form, twice a day for as long as necessary. The herb does not change the composition of breast milk, so appears safe to use.

Chromium

The trace mineral chromium has been lauded as a slimming aid and a muscle builder as well as a treatment for diabetes and a weapon against heart disease. Although chromium is essential for growth and good health, the more spectacular claims for it remain controversial.

Common uses

- Essential for the breakdown of protein, fat and carbohydrates.
- Helps the body to maintain normal blood sugar (glucose) levels.
- May lower total blood cholesterol, LDL ('bad') cholesterol and triglyceride levels.

Forms

- Capsule
- Liquid
- Softgel
- Tablet

CAUTION!

- People with diabetes should consult their doctor before taking chromium. This mineral may alter the dosage for insulin or other diabetes medications.

REMINDER: If you have a medical condition, consult your doctor before taking supplements.

What it is

Chromium is a trace mineral that comes in several chemical forms. As many people do not have enough chromium in their diets, supplements may be worth considering.

What it does

Chromium helps the body to use insulin, a hormone that transfers blood sugar (glucose) to the cells, where it is burned as fuel. With enough chromium the body uses insulin efficiently and maintains normal blood sugar levels. Chromium also aids in breaking down protein and fat.

PREVENTION: A sufficient chromium intake may prevent diabetes in people with insulin resistance. This disorder makes the body less sensitive to the effects of insulin, so the pancreas has to produce more and more of it to keep blood sugar (glucose) levels in check. When the pancreas can no longer keep up with the body's demand for extra insulin, type II diabetes develops. Chromium may avert this outcome by allowing the body to use insulin more effectively in the first place. Chromium also helps to break down fats, so it may reduce LDL ('bad') and increase HDL ('good') cholesterol levels, thus lowering the risk of heart disease.

ADDITIONAL BENEFITS: Chromium can relieve headaches, irritability and other symptoms of low blood sugar (hypoglycaemia) by preventing blood sugar levels from dropping below normal. In people with diabetes it may help to control blood sugar levels. Chromium may also help to lower lipid levels and reduce the risk of coronary artery disease. The most controversial claims associated with the mineral relate to weight loss and muscle building. Although some studies indicate that large doses of chromium picolinate can assist weight reduction or increase muscle mass, others have found no benefit. At best, when combined with a sensible diet and regular exercise, mineral supplements may offer a very slight advantage to someone who wants to lose weight. More research is needed to establish chromium's role in this regard.

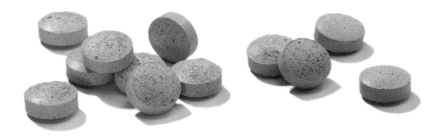

How much you need

No recommended amount has been established for chromium, but scientists believe that 50 to 200 mcg a day can prevent a deficiency in adults. (A daily chromium intake of 200 mcg from food would be hard to achieve even for someone with a healthy, varied diet.)

⊟ **IF YOU GET TOO LITTLE:** A chromium deficiency can lead to inefficient use of glucose. In itself, a lack of chromium is probably not a cause of diabetes, but it can help to bring on the disease in those who are susceptible to it. In addition, anxiety, poor metabolism of amino acids, and high triglyceride and cholesterol levels may occur in individuals who don't get enough chromium.

⊞ **IF YOU GET TOO MUCH:** Chromium supplements do not seem to have any adverse effects even at high doses, although there is some concern that megadoses can impair the absorption of iron and zinc. This can usually be corrected by getting extra iron or zinc through diet or supplements. Supplements containing chromium in the form of chromium picolinate (but not other forms found in supplements) have been linked with cancer and are likely to be banned in the UK.

How to take it

▢ **DOSAGE:** Chromium supplements are generally available in 200 mcg doses. This amount should be taken for general good health, or when following a weight-loss programme or to improve the effectiveness of insulin.

◉ **GUIDELINES FOR USE:** Take chromium in 200 mcg doses with food or a full glass of water to decrease stomach irritation. Chromium is better absorbed when combined with foods high in vitamin C (or taken with a vitamin C supplement). Calcium carbonate supplements or antacids can reduce chromium absorption.

Don't be confused by labels suggesting that one type of chromium – whether picolinate or polynicotinate – is absorbed better than any other. No reliable research supports these claims.

Other sources

Among the foods that contain chromium are whole-grain cereals, potatoes, prunes, peanut butter, nuts, seafood and brewer's yeast. Low-fat diets tend to be higher in chromium than high-fat ones.

CASE HISTORY
Chromium to the rescue

A decade after being diagnosed with diabetes Sarah P. faced the prospect of insulin injections because her pills were not effectively regulating her blood sugar. When she read about chromium she thought, 'Why not try it first?' Her doctor was sceptical and slightly concerned, but he agreed to let her try.

There were no instant results. 'It may seem silly,' Sarah says, 'but I wanted the chromium to work so much that I also began paying extra attention to my diet and forcing myself to take brisk walks twice a day.'

Her blood sugar eventually came down to a healthier level. Was the chromium responsible? Nobody knows for sure. Sarah's doctor, who read the information about chromium that Sarah regularly sent him, acknowledges that he may have dismissed it too soon and would like to see more research done.

Sarah herself has no doubts. 'I've lost a little weight, but I'm still the same person. My blood sugar hasn't been out of control for months. I'm sure it's because of the chromium.'

DID YOU KNOW?
Whole-grain bread is a good source of chromium. Refined grains, found in white bread, contain little of this essential mineral.

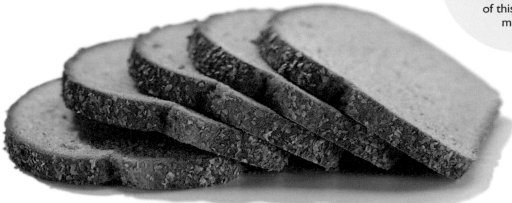

Coenzyme Q$_{10}$

Touted as a wonder supplement, coenzyme Q$_{10}$ is said to enhance stamina, help weight loss, combat cancer and even stave off ageing. These claims are extravagant, but the nutrient does show particular promise in the treatment of heart disease and gum disease.

Common uses

- *Benefits the heart and circulation in cases of heart failure, a weakened heart muscle (cardiomyopathy), high blood pressure, heart rhythm disorders, chest pain (angina) and Raynaud's disease.*

- *Treats gum disease and maintains healthy gums and teeth.*

- *Protects the nerves and may help to slow the progress of Alzheimer's disease and Parkinson's disease.*

- *May help to prevent cancer and heart disease, and may slow down age-related degenerative changes.*

Forms
- Capsule
- Liquid
- Softgel
- Tablet

What it is

Coenzyme Q$_{10}$, a natural substance produced by the body, belongs to a family of compounds called quinones. When it was first isolated, in 1957, scientists called it ubiquinone because it was ubiquitous in nature. In fact coenzyme Q$_{10}$ is found in all living creatures and is also concentrated in many foods, including nuts and oils. In the past decade coenzyme Q$_{10}$ has become one of the most popular dietary supplements around the world. Proponents of the nutrient use it to maintain general good health as well as to treat heart disease and a number of other serious conditions. Some clinicians believe that it is so important in maintaining the normal functioning of the body that it should be dubbed 'vitamin Q'.

What it does

The primary function of coenzyme Q$_{10}$ is as a catalyst for metabolism – the complex chain of chemical reactions during which food is broken down into packets of energy that the body can use. Acting in conjunction with enzymes (hence the name 'coenzyme') the compound speeds up the metabolic process, providing energy that the cells need to digest food, heal wounds, maintain healthy muscles and perform countless other bodily functions. The nutrient has an essential role in energy production, so it is not surprising that it is found in every cell in the body. Especially abundant in the energy-intensive cells of the heart, it helps this organ to beat more than 100,000 times each day. In addition coenzyme Q$_{10}$ acts as an antioxidant, much like vitamins C and E, helping to neutralise the cell-damaging molecules known as free radicals.

⬦ PREVENTION: Coenzyme Q$_{10}$ may have a role in preventing cancer, heart attacks and other diseases linked to free-radical damage. It is also

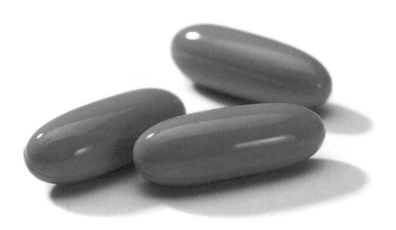

used as an energy enhancer and anti-ageing supplement. Levels of the compound reduce with age (and with certain diseases), so some doctors recommend starting daily supplementation at about the age of 40.

✪ **MAJOR BENEFITS:** Coenzyme Q_{10} has generated much excitement as a possible therapy for heart disease patients, especially those suffering from heart failure or weakened hearts. In some studies patients with poorly functioning hearts improved greatly after adding the supplement to their conventional drugs and therapies. Other studies have shown that people with cardiovascular disease have low levels of this substance in their hearts. Further research suggests that coenzyme Q_{10} may protect against blood clots, reduce blood pressure, diminish irregular heartbeats, treat mitral valve prolapse, lessen symptoms of Raynaud's disease (poor circulation in the extremities) and relieve chest pains (angina). But it is intended as a complement to – not as a replacement for – conventional medical treatments. Do not take this nutrient in place of heart drugs or other prescribed medications.

✤ **ADDITIONAL BENEFITS:** A few small studies suggest that coenzyme Q_{10} may prolong survival in those with breast or prostate cancer, but results remain inconclusive. It also appears to aid healing and reduce pain and bleeding in those with gum disease, and to speed recovery following oral surgery. The supplement shows some promise against Parkinson's and Alzheimer's diseases and fibromyalgia, and it may improve stamina in those with AIDS. Certain practitioners believe that the nutrient helps to stabilise blood sugar levels in people with diabetes.

There are many other claims made for the supplement: that it slows ageing, aids weight loss, enhances athletic performance, combats chronic fatigue syndrome, relieves multiple allergies and boosts immunity. More research is needed to determine the effectiveness of coenzyme Q_{10} for these and other conditions.

How to take it

⊘ **DOSAGE:** The general dosage is 50 mg twice a day. Higher dosages of 100 mg twice a day may be useful for heart or circulatory disorders, or for Alzheimer's disease and other specific complaints.

◉ **GUIDELINES FOR USE:** Take a supplement morning and evening, ideally with food to enhance absorption. Coenzyme Q_{10} should be continued over a long period; it may require eight weeks or longer for results to be noticed.

Possible side effects

Most research suggests that the supplement is harmless, even in large doses. In rare cases it may cause upset stomach, diarrhoea, nausea or loss of appetite. As coenzyme Q_{10} has not been extensively studied, however, it is advisable to consult your doctor before using it, especially if you are pregnant or breastfeeding.

Combination supplements

For many people who feel 'under par' a multivitamin and multimineral combination can help to boost energy levels, improve resistance to disease and enhance a sense of well-being. Some people have more need than others for specific nutrients – those under stress, for example, can benefit from vitamin C and magnesium. But, since many can interact with each other, individual nutrients should be taken alongside a good vitamin and mineral combination.

The hundreds of different combination formulas available can make deciding what is right for you confusing so the table on the right outlines some of the supplements available, their uses, and the nutrients you should look for.

ADDED VALUE

Phytochemicals extracted from plants, such as flavonoids, isoflavones and polyphenols, are now added to many supplements to increase their potency (*see also pages 154-7*). For example, flavonoids are often added to vitamin C formulas, and many antioxidant formulas contain phytochemicals such as rutin or green tea extract. Isoflavones are included in formulas to promote women's health. The addition of phytochemicals has improved the effectiveness of many nutritional supplements and increased the choice.

MINERAL ABSORPTION

Mineral supplements should be taken as a formula containing a mixture of minerals, including calcium, chromium, iron, magnesium, manganese, selenium and zinc.

Different minerals often compete for the same site of absorption within the digestive tract, so a balanced formula will have been put together to ensure that the absorption of one mineral is not reduced by the presence of excessive levels of another, leading to its deficiency.

For specific conditions, such as fatigue or arthritis, it may be necessary to take additional high levels of single minerals, in accordance with the recommendations that are given elsewhere in this book (where due attention to possible interactions has been discussed).

ALL YOU NEED Combine supplements to ensure an adequate intake of essential and non-essential nutrients.

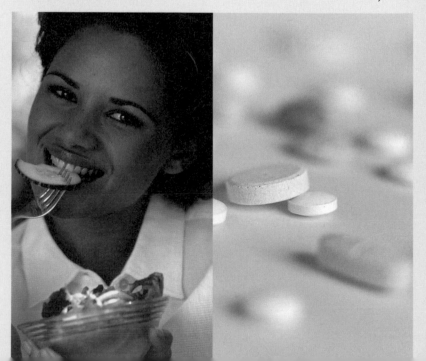

78

FORMS AND INTERACTIONS OF MINERALS

MINERAL	MOST ABSORBABLE FORMS	TO AID ABSORPTION	CAUTION: THESE REDUCE ABSORPTION/ ENHANCE EXCRETION
Calcium	Citrate	Magnesium, vitamin D, lactose	Phytates (from wheat), caffeine, high intakes of zinc, saturated fats, oxalic acid (from rhubarb and spinach), salt, sugar
Magnesium	Citrate, acetate	Calcium, vitamin B_6, vitamin D	Alcohol, caffeine, high calcium or phosphorus, high fat or sugar intake, stress
Iron	Sulphate, fumarate	Vitamin C, fructose, animal protein	Oxalates, phytates, tannin (from tea), phosphates (from cola drinks & food additives) high intake of zinc or calcium
Zinc	Citrate, gluconate, acetate, sulphate	Vitamins B_2 and A	Phytates, oxalates, high calcium, iron or copper, lead, alcohol, smoking, stress
Magnanese	Not known	Vitamin C	Iron, zinc, copper, high intake of calcium
Selenium	Sodium selenate, sodium hydrogen selenite	Not known	Not known
Chromium	Chromium chloride, chromium sulphate	Vitamin B_3	Sugar, high intake of calcium
Copper	Not known	Protein	High intake of zinc. Iron, sulphur, vitamin C

In general, the most potent forms of minerals are the chelates (such as chromium, picolinate, selenomethionine), ascorbates, citrates and gluconates. In these forms the minerals are loosely bound and are readily released during digestion. Inorganic forms, such as carbonates and oxides, tend to be less well absorbed.

Vitamins are also available in a number of forms. For example, vitamin A is available as retinol or its chemical fore-runner beta-carotene. This is because retinol is potentially toxic, so most manufacturers prefer to use beta-carotene, which the body converts to vitamin A as required.

To improve their effects, many formulas now contain 'mixed carotenoids' – mainly beta-carotene with smaller amounts of other health-protective carotenoids added.

COMMON SUPPLEMENT COMBINATIONS

COMBINATION	USES	WHAT THEY SHOULD CONTAIN
A-Z	Multivitamin and multi-mineral complex for general health, which meets most require-ments but not those of calcium or magnesium	**Vitamins** A, D, E, K, C, B_1 (thiamin), B_2 (riboflavin), B_3 (niacin), B_5 (pantothenic acid), B_6, B_{12}, folic acid, biotin. **Minerals** boron, chromium, iron, manganese, potassium, selenium, zinc
Bone formula	Supports bone health and helps prevent osteoporosis	Calcium, magnesium, boron, vitamins D, C and K
Women's health formula	Maintains hormonal balance	Vitamins C, B_6 and E, folic acid, iron, zinc and magnesium
Children's formula	Multivitamin and multi-mineral suitable for children: available as powders, chewable tablets or liquid drops.	A broad range of nutrients and including carotenoids, vitamin B complex, vitamins C, D, E, iron, zinc, manganese, chromium and selenium
Pregnancy	Promotes health and development of mother and baby	A good combination for pregnancy should include at least folic acid, vitamin C, magnesium and iron
Antioxidant	Prevents damage to cells by free radicals	Beta-carotene (as mixed carotenoids), vitamins C and E and selenium. Other nutrients that may also be present include zinc, manganese, copper, lutein, lycopene, resveratrol, bilberry extract, green tea extract, quercetin, L-glutathione, L-cysteine, anthocyanosides
Echinacea and goldenseal	To boost the immune system	Echinacea: *see page 89* Goldenseal: *see page 119*

Copper

Essential in preventing cardiovascular disease, maintaining good skin and hair colour and promoting fertility, copper is found in at least 15 proteins in the human body. But some nutritionists believe that many people may be marginally deficient in this important nutrient.

Common uses

- Strengthens blood vessels, bones, tendons and nerves.
- Helps to maintain fertility.
- Ensures healthy hair and skin pigmentation.
- Promotes blood clotting.

Forms

- Capsule
- Tablet

CAUTION!

REMINDER: *If you have a medical condition, consult your doctor before taking supplements.*

What it is

Copper, the reddish brown malleable metal commonly used in cookware and plumbing, is also present as a trace element throughout the human body. This mineral is available in nutritional supplement form as copper carbonate, copper citrate and copper gluconate. Although copper can be obtained from a wide variety of foods, the typical British diet is low in it because the foods that are the best sources, such as shellfish, liver, whole grains, beans, nuts and seeds, are not eaten frequently.

What it does

Copper is essential in the formation of collagen, a fundamental protein in bones, skin and connective tissue. It plays an important role in the development of red blood cells, and may also help the body to use its stored iron and play a role in maintaining immunity and fertility. Involved in the formation of melanin (a dark natural colour found in the hair, skin and eyes), copper also promotes consistent pigmentation.

🛡 **PREVENTION:** Evidence suggests that copper can be a factor in preventing high blood pressure and heart rhythm disorders (arrhythmias). And some researchers believe that it may protect tissues from damage by free radicals, helping to prevent cancer, heart disease and other ailments. Getting enough copper may also help keep to cholesterol levels low.

✳ **ADDITIONAL BENEFITS:** Copper is necessary for the manufacture of many enzymes, especially superoxide dismutase (SOD), which appears to be one of the body's most potent antioxidants. It may also help to stave off bone loss that can lead to osteoporosis.

How much you need

Although there is no daily RDA for copper, adults are advised to obtain 1.5 to 3 mg daily to keep the body functioning normally.

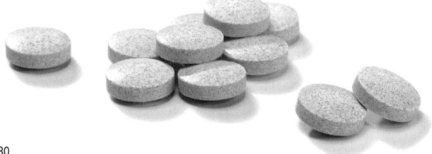

⊟ **IF YOU GET TOO LITTLE:** A true copper deficiency is rare. It usually occurs only in individuals with illnesses such as Crohn's disease or coeliac disease, or in those with inherited conditions that inhibit copper absorption, such as albinism. Symptoms of deficiency are: fatigue; heart rhythm disorders; brittle, discoloured hair; high blood pressure; anaemia; skeletal defects; and infertility.

But even a mild deficiency may have some adverse health effects. For example, a preliminary study involving 24 men found that a diet low in copper caused a significant increase in LDL ('bad') cholesterol and a decrease in HDL ('good') cholesterol. These changes in their cholesterol profiles increased the participants' risk of heart disease.

⊞ **IF YOU GET TOO MUCH:** Just 10 mg of copper taken at one time can produce nausea, muscle pain and stomachache. Severe copper toxicity from oral copper supplements has not been noted to date. However, some people who work with pesticides containing copper have suffered liver damage, coma and even death.

How to take it

▱ **DOSAGE:** Unless a practitioner advises otherwise, copper should only be taken in the form of a multivitamin or multimineral supplement that provides no more than 1 mg of copper daily.

◐ **GUIDELINES FOR USE:** It is advisable to take a supplement at the same time every day, preferably with a meal to decrease the chance of stomach irritation.

Other sources

Shellfish (oysters, lobsters, crabs) and offal are excellent sources of copper. However, if you are concerned about your cholesterol levels, there are many vegetarian foods rich in copper as well. These include legumes; whole grains, such as rye and wheat, and products made from them (bread, cereal, pasta); nuts and seeds; vegetables such as peas, artichokes, avocados, radishes, garlic, mushrooms and potatoes; fruits such as tomatoes, bananas and prunes; and soya products.

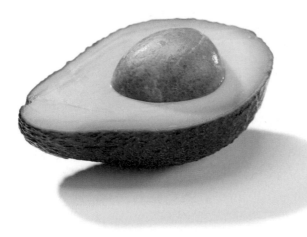

Cranberry

Tangy, ruby-red cranberries, often used for making sauce or jelly to accompany roast turkey, have long been considered nature's cure for urinary tract infections, which particularly afflict women of all ages. Modern science has confirmed the merit of this folk wisdom.

Vaccinium macrocarpon

Common uses

- Treats lower urinary tract infections (also called bladder infections or cystitis).
- May prevent recurrence of urinary tract infections.
- Helps to deodorise urine.

Forms

- Capsule
- Fresh or dried fruit
- Juice
- Liquid/tincture
- Powder
- Softgel
- Tablet
- Tea

CAUTION!

- Cranberry is not a substitute for antibiotics in treating an acute urinary tract infection. Consult your doctor if you don't feel better after 24 to 36 hours of using cranberry for a suspected infection.

- Consult your doctor at once if symptoms include fever, shivering, back pain or blood in the urine, which may be signs of a kidney infection requiring medical attention.

REMINDER: *If you have a medical condition, consult your doctor before taking supplements.*

What it is

The cranberry, a native American plant closely related to the blueberry, has been used for centuries in both healing and cooking. The name is a shortened form of craneberry – the flowers of the low-growing shrub were thought to resemble the heads of the cranes that frequented the bogs where it grew. The berries are now widely cultivated throughout the USA. As a traditional medicine, cranberries were crushed and used as poultices for treating wounds and tumours, and also as a remedy for scurvy, a gum and bleeding disorder caused by a deficiency of vitamin C. More recently, medical interest in the cranberry has focused on its role in preventing and treating urinary tract infections (UTIs), which are caused by E. *coli* and other types of bacteria.

What it does

In the 1920s it was discovered that people who consumed large amounts of cranberries produced a more acidic, 'purer' urine. The effect of the cranberries was to stimulate the creation of a powerful substance called hippuric acid, which proved to have a strong antibiotic effect on the urinary tract. It was realised that hippuric acid

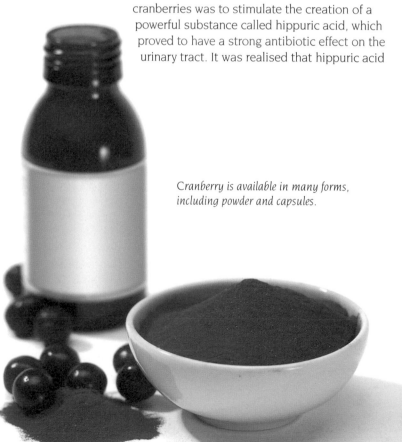

Cranberry is available in many forms, including powder and capsules.

discouraged and sometimes even eliminated infection-causing bacteria. However, more recent studies show that cranberry's main infection-fighting capabilities may be the result of a different property of the fruit. Cranberry appears to inhibit the adhesion of harmful microorganisms to certain cells lining the urinary tract. This makes the environment a less hospitable place for E. *coli* and other disease-causing bacteria to breed, and thereby reduces the likelihood of infection. It is believed that the substances responsible for this effect are a group of phytochemicals known as proanthocyanidins; they are present in cranberry juice but absent from grapefruit, orange, guava, mango and pineapple juices.

✿ **MAJOR BENEFITS:** Scientists have now confirmed the effectiveness of cranberry in preventing and treating urinary tract infections. Several studies have shown that daily consumption of cranberry, in either juice or capsule form, dramatically reduces the recurrence of such infections. Women are ten times more likely to develop these infections than men – 25% to 35% of women aged 20 to 40 have had at least one – but there is no reason why men should not benefit from cranberry as well.

Cranberry also appears to shorten the course of urinary tract illness, helping to alleviate pain, burning, itching and other symptoms. It is important to remember, though, that persistent urinary tract infections should be treated promptly with antibiotics to prevent complications. However, cranberry juice can be safely taken in combination with conventional drugs. It may even hasten the healing process.

✿ **ADDITIONAL BENEFITS:** Cranberry helps to deodorise urine, so it should be included in the diet of anyone suffering from the embarrassing odours associated with incontinence. In addition, cranberry's high vitamin C content makes it a natural vitamin supplement. Research also indicates that cranberry may help to reduce cholesterol levels in the blood. A recent US study showed that drinking three glasses of cranberry juice each day significantly raises HDL (good) cholesterol and increases antioxidant levels in the blood, and may reduce the risk of heart disease.

How to take it

⊘ **DOSAGE:** *To treat urinary tract infections*: Take about 800 mg of cranberry extract a day (two 400 mg capsules), or you can drink at least 500 ml of undiluted juice a day or take it in tincture form; follow the instructions on the packet. *To prevent recurrences*: The dose can be halved to 400 mg of cranberry extract a day, or at least 250 ml of juice.

◉ **GUIDELINES FOR USE:** Cranberry can be taken with or without food. Drinking plenty of water or other fluids in addition to cranberry and throughout the day should speed recovery. Cranberry has no known interactions with antibiotics or other medications, but by acidifying the urine it may lessen the effect of another herb, uva ursi (also known as bearberry), which is sometimes used for urinary tract infections.

Possible side effects

There are no known side effects from either short-term or long-term use of cranberry. It also appears to be safe for consumption by pregnant or breastfeeding women.

Dandelion

Taraxacum officinale

Known mostly as a persistent and prolific weed, dandelion is grown commercially in several countries. Its leaves and roots are a rich source of vitamins and minerals, and its active ingredients are particularly useful for treating digestive and liver problems.

Common uses

- *The root strengthens liver function: useful in cases of hepatitis (liver inflammation) and jaundice.*
- *The root aids digestion by stimulating the release of bile from the liver and gallbladder; may help to prevent gallstones.*
- *The root helps to reduce oestrogen dominance in endometriosis and breast pain.*
- *The leaves help to reduce fluid retention.*

Forms

- Capsule
- Dried or fresh herb/tea
- Liquid
- Tablet
- Tincture

CAUTION!

- Dandelion should not be used during acute attacks of gallstones. Seek medical advice.

REMINDER: If you have a medical condition, consult your doctor before taking supplements.

What it is

Dandelion grows wild throughout much of the world and is cultivated in parts of Europe for medicinal uses. Closely related to chicory, the plant can grow 30 cm high; its spatula-shaped leaves are shiny, hairless and deeply serrated. The solitary yellow flower blooms for much of the growing season, opening at daybreak and closing at dusk and in wet weather (some cultures have used dandelions to signal the approach of rain). After the flower matures, the plant forms a puffball of seeds that are dispersed by the wind (or by playful children). Supplements usually contain the root (which is tapered and sweet tasting) or leaves, though the whole plant and flowers are also valued for their healing properties.

What it does

Folk healers have long prescribed dandelion root for liver and digestive problems, and the leaf for fluid retention. Dandelion's various active ingredients enhance the performance of the liver and kidneys, so the plant is useful for a wide range of disorders where the elimination of toxins is indicated.

✚ **MAJOR BENEFITS:** Studies of dandelion's beneficial effects on the liver have shown that the herb increases the production and flow of bile (a digestive aid) from the liver and gallbladder, helping to treat such conditions as gallstones, jaundice and hepatitis. The leaf has a strong diuretic action which has been ascribed to its content of potassium, a natural diuretic. Dandelion is sometimes mixed with other nutritional supplements that reinforce liver function, including milk thistle, black radish, celandine, beet leaf, fringe tree bark, inositol, methionine and choline. Such combinations are usually sold as liver or lipotropic ('fat-metabolising') formulas in health-food shops.

Its capacity to improve liver function means that dandelion root (in combination with other liver-strengthening nutrients) may be effective for relieving the symptoms of oestrogen excess, such as endometriosis and cyclical breast pain. By enhancing the liver's ability to remove excess oestrogen from the body, it helps to restore a healthy balance of hormones in women who are afflicted with these disorders.

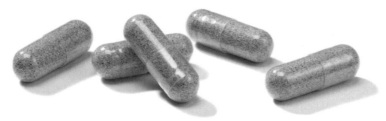

ADDITIONAL BENEFITS: Dandelion root acts as a mild laxative, so a tea made from it may provide a gentle remedy for constipation. The herb can also enhance the body's ability to absorb iron from either food or supplements, which makes it useful in some cases of anaemia. Early research suggests that dandelion may be of value in treating cancer: the Japanese have patented a freeze-dried extract of dandelion root to use against tumours, and the Chinese are using dandelion extracts to treat breast cancer (an approach supported by positive effects in animal studies). But additional studies need to be conducted in humans to determine the herb's true effectiveness against specific types of cancer.

Researchers have found that dandelion can lower blood sugar levels in animals, which suggests that it may have a role to play in the treatment of diabetes. The diuretic effect of the leaves makes them a useful treatment for water retention and bloating.

How to take it

DOSAGE: *To strengthen liver function in cases of hepatitis, gallstones and endometriosis:* Take 500 mg of a powdered solid dandelion-root extract twice a day. This amount may also be found in some lipotropic (liver) combinations. Or take 1 or 2 teaspoons of a liquid dandelion extract three times a day. *For constipation:* Drink one cup of dandelion root tea three times a day. *For anaemia:* Have 1 teaspoon of fresh dandelion juice or tincture each morning and evening with half a glass of water. *For water retention:* Drink one cup of dandelion leaf tree three times a day.

GUIDELINES FOR USE: Drink fresh dandelion juice or liquid extract with water. Capsules and tablets containing dandelion root extract can be consumed with or without food. No adverse effects have been reported in pregnant or breastfeeding women.

Possible side effects

Dandelion has no serious side effects. In large doses it may cause a skin rash, upset stomach or diarrhoea. Stop using it if this happens, and discuss the reaction with your doctor.

FACTS & TIPS

■ To make dandelion tea, use the dried chopped root or leaves of the dandelion. Pour a cup of very hot water over 1 or 2 teaspoons of the herb and allow it to steep for about 15 minutes. The tea can be blended with other herbs, such as liquorice, and sweetened with honey.

■ Dandelion is a health-giving and nutritious food or drink. Both the leaves and the flowers taste good when steamed like spinach, and the pleasantly bitter greens make a tangy addition to salads. Juice can be extracted from the leaves, and the root can be roasted and used to brew a drink that substitutes for coffee (without the stimulant effects).

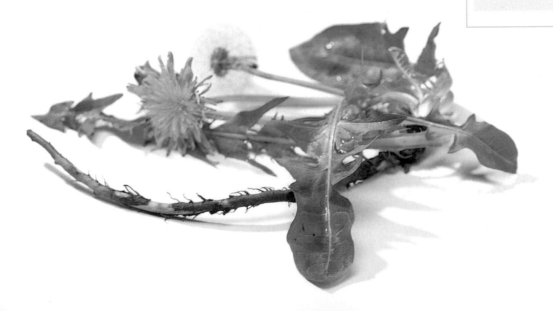

Dong quai

Angelica sinensis
A. acutiloba

An ingredient in many herbal 'women's supplements', dong quai, or Chinese angelica, is a traditional tonic used in Asia to aid the female reproductive system. Its popularity is second only to ginseng's in China and Japan, but Western experts continue to debate the effectiveness of this herb.

Common uses

- May *help to ease menstrual cramps.*

- May *reduce hot flushes associated with the menopause.*

Forms

- Capsule
- Dried herb/tea
- Liquid
- Softgel
- Tablet
- Tincture

What it is

Although dong quai grows wild in Asia, it is also widely cultivated for medicinal purposes in China (the species *Angelica sinensis*) and in Japan (*A. acutiloba*), where many women take it daily to maintain overall good health. The most widely available therapeutic form is derived from the root of *A. sinensis*, a plant with hollow stems that grows up to 2.5 m tall and has clusters of white flowers. When in bloom, angelica resembles Queen Anne's lace, its botanical relative. Other names for dong quai include dang gui, tang kuie and Chinese angelica.

What it does

Dong quai is believed to keep the uterus healthy and to regulate the menstrual cycle. It may also widen blood vessels and increase blood flow to various organs. Even among herbal experts, however, questions linger about its benefits. One reason dong quai has been difficult to assess is that it is often taken in combination with other herbs.

MAJOR BENEFITS: Traditionally, dong quai has been used in the treatment of menstrual and menopausal problems. The herb has been claimed to correct abnormal bleeding patterns, to alleviate symptoms of premenstrual syndrome (PMS), to ease menstrual cramps, to reduce menopausal hot flushes and to lessen the vaginal dryness associated with the menopause.

There are two theories about how dong quai helps to combat these ailments. Some herbalists believe that it contains plant oestrogens (phytoestrogens), which are weaker than oestrogens produced by the body but which form chemical bonds with oestrogen receptors in human cells. Phytoestrogens are effective in restoring hormonal equilibrium; for example, they can prevent hot flushes by compensating for the decline in oestrogen levels that occurs after the menopause.

Other researchers attribute the effectiveness of dong quai to its abundance of coumarins. This group of natural chemicals dilates blood

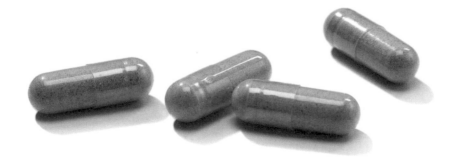

vessels, increases blood flow to the uterus and other organs, and stimulates the central nervous system. Coumarins also appear to reduce inflammation and muscle spasms, which may account for dong quai's ability to reduce the severity of menstrual cramps.

⊕ **ADDITIONAL BENEFITS:** Although dong quai is not typically used to lower blood pressure, it does have this effect because it dilates blood vessels, making it easier for the heart to pump blood through the body. This has the additional benefit of improving peripheral circulation.

How to take it

▨ **DOSAGE:** For PMS, *menstrual irregularities, menstrual cramps or hot flushes*: Take 600 mg of dong quai extract daily. The same effect can be obtained from taking 30 drops of tincture three times a day. In capsule, tablet or liquid form, extracts should be standardised to contain 0.8% to 1.1% ligustilide. Alternatively you can also use a preparation in which dong quai is combined with such menstrual-regulating herbs as chasteberry, liquorice and Siberian ginseng.

◉ **GUIDELINES FOR USE:** For symptoms of PMS, use dong quai on the days when you are not menstruating. If you also suffer from menstrual cramps, continue using dong quai until menstruation stops. For cramps without PMS, begin taking dong quai the day before your period is due. For hot flushes, use it daily. Continue the herb for two months before deciding whether it has achieved the desired effect.

Possible side effects

Dong quai may have a mild laxative effect and may cause heavy menstrual bleeding. Protect yourself from the sun when using dong quai, because its root contains compounds called psoralens that can make some people more sensitive to sunlight and cause severe sunburn.

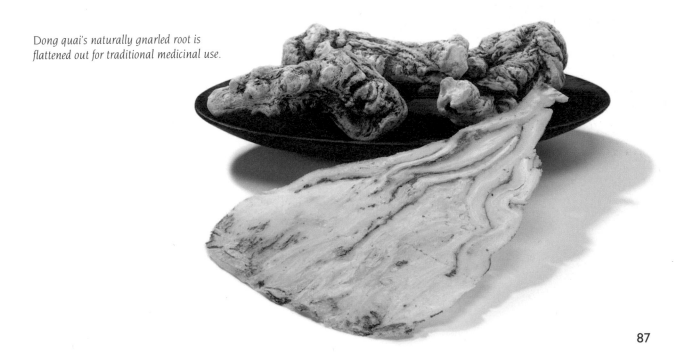

Dong quai's naturally gnarled root is flattened out for traditional medicinal use.

Echinacea

Echinacea angustifolia
E. pallida
E. purpurea

A plant native to the USA, long used by traditional healers and earlier generations of doctors, echinacea fell out of favour with the advent of modern antibiotics. But it is regaining popularity as a safe and powerful immune-system booster to fight colds, flu and other infections.

Common uses

- *Reduces the body's susceptibility to colds and flu.*
- *Limits the duration and severity of infections.*
- *Helps to fight thrush and recurrent respiratory, middle-ear and urinary tract infections.*
- *Speeds the healing of skin wounds and inflammations.*

Forms

- Capsule
- Dried herb/tea
- Liquid
- Lozenge
- Softgel
- Tablet
- Tincture

CAUTION!

- If you are taking antibiotics or other drugs for an infection, use echinacea in addition to, rather than as a replacement for, those medications.

- In progressive infections such as tuberculosis, echinacea may not be effective.

REMINDER: *If you have a medical condition, consult your doctor before taking supplements.*

What it is

Also known as the purple, or prairie, coneflower, echinacea (pronounced ek-in-NAY-sha) is a wild flower with daisy-like purple blossoms, native to the grasslands of the central USA. For centuries the Plains tribes used the plant to heal wounds and to counteract the toxins of snakebites. The herb also became a favourite among European pioneers in America and their doctors as an all-purpose fighter of infections. It is popularly grown in the UK as a garden plant.

Of the nine echinacea species, three (E*chinacea angustifolia*, E. *pallida* and E. *purpurea*) are used medicinally. They appear in literally hundreds of commercial preparations, which utilise different parts of the plant (flowers, leaves, stems or roots) and come in a variety of forms. Echinacea contains many active ingredients thought to strengthen the immune system, and in recent years it has become one of the most extensively used herbal remedies in the world.

What it does

A natural antibiotic and infection fighter, echinacea helps to kill bacteria, viruses, fungi and other disease-causing microbes. It acts by stimulating various immune-system cells that are key weapons against infection. In addition, the herb boosts the cells' production of an innate virus-fighting substance called interferon. These effects are relatively shortlived, however, so it is advisable to take the herb at frequent intervals – as often as every couple of hours during acute infections. Echinacea normalises immune response even in autoimmune conditions such as eczema (for which it is a traditional treatment).

PREVENTION: Echinacea can help to prevent the two most common viral ailments – colds and flu. It is most effective when taken at the first hint of illness. In one study of people who were susceptible to colds, those who used the herb for eight weeks were 35% less likely to come down with a cold than those given a placebo. Furthermore, they caught colds less often – 40 days elapsed between infections, versus 25 days for the placebo group. Studies confirm that echinacea is also useful if you are already suffering from the aches, pains, congestion or fever of colds or flu. Overall, symptoms are less severe and subside sooner.

ADDITIONAL BENEFITS: Echinacea may be of value for recurrent ailments, including thrush and infections of the urinary tract or middle ear. It is also sometimes used to treat streptococcal and staphylococcal infections, herpes infections (including genital herpes, cold sores and shingles), bronchitis and sinus infections. Autoimmune conditions which may respond to echinacea include lupus, multiple sclerosis, rheumatoid arthritis and similar disorders. The herb is also being studied as a treatment for chronic fatigue syndrome and AIDS, and it may prove effective against some types of cancer, particularly in patients whose immune systems have been depressed by radiotherapy or chemotherapy.

Echinacea can be applied to the skin. Its juice promotes the healing of all kinds of wounds, boils, abscesses, eczema, burns, mouth ulcers or cold sores, and bedsores. To treat a sore throat or tonsillitis, the tincture can be diluted and used as a gargle.

How to take it

☑ **DOSAGE:** Because echinacea comes in many different forms, check the product's label for the proper dosage; most tablets are of powdered root rather than extract. *For colds and flu*: A high dose is needed – up to 200 mg five a times a day. In one major study, patients with flu who were given 900 mg of echinacea a day did better than those who received either a lower dosage of 450 mg a day or a placebo. *For other infections*: The recommended dose is 200 mg three or four times a day. *For long-term use as a general immune booster*: To derive the most benefits, especially for those prone to chronic infections, alternate echinacea every three weeks with other herbs that enhance the immune system, including goldenseal, astragalus, pau d'arco and medicinal mushrooms. Echinacea teas, often blended with other herbs, are available as well.

◉ **GUIDELINES FOR USE:** It is sometimes advised that echinacea should be used for no longer than eight weeks, followed by a one-week interval before you resume taking it. However, medical herbalists often use the herb continuously for the treatment of autoimmune conditions such as eczema. You can take it with or without food.

Possible side effects

At recommended doses, echinacea has no known side effects, and no adverse reactions have been reported in pregnant or breastfeeding women. However, people who are allergic to flowers in the daisy family may also be allergic to this herb. If you develop a skin rash or have trouble breathing, consult your doctor straightaway.

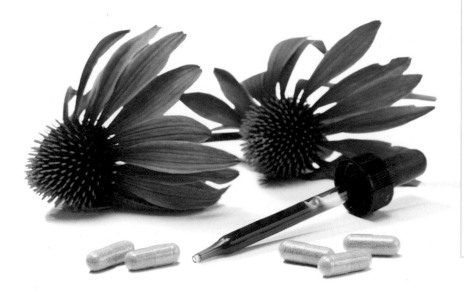

Evening primrose oil

Native Americans introduced the early settlers to the healing powers of the evening primrose. Modern research focuses on the therapeutic effect of the oil from its seeds, which contain a special fatty acid called gamma-linolenic acid (GLA).

Oenothera biennis

Common uses

- *Eases rheumatoid arthritis pain.*
- *Can minimise symptoms of diabetic nerve damage.*
- *Relieves eczema symptoms.*
- *Helps to treat premenstrual syndrome (PMS), endometriosis and menstrual cramps.*
- *Lessens inflammation of acne, rosacea and muscle strains.*

Forms

- Capsule
- Oil
- Softgel

CAUTION!

■ People with a history of epilepsy should consult their doctor before taking evening primrose oil. Some reports indicate that high doses may precipitate an attack.

REMINDER: If you have a medical condition, consult your doctor before taking supplements.

What it is

Called evening primrose because its light yellow flowers open at dusk, this wild flower is native to North America. The plant and its root have long been used for medicinal purposes – to treat bruises, haemorrhoids, sore throats and stomach aches – but the use of its seed oil, which contains gamma-linolenic acid (GLA), is relatively recent. GLA is an essential fatty acid that the body converts to hormone-like compounds called prostaglandins, which regulate a number of bodily functions.

Although the body can make GLA from other types of fat, there is no one food that has appreciable amounts of GLA. Evening primrose oil provides a concentrated source: 7% to 10% of its fatty acids are in the form of GLA. But there are other sources of GLA. Borage seed oil and blackcurrant seed oil contain larger quantities of GLA – 20% to 26% for borage; 14% to 19% for blackcurrant – than evening primrose oil, but they also have higher percentages of other fatty acids that may interfere with GLA absorption. Most of the studies investigating the effects of GLA have used evening primrose oil, and for this reason it is the preferred source of GLA. Borage oil may nevertheless be a good substitute: it is cheaper than evening primrose oil, and a lower dose is required to produce a therapeutic effect.

What it does

The body produces several types of prostaglandin; some promote inflammation, others control it. The GLA in evening primrose oil is directly converted to important anti-inflammatory prostaglandins, which accounts for most of the supplement's therapeutic effects. In addition, GLA is an important component of cell membranes.

◙ **PREVENTION:** The GLA in evening primrose oil appears to inhibit the development of diabetic neuropathy, the nerve damage that is a common complication of diabetes. In a study of people with a mild form of the condition, one year of treatment with evening primrose oil reduced numbness and tingling, loss of sensation and other symptoms of the disorder better than a placebo did, suggesting that evening primrose may be effective in reversing neuropathy.

✺ **ADDITIONAL BENEFITS:** One of the leading uses for evening primrose oil is to treat eczema, an allergic skin condition that may develop if the body has trouble converting fats from food into GLA. Some studies of people with eczema have indicated that taking evening primrose oil for three to four months can alleviate itching and reduce the need for topical steroid creams and drugs with unpleasant side effects.

Some studies have indicated that evening primrose oil can be effective in treating menstrual disorders such as PMS, menstrual cramps and endometriosis. In particular, the oil blocks the inflammatory prostaglandins that cause menstrual cramps. It also appears to ease the breast tenderness that some women experience just before their periods, and may play a role in reversing infertility in some women.

Rheumatoid arthritis is characterised by joint pain and swelling, and studies have found that these symptoms improve with supplements of evening primrose oil or another source of GLA. Conditions that involve inflammation, such as rosacea, acne and muscle strain, may also benefit from evening primrose oil.

How to take it

☑ **DOSAGE:** The recommended therapeutic dose for evening primrose oil is generally 1000 mg three times a day. This supplies 240 mg of GLA a day. To get an equivalent amount of GLA from other sources you would need to take 1000 mg of borage oil or 1500 mg of blackcurrant oil each day. Evening primrose oil or borage oil can also be applied topically to the fingers to ease the symptoms of Raynaud's disease.

◉ **GUIDELINES FOR USE:** Take evening primrose oil or other sources of GLA with meals to enhance absorption.

Possible side effects

In studies, about 2% of the participants using evening primrose oil experienced bloating or abdominal upset. However, consuming it with food may lessen this effect.

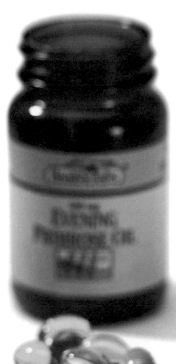

Although evening primrose oil is available as a liquid, it may be more convenient to take it in softgel form.

RECENT FINDINGS

In a study of 60 people with eczema, GLA – the essential fatty acid in evening primrose oil – was found to be superior to a placebo in reducing the itching and oozing of the condition. Those in the GLA group took 274 mg twice a day (an amount found in approximately seven 1000 mg evening primrose capsules) for 12 weeks. Examinations by a dermatologist every four weeks confirmed the gradual improvement of symptoms reported by these patients.

A study from the University of Massachusetts Medical Center showed that very high doses of GLA in the form of borage oil (2.4 grams of GLA a day) reduced damage to joint tissue in people with rheumatoid arthritis. As a result they had less joint pain and swelling.

Feverfew

Tanacetum parthenium

In the Middle Ages feverfew was believed to purify the air and prevent malaria and other life-threatening diseases. It has since been relied on to treat headaches, stomach problems and menstrual irregularities. Most recently the herb has been hailed as a migraine preventative.

Common uses

■ *Helps to prevent or reduce the intensity of migraines.*

■ *May ease menstrual complaints.*

Forms

■ Capsule
■ Dried herb/tea
■ Tablet

CAUTION!

■ Pregnant women should avoid feverfew because it may cause contractions of the uterus. Women who are breastfeeding should not use the herb.

■ Feverfew may inhibit blood clotting, so consult your doctor before using it if you are taking anticoagulant drugs.

REMINDER: If you have a medical condition, consult your doctor before taking supplements.

What it is

Feverfew – also known as featherfew or febrifuge – is a member of the botanical family that includes daisies and sunflowers. With its bright yellow-and-white blossoms and feathery yellow-green leaves, the herb resembles chamomile and is often mistaken for it. The leaves are used medicinally, and although the flowers have no health benefits they emit a strong aroma. The odour of feverfew is apparently offensive to insects, so if you plant the herb in your garden it will act as a natural repellent.

What it does

The active compound in feverfew, called parthenolide, seems to block substances in the body that widen and constrict blood vessels and cause inflammation.

PREVENTION: Although the exact cause of migraines is unknown, some doctors think that these headaches occur when blood vessels in the head constrict and then rapidly dilate. Such a dramatic change can trigger the release of chemicals that cause pain and inflammation which are stored in platelets (the small blood cells involved in blood clotting). Researchers speculate that feverfew prevents the sudden dilation of blood vessels, and thereby inhibits the release of those chemicals. Although this action makes feverfew a good migraine preventative, the herb cannot relieve a migraine once it occurs.

Word of mouth among people with chronic migraines led to wide-

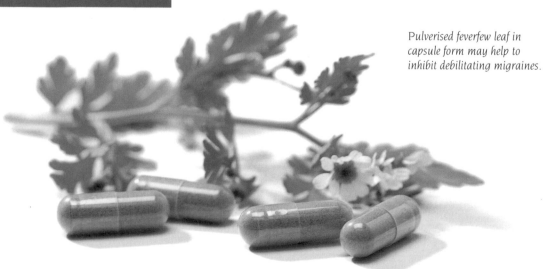

Pulverised feverfew leaf in capsule form may help to inhibit debilitating migraines.

spread use of feverfew beginning in the 1970s. To determine the herb's effectiveness British researchers recruited migraine sufferers who had already been using feverfew regularly. The researchers divided the subjects into two groups: one group continued to take feverfew; the other was given a placebo. Those taking the placebo pills soon experienced more frequent and more intense headaches, but those in the feverfew group had no increase in migraine occurrences. Another study showed that feverfew reduced the number of migraines by 24%, and that, even when the headaches did occur, they were much less severe. The results of these and other studies have led health authorities in Canada and other countries to approve the use of feverfew for migraine prevention.

✴ **ADDITIONAL BENEFITS:** Feverfew has long been used to treat menstrual complaints, in particular menstrual cramps, which result from an excess of prostaglandins produced by the lining of the uterus. Prostaglandins are hormone-like substances that can cause pain and inflammation. Feverfew inhibits the production of them.

The anti-inflammatory action of the herb also encouraged its use as a treatment for the inflamed, sore joints that occur in rheumatoid arthritis. However, a study of arthritis patients found no additional benefit from taking feverfew in conjunction with medications commonly prescribed for the condition. No studies have been done to establish how the herb might work when taken on its own, or in combination with other herbal treatments for rheumatoid arthritis.

How to take it

🗹 **DOSAGE:** For migraines, a dose of 250 mg a day of a feverfew product standardised to contain at least 0.4% parthenolide is typical.

◉ **GUIDELINES FOR USE:** The experience of the migraine sufferers in the British study cited above underlines the importance of taking feverfew daily over a long period. If you stop taking the herb after a short time, the headaches may resume.

Possible side effects

Few side effects have been noted, even when feverfew is used long term. There have been reports of sores and inflammation of the mucous membranes of the mouth, but this reaction seems to be limited to people who chew the fresh leaves (a common practice before feverfew supplements became available). Some people experience stomach upsets from both the fresh leaves and supplements. Skin contact with the plant can cause a rash; anyone who develops a rash after touching feverfew should not use the product internally.

CASE HISTORY
A migraine preventative

For a while Nick L. put all his faith in the new migraine drugs because of their amazing ability to stop the dizzying pain of his headaches. But what he really wanted was something that could prevent a migraine from starting. His doctor suggested other drugs, but their side effects were troublesome. 'The beta-blockers saw off my migraines,' Nick remembers, 'but my sex life vanished too.' He tried several types, but the result was always the same.

During a trip to Manchester he saw a shop sign: 'Migraine Sufferers – We have feverfew in stock.' Although he was sceptical of herbal therapies he bought a bottle, which sat unopened in his medicine chest for six months.

Then he read an article affirming the safety and effectiveness of feverfew. He decided to give it a try and took two capsules with his daily vitamin supplement. 'From that point on it was a migraine-free year,' he says, 'my first since childhood.'

Fibre

Hippocrates praised wholemeal bread 'for its salutary effect upon the bowel' but only in the past 30 years has the health significance of fibre been fully recognised. The shift began after two British doctors working in Africa realised that a high-fibre diet could counteract certain Western diseases.

Common uses

- *Promotes good digestion and healthy bowels.*
- *Lowers blood cholesterol.*
- *Can relieve constipation, diarrhoea, irritable bowel syndrome and haemorrhoid pain.*
- *Stabilises blood glucose levels.*
- *Can facilitate weight loss.*
- *May help to prevent gallstones.*

Forms
- Bran-rich cereals
- Granules
- Powder

CAUTION!

■ High intakes of fibre can reduce the effectiveness of some drugs, including oral contraceptives and the anti-cholesterol drug lovastatin.

■ Swallowing fibre tablets or capsules can be dangerous. When they become hydrated they can expand and create an obstruction in the throat or further down the intestine.

■ If you have a rare allergic reaction to psyllium, such as a rash or breathing difficulties, seek immediate medical help.

REMINDER: If you have a medical condition, consult your doctor before taking supplements.

What it is

Fibre provides almost no nutritional value, but both soluble fibre and insoluble fibre play an important role in maintaining good health. Soluble fibre – found in fruit, vegetables, oats, nuts and pulses – is made up of gums and other constituents of plant cells and plant cell walls that swell in water. It is broken down into simpler components by the action of bacteria in the large intestine. Psyllium seeds are a commonly used source of soluble fibre. Insoluble fibre – found in cereals and grains – consists mainly of the cellulosic constituents of plant cell walls, which bind with water but do not swell appreciably. It passes undigested through the intestines because it cannot be absorbed or broken down by the body's own enzymes.

What it does

Fibre absorbs excess water from the intestine to make larger, softer stools. It also binds to cholesterol which is then expelled, and so is useful for reducing cholesterol levels in the bloodstream. Insoluble fibre, such as cellulose, assists the function of the gut as well as binding with cancer-causing substances and toxins and aiding their excretion. Although soluble fibre cannot be digested, it is fermented by friendly bacteria in the gut, producing fatty acids that are important for nourishing the cells of the intestine.

❂ **MAJOR BENEFITS:** A shortage of fibre in the diet has been linked to a number of degenerative, chronic diseases including heart disease, diverticular disorders and diabetes. Although a healthy diet should contain 18 grams of fibre a day, most people in the UK have an average intake of only 12 grams. Eating just one slice of wholemeal bread provides an extra 5 grams of fibre.

A fibre-rich diet can help to prevent constipation and haemorrhoids by increasing the water content of stools, making it easier for them to be passed out of the body. A diet high in soluble fibre can help to reduce the body's need for insulin and assist diabetics by slowing down the absorption of blood sugar. Soluble fibre also reduces the removal of cholesterol from the gut into the bloodstream, leading to lower levels of blood cholesterol. In one study people with high levels of cholesterol were given a minimum of 10 grams of psyllium daily for six weeks or longer. They showed a significantly higher reduction (between 6 and 20%) of LDL ('bad') cholesterol than those on a low-fat diet.

Being a rich source of soluble fibre, psyllium helps to regulate bowel function in people suffering from diarrhoea, as well as constipation. Hence it may be helpful to those with irritable bowel syndrome, where the symptoms can alternate between these extremes.

✤ **ADDITIONAL BENEFITS:** In some studies, fibre has been shown to help weight loss by filling the stomach with absorbed water and decreasing appetite as well as delaying the moment when food leaves the stomach. High-fibre foods, especially linseed, contain plant oestrogens known as lignans which have been linked to a reduced risk of cancer, and of breast cancer in particular. Psyllium may have a role to play in preventing gallstones; a Mexican study of obese patients with an increased risk of gallstones found that psyllium helped to avert the condition.

How to take it

✐ **DOSAGE:** Start with a small dose of between 1 and 2 grams with each meal. This can be increased gradually to between 1 and 3 tablespoons (up to 10 grams) of powder two or three times a day with 250 ml of juice or water. Never take more than 30 grams in one day.

◉ **GUIDELINES FOR USE:** If you are taking fibre supplements ensure that you also have a high intake of liquids because fibre absorbs large quantities of water. After taking fibre supplements it it advisable to wait two hours before taking any medication because the supplements may delay their absorption. Pregnant women should seek medical advice before taking fibre supplements.

Possible side effects

A sudden high intake of fibre may create bloating and abdominal pain. Beans and pulses in particular can cause wind and flatulence. Some people develop gastric irritation when they consume fibre, especially wheat.

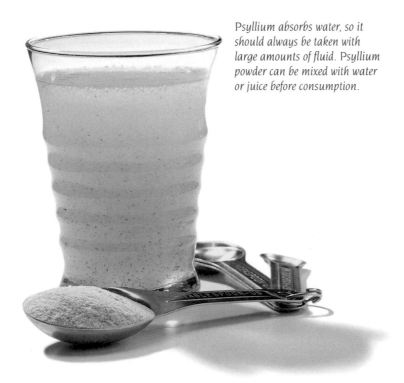

Psyllium absorbs water, so it should always be taken with large amounts of fluid. Psyllium powder can be mixed with water or juice before consumption.

Fish oils

Scientists noticed a curiously low incidence of heart disease among Greenland's Inuits despite their high-fat diet. The reason? They were eating fish rich in omega-3 fatty acids. Later studies confirmed the cardio-protective effect of fish oils while uncovering other benefits as well.

Common uses

- *Help to prevent cardiovascular disease; useful for other circulatory conditions, including lowering levels of triglycerides (blood fats).*
- *Block disease-related inflammatory responses in the body.*
- *May lower blood pressure.*

Forms

- Capsule
- Liquid
- Powder
- Softgel

What they are

The fat in fish contains a class of polyunsaturated fatty acid called omega-3s. These fatty acids differ from the polyunsaturated fatty acids found in vegetable oils, called omega-6s, and have different effects on the body. (Fish do not manufacture such fats but obtain them from the plankton they eat; the colder the water, the more omega-3s the plankton contains.) The two most potent forms of omega-3s – eicosapentaenoic acid (EPA) and docosahexanoic acid (DHA) – are found in abundance in cold-water fish such as salmon, trout, mackerel and tuna. The sources of a third type of omega-3, alpha-linolenic acid (ALA), are certain vegetable oils (such as flaxseed oil) and leafy greens (such as purslane). However, ALA may not be as effective as EPA and DHA; this is still being researched.

What they do

Omega-3s play a key role in a range of vital body processes, from regulating blood pressure and blood clotting to boosting immunity. They may be useful for preventing or treating many diseases and disorders.

PREVENTION: Fish oils appear to reduce the risk of heart disease. They do this in several ways. Most importantly, the presence of omega-3s makes platelets in the blood less likely to clump together and form the clots that lead to heart attacks. Next, omega-3s can reduce triglycerides (blood fats carried with cholesterol) and may lower blood pressure. In addition, recent research has shown that omega-3s strengthen the heart's electrical system, preventing heart-rhythm abnormalities. However, the strongest evidence for the cardiovascular benefits of fish oils comes from studies in which the participants ate fish rather than taking fish oil supplements.

Within the artery walls, omega-3s inhibit inflammation, which is a factor in plaque build-up. Therapeutic doses of fish oils are one of the few successful ways to prevent the reblockage of arteries that often occurs after angioplasty (a procedure in which a small balloon is guided through an artery to a blockage and is inflated to compress plaque, widen the vessels and improve blood flow to the heart). This effect on blood vessels makes fish oils helpful for Raynaud's disease as well.

ADDITIONAL BENEFITS: Omega-3s are also effective general anti-inflammatories, useful for joint problems, lupus and psoriasis. Studies indicate that people with rheumatoid arthritis experience less joint swelling and stiffness, and may even be able to manage on lower doses of anti-inflammatory drugs, when they take fish oil supplements. In a study of people with Crohn's disease (a painful type of inflammatory bowel disease), 69% of those taking enteric-coated fish oil supplements (about 3 grams of fish oils a day) experienced no symptoms of their illness, compared with just 28% of those receiving a placebo. Fish oils may also help to ease menstrual cramps. In addition, omega-3s may play a role in mental health: some nutritionists believe that there is a correlation between the increasing incidence of depression in Australia and the declining consumption of fish, and preliminary studies suggest that omega-3 fatty acids may reduce the severity of schizophrenia by about 25%, and also help to correct dyslexia in children.

How to take them

⊘ **DOSAGE:** *For heart disease, Raynaud's disease, lupus and psoriasis*: Take 3000 mg of fish oils a day. *For rheumatoid arthritis*: Take 6000 mg a day. *For inflammatory bowel disease*: Take 5000 mg a day.

◉ **GUIDELINES FOR USE:** Fish oil supplements are not necessary for heart disease prevention or treatment if you eat oily fish at least twice a week. However, supplements are recommended for rheumatoid arthritis and other inflammatory conditions. Take capsules with meals. Supplements may be easier to tolerate if you take them in divided doses: for example, 1000 mg three times a day, instead of 3000 mg at one time. When taking supplementary fish oil, ensure that you get extra antioxidant protection by eating plenty of fruit and vegetables or taking extra vitamin E.

Possible side effects

Fish oil capsules may cause belching, flatulence, bloating, nausea and diarrhoea. Very high doses may result in a slightly fishy body odour. There is some concern that high doses can lead to internal bleeding, but a study of people with heart disease who took 8000 mg of fish oil supplements in addition to aspirin (an anticoagulant) found no increase in the incidence of internal bleeding. Some studies have found that high doses of fish oils worsen blood sugar control in people with diabetes; others have shown no effect. To be safe, diabetics should not take more than 2000 mg of fish oil supplements a day except on medical advice.

Individuals with high levels of triglycerides should be careful if they also have high LDL ('bad') cholesterol: therapeutic doses of fish oils can increase LDL. Garlic supplements may be the remedy. One study found that garlic reversed the fish oils' LDL-raising effect. For rheumatoid arthritis and other inflammatory conditions, eating fish is probably not sufficient, and fish-oil supplements are recommended.

BUYING GUIDE

■ If you find that you cannot tolerate a particular brand of fish oil supplements, try a different one. The side effects that can be experienced vary from brand to brand.

■ Don't try to save money by buying fish oil supplements in bulk because they can become rancid in a very short amount of time.

■ Cod-liver oil preparations are a good source of omega-3s, but they contain vitamin A, so pregnant women should use an alternative source of fish oil.

RECENT FINDINGS

A study involving 120 children in County Durham found that supplements of omega-3s can help to improve the reading and writing abilities and concentration of children with learning difficulties.

Fish oils may help to prevent breast cancer. A French study indicated that women with a high intake of omega-3s had a significantly reduced risk of breast cancer. Further work suggested that omega-3s may increase the production of one of the genes that is known to suppress breast cancer.

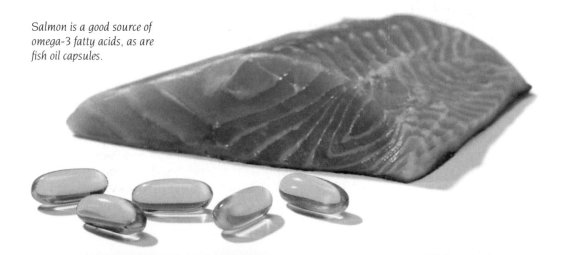

Salmon is a good source of omega-3 fatty acids, as are fish oil capsules.

5-HTP

People suffering from depression, insomnia, migraines or obesity have a new supplement to consider: 5-HTP. Unlike the amino acid tryptophan, which was recalled owing to safety concerns, 5-HTP appears to be safe – and it may be even more effective than its close chemical cousin.

Common uses

- *Relieves depression.*
- *Helps to overcome insomnia.*
- *Aids in weight control.*
- *Treats migraines.*
- *May ease pain of fibromyalgia.*

Forms

- Capsule
- Tablet

CAUTION!

■ Consult your doctor if you are taking antidepressants. The combination of 5-HTP with an antidepressant can cause anxiety, confusion, rapid heart rate, sweating, diarrhoea or other adverse reactions.

■ Do not drive or do hazardous work until you determine how 5-HTP affects you. It can cause drowsiness in some people.

■ 5-HTP may be toxic in high doses, cause liver problems and aggravate asthma. Avoid if pregnant or planning a pregnancy.

REMINDER: If you have a medical or psychiatric condition, consult your doctor before taking supplements.

What it is

The nutrient 5-HTP, short for 5-hydroxytryptophan, is a derivative of the amino acid tryptophan which is found in such high-protein foods as beef, chicken, fish and dairy products. The body makes 5-HTP from the tryptophan present in our diets. Tryptophan is also found in the seeds of an African plant called *Griffonia simplicifolia*, which is the source of the 5-HTP supplements sold in health-food shops.

The focus of much recent interest, 5-HTP acts on the brain, helping to elevate mood, promote sleep, aid weight loss and relieve migraines, among other uses. Unlike many other supplements (and drugs) that contain substances with molecules too large to pass from the bloodstream into the brain, 5-HTP is small enough to enter the brain. Once there it is converted into a vital nervous-system chemical, or neurotransmitter, called serotonin. Although it affects many parts of the body, serotonin's most important actions take place in the brain, where it influences everything from mood to appetite to sleep.

Its close relationship with the amino acid tryptophan makes 5-HTP somewhat controversial. In 1989 the sale of L-tryptophan and other tryptophan supplements was banned in the UK and other countries after reports of a fatal illness among those taking it. The illness was later found to be caused by contamination of the supplement during the manufacturing process, not by the tryptophan itself. In 1994 5-HTP began to be sold in the USA as an over-the-counter alternative to tryptophan, and it is now available in the UK. 5-HTP is not made in the same way as tryptophan, and so it avoids the contamination problems of its predecessor. Though safety concerns have been raised, many researchers believe it is safe and effective.

What it does

In recent years 5-HTP has been studied as a treatment for such mood disorders as depression, anxiety and panic attacks because it can boost levels of serotonin in the brain. Scientists are also investigating whether

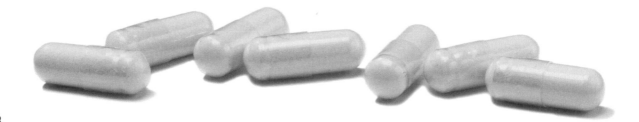

it may work for an array of additional complaints linked to low serotonin levels, including migraines, fibromyalgia, obesity, eating disorders, PMS and even violent behaviour. Although additional research is needed to determine its effectiveness against many of these conditions, preliminary studies suggest it may be very beneficial for some.

✪ **MAJOR BENEFITS:** For decades doctors have been prescribing 5-HTP for the treatment of depression and insomnia. In some cases it may be more effective, lift depression more quickly and produce fewer side effects than standard antidepressant drugs. In one study, more than half the patients with long-term depression who were resistant to all other antidepressants felt better after taking 5-HTP. The nutrient has also been shown to promote sleep, and to improve the quality of sleep, by increasing the amount of time people spend in two key sleep stages: deep sleep and REM sleep (the dreaming stage). After dreaming for longer, those on 5-HTP awaken feeling more rested and refreshed.

✪ **ADDITIONAL BENEFITS:** Individuals trying to lose weight or suffering from migraines may benefit from 5-HTP. In one study, overweight women who took the supplement ate fewer calories, lost more weight and were more likely to feel full while on a diet than those given a placebo. It may also be useful in relieving severe headaches, including migraines, reducing not only their frequency but also their intensity and duration.

The supplement may also work to increase pain tolerance in those with fibromyalgia, a chronic condition marked by aches and fatigue, in part by helping to relieve any underlying depression. In an Italian study of 200 fibromyalgia sufferers, those who took 5-HTP with conventional antidepressants had less pain than those taking either 5-HTP or the drugs alone. If you are taking antidepressants, don't try 5-HTP without consulting your doctor first: adverse reactions can occur.

How to take it

☑ **DOSAGE:** The recommended dose for depression and most other ailments is 50 to 100 mg three times a day. *For migraines*: Take up to 100 mg three times a day if necessary. *For insomnia*: Take a single 100 mg dose half an hour before bedtime. When using 5-HTP it is advisable to start with a low dose (such as 50 mg) and gradually increase it if needed.

◈ **GUIDELINES FOR USE:** To ensure rapid absorption, take 5-HTP on an empty stomach. For weight control, take the supplement 30 minutes before meals. Don't use 5-HTP for more than three months except on medical advice. Some doctors combine it with the mood-enhancing herb St John's wort, but you should not take it with that herb or with conventional antidepressants without checking with your doctor first.

Possible side effects

The generally mild side effects include nausea, constipation, flatulence, drowsiness and a reduced sex drive. Nausea usually diminishes within a few days.

Flaxseed oil

A rich source of healing oil, flaxseed (or linseed) has been cultivated for more than 7000 years. The oil is used to prevent and treat heart disease and to relieve a variety of inflammatory disorders and hormone-related problems, including infertility.

Linum usitatissimum

Common uses

- Helps to protect against heart disease.
- Promotes healthy skin, hair and nails.
- May reduce inflammation.
- May be useful for infertility, impotence, menstrual cramps and endometriosis.
- May help to alleviate nerve disorders.
- Relieves constipation and diverticular disorders.

Forms
- Capsule
- Oil
- Powder
- Softgel

CAUTION!

■ Some people are allergic to flaxseed. If you experience difficulty breathing after taking the supplement, seek immediate medical attention.

■ Always take ground flaxseed with plenty of water (a large glass per tablespoon) to prevent it from swelling up and blocking your throat or digestive tract.

REMINDER: *If you have a medical condition, consult your doctor before taking supplements.*

What it is

The flax plant was first used as a fibre for weaving – and it remains the source of natural linen fabric. However, it has also been renowned for centuries for its medicinal properties. The slender annual grows up to a metre in height and bears blue flowers from February to September. Both the oil from the seeds (also known as linseeds) and the seeds themselves are used for therapeutic purposes.

What it does

Flaxseeds are a source of essential fatty acids (EFAs) – fats and oils critical for health which the body cannot make on its own. One EFA found in flaxseeds, alpha-linolenic acid, is known as an omega-3 fatty acid; it is also found in many other seed oils, including rape, soya, blackcurrant and walnut. However, alpha-linolenic acid is not as potent as the omega-3 fatty acids found in fish oils, which have been acclaimed in recent years for protecting against heart disease and for treating many other ailments.

   Flaxseeds also contain omega-6 fatty acids (in the form of linolenic acid), the same healthy fats that are present in many vegetable oils. In addition, flaxseeds provide substances called lignans which appear to have beneficial effects on various hormones and may help to fight cancer, bacteria, viruses and fungi. Weight for weight, flaxseeds contain up to 800 times the lignans found in most other foods.

✪ **MAJOR BENEFITS:** EFAs work throughout the body to protect cell membranes – the outer coverings that are gatekeepers for all cells,

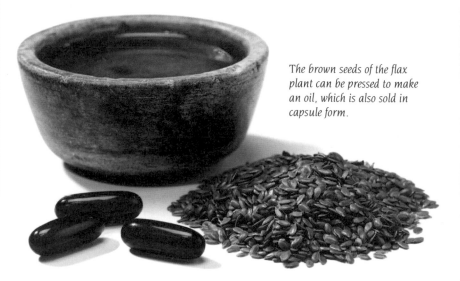

The brown seeds of the flax plant can be pressed to make an oil, which is also sold in capsule form.

admitting healthy nutrients and barring damaging substances. That function explains why flaxseed oil may have such far-reaching effects.

Flaxseed oil works to lower cholesterol, and so protects against heart disease. It may also prove beneficial against angina and high blood pressure. A recent five-year study at Simmons College in Boston, Massachusetts, indicated that it might be useful in preventing second heart attacks. As a digestive aid it can prevent or even dissolve gallstones, and it also promotes healthy hair and nails. In addition it may facilitate the transmission of nerve impulses, which makes it potentially useful for numbness and tingling as well as for chronic brain and nerve ailments such as Alzheimer's disease, or nerve damage from diabetes. It may help to fight fatigue, but more research is needed.

Crushed flaxseeds are an excellent natural source of fibre. They add bulk to stools, and their oil lubricates the stools, making flaxseeds useful for the relief of constipation and diverticular complaints.

✲ **ADDITIONAL BENEFITS:** Flaxseeds contain plant-based oestrogens, called phytoestrogens, which mimic the female sex hormone oestrogen, so the oil can have beneficial effects on the menstrual cycle, balancing the ratio of oestrogen to progesterone. It helps to improve uterine function and can therefore treat fertility problems. It may help to reduce menopausal symptoms such as hot flushes. Also, possibly because of anti-inflammatory action, flaxseed oil can reduce menstrual cramps or the pain of fibrocystic breasts.

The oil can promote well-being in men as well: it has shown some promise in treating male infertility and prostate problems. In some studies flaxseeds were also found to possess antibacterial, antifungal and antiviral properties, which may partly explain why flaxseed oil is effective against ailments such as cold sores and shingles.

How to take it

⊘ **DOSAGE:** Liquid flaxseed oil is the easiest way to take a therapeutic amount, which ranges from 1 teaspoon to 1 tablespoon once or twice a day. For the equivalent of 1 tablespoon of the oil in capsule form you need to swallow about 14 capsules, each containing 1000 mg of oil. For flaxseed fibre, mix 1 or 2 tablespoons of ground flaxseeds with a glass of water and drink it up to three times a day; the treatment may take a day or so to be effective.

◐ **GUIDELINES FOR USE:** Take flaxseed oil with food, which enhances absorption by the body. You can also mix it with juice, yoghurt, cottage cheese or other foods and drinks.

Possible side effects

Flaxseed oil appears to be very safe. Those using the ground seeds may experience some flatulence initially, but this should soon disappear.

Folic acid

Folic acid is necessary for every function in the body that requires cell multiplication. It is especially important in foetal development, and helps to produce key chemicals for the brain and nervous system. Yet nine out of ten adults consume too little of this vital nutrient.

Common uses

- *Protects against birth defects.*
- *Reduces heart disease and stroke risk.*
- *Lowers risk for several cancers.*
- *Can alleviate depression, especially in elderly people.*

Forms

- Capsule
- Liquid
- Powder
- Tablet

CAUTION!

Folic acid supplements may mask a type of anaemia caused by a vitamin B_{12} deficiency. Unchecked, this anaemia can cause irreversible nerve damage and dementia. If you take folic acid supplements, be sure to take extra vitamin B_{12} as well.

REMINDER: If you have a medical or psychiatric condition, consult your doctor before taking supplements.

What it is

A water-soluble B vitamin, also called folacin or folate, folic acid was identified in the 1940s, when it was extracted from spinach. The body cannot store it for very long, so you need to replenish your supply daily. Cooking, or even long storage, can destroy up to half the folic acid in foods, so supplements may be the best way to ensure that your body is getting enough.

What it does

Folic acid is utilised in the body thousands of times a day to make blood cells, heal wounds, build muscle – and in every other process that requires cell division. Folic acid is critical to DNA and RNA formation and ensures that cells duplicate normally.

PREVENTION: Adequate folic acid at conception and for the first three months of pregnancy greatly reduces the risk of serious birth defects, including spina bifida and cleft palate, so women should take folic acid if they are trying to conceive as well as during pregnancy. The B vitamin appears to regulate the body's production and use of homocysteine, an amino acid-like substance that at high levels may damage the lining of blood vessels, making them more susceptible to plaque build-up. This makes folic acid an important weapon against heart disease. It may also ward off cancers, especially those of the lungs, cervix, colon and rectum.

ADDITIONAL BENEFITS: People who are depressed often suffer from a deficiency of folic acid. Supplements of the B vitamin may relieve depression by reducing homocysteine, high levels of which are believed to contribute to the condition. Studies also show that taking folic acid improves the effectiveness of antidepressants in people with low folic

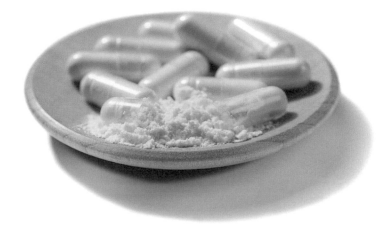

acid levels. Folic acid supplements have been useful in treating gout and irritable bowel syndrome as well. High homocysteine levels are thought to be a factor in the development of osteoporosis, so folic acid may even help to keep bones strong.

How much you need

The current recommended target for folic acid is 200 mcg a day for adults, but women who are pregnant or likely to become pregnant are advised to take 400 mcg daily, in addition to the recommended dietary target of 200 mcg daily. Supplements are important for older people, who may not get enough of the vitamin in food.

⊟ **IF YOU GET TOO LITTLE:** Though relatively rare, a severe folic acid deficiency can cause a form of anaemia (megaloblastic anaemia), a sore red tongue, chronic diarrhoea and poor growth (in children). Alcoholics and people who are on certain medications (for cancer or epilepsy) or who have malabsorption diseases (Crohn's, coeliac, sprue) are susceptible to severe deficiency. Much more common is a low level of folic acid, which causes no symptoms but raises the risk of heart disease or birth defects.

⊞ **IF YOU GET TOO MUCH:** Very large doses – 5000 to 10,000 mcg – offer no benefit and may be dangerous for people with hormone-related cancers, such as those of the breast or prostate. High doses may also cause seizures in those with epilepsy. The advised upper safe limit for folic acid in the UK is 1000 mcg for adults.

How to take it

▨ **DOSAGE:** *For overall good health and the prevention of heart disease*: Take a dose of 200 mcg of folic acid a day. *For pregnant women and women who might become pregnant*: Take 400 mcg a day. (Adequate folic acid stores are important because the vitamin plays a role in a baby's development from conception.) *For people with depression*: Take 400 mcg a day, as part of a vitamin B-complex supplement.

◉ **GUIDELINES FOR USE:** Folic acid can be taken at any time of the day, with or without food. When taking individual folic acid supplements for any reason, combine it with an additional 1000 mcg of vitamin B_{12} to prevent a B_{12} deficiency.

Other sources

Excellent food sources of folic acid include green vegetables, beans, whole grains and orange juice. Some refined grain products are now fortified with folic acid.

RECENT FINDINGS

For prevention of disease, the best way to obtain enough folic acid may be through supplements. In a small study, people taking 400 mcg of folic acid a day in pills or in specially fortified foods increased their folic acid level. But those who just ate foods naturally rich in folic acid showed no increase. Scientists speculate that the folic acid found naturally in foods may not be absorbed well enough to have a therapeutic effect.

——⌇⌇——

A preliminary study by Oxford University hints that folic acid may play a role in preventing Alzheimer's disease. People with the disease tended to have lower blood levels of folic acid and vitamin B_{12} than healthy people of the same age.

DID YOU KNOW?

To get the daily 200 mcg of folic acid recommended for good health, you'd need to eat 12 spears of asparagus a day.

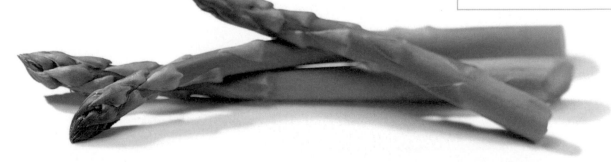

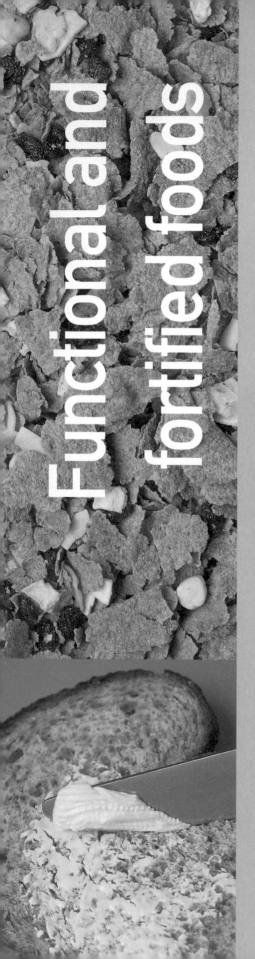

Functional and fortified foods

Enhanced foods – such as bioyoghurts and cereals with added nutrients – are growing in popularity. Some can boost vitamin and mineral levels; others show promise in preventing or treating ailments, but more research is needed to prove their worth. The big advantage of these 'functional' or 'fortified' foods lies in the amounts of 'macronutrients', such as calcium and omega-3 fatty acids, that they contain – much more than tablets.

■ Functional foods are foods meant to offer a specific health benefit over and above the level of nutrients found in their conventional counterparts.

■ Fortified foods have had extra vitamins and/or minerals added so that one portion of the food will provide a substantial percentage of the recommended daily intake of that nutrient.

■ Many fortified foods can be considered functional foods – for example, bread fortified with folic acid, which may help to prevent heart disease and protect women from having babies with neural-tube defects such as spina bifida.

■ Examples of functional foods include bioyoghurts containing specially selected bacteria, and spreads with added fish oils or cholesterol-lowering agents.

CAN FOODS ACT AS MEDICINES?

The purpose of 'enhancing' foods is to aid in the prevention of certain diseases, or in the treatment of certain conditions. For example, 'friendly' bacteria are used to help to relieve bowel problems, and plant sterols to reduce cholesterol levels. However, functional foods are categorised as foods rather than medicines, so under food labelling law no claims that they 'prevent' or 'cure' specific diseases can be made for them.

REGULAR INTAKE

To be effective, functional foods must be taken regularly, just like dietary supplements. Some manufacturers are producing functional foods with the same nutritional objective but in different formats, in order to provide variety in the diet.

PROBIOTICS AND PREBIOTICS

The gut contains billions of bacteria. These play a vital role in the normal functioning of the digestive system, the lowering of blood cholesterol levels, the promotion of the immune response, protection from colon cancer, and the synthesis of certain vitamins. They also prevent colonisation of the gut by harmful bacteria that may cause food poisoning.

Stress, antibiotics, certain drugs and female hormones can cause a proliferation of disease-causing bacteria at the expense of numbers of the bacteria that keep us healthy. However, the balance of microbes in the intestines may be improved by taking probiotics: probably the most widely available functional foods.

Probiotics come in the form of bioyoghurts, milk-based drinks – such as Yakult and Actimel – and fruit juices with added 'friendly' bacteria. The most commonly used friendly bacteria are the lactobacilli (acidophilus) and bifido-bacteria (bifidus) families. To be effective they may have to be eaten daily, or the improved colonisation of the gut may not be sustained.

Prebiotics – also used to improve intestinal health – are carbohydrates that pass unchanged through the digestive system and enter the large bowel, where they act as nutrients for 'friendly' bacteria, including those that may have been taken in probiotics.

The 'friendly' bacteria are then able to compete more successfully against the harmful micro-organisms, resulting in a healthier gut function.

PHYTOESTROGENS

High intakes of isoflavones, the most active phytoestrogens in the human diet (see *page 153*), may reduce the risk of coronary heart disease and some cancers, including breast, prostate and bowel cancer. They may also help to reduce menopausal symptoms and the risk of osteoporosis. Functional foods containing soya protein or the pure isoflavones are being developed.

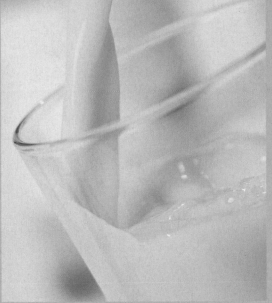

PLANT STEROLS

A group of plant chemicals with a structure similar to cholesterol is plant sterols. They are not absorbed by the gut, but have been found to reduce the absorption of cholesterol both from foods and from the bile that the liver discharges into the intestine.

Plant sterols can lower blood cholesterol levels and thereby reduce the risk of heart disease. For this reason they are added to some margarines and sold as functional foods; a certain amount of the margarine must be eaten each day for the desired effect to be achieved.

FOLIC ACID

A low folic acid intake has been linked to increased blood levels of homocysteine, and possibly to incidence of cancer of the colon and Alzheimer's disease.

Homocysteine is a product of protein metabolism found in the blood; in some people its level can rise, and this is believed to increase the risk of heart disease. Levels of homocysteine are usually controlled by three enzymes, two of which are dependent on the presence of folic acid, or folate.

Many foods, such as bread and breakfast cereals, are fortified with this B vitamin to help to reduce the incidence of these diseases and to protect unborn babies from developing neural-tube defects.

FISH OILS

Fish oils containing omega-3 essential fatty acids (EFAs) have been shown to reduce both the risk of death following a heart attack and the incidence of heart disease. Intakes of omega-3 EFAs in the European Union are currently at only 50% of recommended levels.

Margarines enriched with fish oils have been available in the UK, but did not prove popular. Manufacturers are developing other foods rich in omega-3 fats, but masking their taste is a major problem.

BONE HEALTH

Calcium, magnesium and vitamin D are believed to be the most important nutrients for bone health. For decades white flour has been fortified with calcium, and margarines fortified with vitamin D. Functional foods containing nutrients to aid bone health have also now become available. They include fortified orange juice, cereal bars and chocolate drinks.

Fungi

Ganoderma lucidum (reishi)
Grifola frondosa (maitake)
Lentinus edodes (shiitake)

Common uses

- Build immunity.
- Help to prevent cancer.
- Enhance cancer treatments.
- Alleviate bronchitis, sinusitis.
- Treat chronic fatigue syndrome.
- Help to prevent heart disease.

Forms

- Capsule
- Dried mushrooms
- Fresh mushrooms
- Liquid
- Powder
- Tablet
- Tea

CAUTION!

- If you are taking anticoagulant drugs, it is advisable to avoid reishi supplements because the mushrooms contain compounds that also 'thin' the blood.

REMINDER: If you have a medical condition, consult your doctor before taking supplements.

Shiitake and maitake are more than just exotic-sounding items on a Japanese menu. In fact, they are members of a special group of medicinal fungi, or mushrooms, that have been heralded in Asia for centuries as longevity tonics and immune-system boosters.

What they are

Traditional Asian medicine has long cherished certain species of mushroom – including maitake, reishi and shiitake – for their health-promoting effects. Reishi mushrooms, in particular, are one of the major Chinese tonics, and were first described in Chinese writings of 200 BC. Although other mushrooms – tree ear and oyster mushrooms, for instance – may also provide some health benefits, most research has focused on the three types mentioned above.

The mushrooms are available as powders (in loose form, to be brewed as a tea, or in capsules or tablets) or as liquid extracts, in which their potency is concentrated. Dried reishi and fresh and dried shiitake and maitake mushrooms may be found in Asian supermarkets and in some gourmet shops, but for therapeutic purposes supplements are preferred. Maitake, reishi and shiitake mushroom powders are sometimes combined in one capsule.

What they do

Medicinal mushrooms have various effects, including boosting the body's immune system, lowering cholesterol, acting as an anticoagulant and playing a supportive role in the treatment of cancer.

✤ **MAJOR BENEFITS:** Maitake mushrooms are commonly used in Japan to strengthen the immune systems of people undergoing chemotherapy treatment for cancer. Studies have shown that maitake extracts increase the effectiveness of lower chemotherapy doses while protecting healthy cells from the damage such drugs can cause.

Medicinal mushrooms boost the immune system, aiding in the battle against disease-causing organisms. Some studies show that they may be powerful enough to help people with HIV infection and AIDS, who have very weak immune systems. For example, shiitake mushrooms contain a carbohydrate compound called lentinan, which promotes the body's production of T cells and other immune-system components. Other people with compromised immune systems, such as those with chronic fatigue syndrome, may benefit from medicinal mushrooms too.

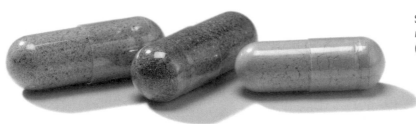

Supplements made from shiitake, reishi and maitake mushrooms (left to right) come in capsule form.

✳ **ADDITIONAL BENEFITS:** Traditionally, reishi mushrooms (known to the Chinese as 'spirit plants') are used to encourage relaxation, which makes them suitable for the treatment of stress and fatigue. Reishi also contain anti-inflammatory compounds that are beneficial for bronchitis and possibly for other respiratory ailments. In a Chinese study of 2000 people with bronchitis, 60% to 90% of those given reishi tablets improved within two weeks. Maitake, reishi and shiitake mushrooms may also help to fight heart disease by reducing the tendency of blood to clot, lowering blood pressure and possibly reducing cholesterol levels.

How to take them

✐ **DOSAGE:** *For immune-system support for cancer:* Take 200 mg maitake, 500 mg of reishi and 400 mg shiitake mushrooms three times a day. For *heart disease or* HIV/AIDS: Take 1500 mg of reishi and 600 mg maitake daily. For *bronchitis or sinusitis:* Take 1500 mg of reishi and/or 600 mg of maitake daily during the illness.

◐ **GUIDELINES FOR USE:** The effects of medicinal mushrooms are not dramatic, and may need several months to become apparent. For best results, divide the supplements into two or three daily doses and take with or without food. As these medicinal mushrooms are also traditional foods, the dried fungi can be added to soups or infused with hot water to make teas. Reishi mushrooms occur in six different colours; the red and purple varieties are most commonly used medicinally.

Possible side effects

Maitake, reishi and shiitake mushrooms are all safe when used in appropriate doses. In rare cases, long-term use of reishi – three to six months of daily use – may cause dryness in the mouth, a skin rash and itchiness, an upset stomach, nosebleeds or bloody stools. If any of these symptoms occur, stop taking reishi. Pregnant or breastfeeding women should consult a doctor before trying any of the mushrooms medicinally.

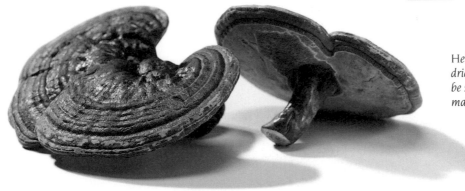

Helpful in combating stress, dried reishi mushrooms can be simmered in water to make a calming tea.

Garlic

Allium sativum

Prized by the ancient Egyptians for its strength-enhancing properties, garlic has since been used to treat every type of ailment, from leprosy to haemorrhoids. Modern research has focused on exploiting its potential to reduce the risk of heart disease and cancer.

Common uses

- *May lower cholesterol levels.*
- *Reduces blood clotting.*
- *Fights infections.*
- *Acts to boost immunity.*
- *May prevent some cancers.*
- *May produce a slight drop in blood pressure.*
- *Combats fungal infections.*

Forms

- Capsule
- Fresh herb
- Liquid
- Oil
- Powder
- Softgel
- Tablet

CAUTION!

■ Consult your doctor if you are taking drugs to prevent blood clots (anticoagulants or aspirin) or to reduce high blood pressure (antihypertensives). Garlic may intensify the effects of these drugs.

REMINDER: If you have a medical condition, consult your doctor before taking supplements.

What it is

For thousands of years garlic has been valued for its therapeutic powers. Egyptian pyramid builders took it for strength and endurance; in the 19th century Louis Pasteur investigated its antibacterial properties; and physicians in the two world wars used it to treat battle wounds. Garlic is related to the onion, the shallot and other plants in the genus *Allium*. The entire plant is odoriferous, but the strongest aroma is concentrated in the bulb, the site of garlic's healing powers and flavour.

Most of garlic's health benefits derive from its more than 100 sulphur compounds. When the bulb is crushed or chewed, alliin, one of these compounds, becomes allicin, the chemical responsible for garlic's odour and health-giving effects. In turn, some of the allicin is rapidly broken down into other sulphur compounds, such as ajoene, which can also have medicinal properties. Cooking garlic inhibits the formation of allicin and eliminates some of the other therapeutic chemicals.

What it does

Traditionally, garlic has been employed to treat a wide range of ailments and diseases. Today researchers are focusing on its potential to reduce the risk of heart disease and cancer.

⊙ **PREVENTION:** The liberal use of garlic in Mediterranean cooking may partly explain why countries such as Italy and Spain have such a low incidence of hardening of the arteries (atherosclerosis).

Several studies suggest that garlic can prevent heart disease in various ways. For example, garlic makes platelets (the cells involved in blood clotting) less likely to clump and stick to artery walls, and so reduces the risk of a heart attack. There is evidence that the herb dissolves clot-forming proteins which can affect plaque development. Garlic also lowers blood pressure slightly, mainly through its ability to widen blood vessels and help blood to circulate more freely. Results of recent studies examining garlic's effect on cholesterol are not clear-cut,

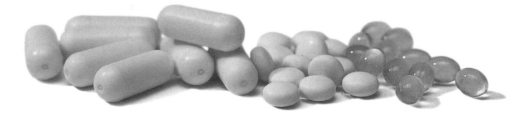

Garlic supplements come in many forms, including capsules, tablets and softgels.

but most doctors who favour nutritional remedies think that garlic, perhaps in combination with other cholesterol-lowering supplements, is worth a try. The herb may affect the metabolism of cholesterol in the liver; as a result, less cholesterol is released into the blood.

❋ **ADDITIONAL BENEFITS:** Garlic may have anticancer properties. It has been found to be particularly effective in preventing digestive cancers and possibly even breast and prostate cancers, but is not clear how garlic produces these benefits. Several mechanisms may be involved; for example, the herb acts to increase the level of enzymes that can detoxify cancer triggers. Garlic also blocks the formation of nitrites linked to stomach cancer, and it stimulates the immune system. Its antioxidant properties are important as well.

Garlic is often effective against infectious organisms – viruses, bacteria and fungi – because allicin can block the enzymes that give the organisms their ability to invade and damage tissues. The herb has also been shown to inhibit the fungi responsible for athlete's foot and swimmer's ear.

How to take it

▱ **DOSAGE:** Look for supplements that supply 4000 mcg of allicin potential per tablet, approximately the same amount of allicin potential found in one clove of fresh garlic. For *general health or to help high cholesterol*: Take a 400 to 600 mg garlic supplement each day. For *colds and flu*: Take a 400 to 600 mg garlic supplement four times a day. For *topical benefits*: Apply garlic oil two or three times a day. Some skin conditions, including warts and insect bites, may respond to garlic oil, or a crushed raw garlic clove, applied directly to the affected area.

◉ **GUIDELINES FOR USE:** Garlic can be taken indefinitely. However, if you are using the herb for cholesterol problems, have your levels checked after three months to see if they have changed; if you have derived no benefits from garlic, talk to your doctor about other remedies.

Possible side effects

Some people develop indigestion, intestinal gas and diarrhoea when taking high doses of garlic. Using enteric-coated supplements may reduce such side effects. Skin rashes have also been reported.

To get the full medicinal benefits of fresh garlic, it should be eaten raw.

RECENT FINDINGS

In a study 34 Venezuelan soldiers with athlete's foot were treated with topical applications of ajoene cream, twice daily for seven days. The treatment completely cured 79% of the soldiers and an additional seven-day course cured the remainder.

Garlic may prevent stiffening of the aorta – the artery that carries blood from the heart to the rest of the body – which occurs naturally with age. In one study, 200 people took either garlic supplements or a placebo daily for two years. At the end of the study the aortas of the 70-year-olds in the garlic group were as supple as those of the 55-year-olds who didn't take the supplement. A flexible aorta may help to reduce age-related damage.

Ginger

Zingiber officinale

From ancient India and China to Greece and Rome, ginger was revered as a culinary and medicinal spice. Medieval Europeans traced the herb to the Garden of Eden. Valued by traditional healers, ginger is still widely used to prevent motion sickness and as a remedy for digestive problems.

Common uses

- *Alleviates nausea and dizziness.*
- *May relieve the pain and inflammation of arthritis.*
- *Eases muscle aches.*
- *Relieves cold and flu symptoms.*
- *Reduces flatulence.*

Forms

- Capsule
- Crystallised herb
- Fresh or dried root/tea
- Liquid
- Oil
- Softgel
- Tablet
- Tincture

CAUTION!

■ Up to 250 mg of ginger four times a day may relieve morning sickness during the first two months of pregnancy, but higher doses or longer use require medical supervision.

■ Chemotherapy patients should not take ginger on an empty stomach because it can irritate the stomach lining.

REMINDER: If you have a medical condition, consult your doctor before taking supplements.

What it is

Renowned for its stomach-settling properties, ginger is native to parts of India and China as well as Jamaica and other tropical areas. This warm-climate perennial is closely related to turmeric and cardamom, and its roots are used for culinary and therapeutic purposes. As a spice, ginger adds a hot and lemony flavour to foods as disparate as biscuits and roast pork. Medicinally, it continues to play a major role in traditional healing.

What it does

For thousands of years, all around the globe, this pungent spice has been popular as a treatment for digestive problems ranging from mild indigestion and flatulence to nausea and vomiting. It has also been used to relieve colds and arthritis. Modern research into ginger's active ingredients confirms the effectiveness of many of these ancient remedies.

MAJOR BENEFITS: What can you do with a seasick sailor? The answer is: try ginger. In a Danish study a group of 40 naval cadets took 1 gram of powdered ginger a day; they were much less likely to break out in a cold sweat and to vomit (classic symptoms of seasickness) than were 39 others who took a placebo.

Ginger works primarily in the digestive tract, boosting digestive fluids and neutralising acids, so it is sometimes used as an alternative to antinausea drugs that can affect the central nervous system and cause grogginess. Studies of women undergoing exploratory surgery (laparoscopy) or major gynaecological surgery show that taking 1 gram of ginger before an operation can significantly reduce postoperative nausea and vomiting, a common side effect of anaesthetics and other drugs used in surgery. Ginger also appears to counter the nausea created by chemotherapy, though it is advisable to take it with food to minimise any stomach irritation.

Ginger's antinausea effects make it useful for reducing dizziness, a common problem in older patients, as well as for treating morning sickness. For years ginger has been a staple of folk medicine, primarily as a digestive aid to counter stomach upset. Ginger supplements (or fresh pulp mixed with lime juice) are also a good remedy for flatulence.

ADDITIONAL BENEFITS: Ginger's anti-inflammatory and pain-relieving properties may help to relieve the muscle aches and chronic pain associated with arthritis. In a study of seven women with rheumatoid arthritis (an autoimmune disease characterised by severe inflammation) a daily dose of just 5 to 50 grams of fresh ginger or capsules containing up to 1 gram of powdered ginger was shown to lessen joint pain and inflammation. Its anti-inflammatory properties suggest that ginger may ease bronchial constriction brought on by colds or flu.

How to take it

⬚ **DOSAGE:** *To prevent motion sickness, dizziness and nausea, reduce flatulence, and relieve chronic pain or rheumatoid arthritis:* Take ginger up to three times a day, or every four hours as needed. The usual dose is 100 to 200 mg of standardised extract in capsule or tablet form, or 1 or 2 grams of fresh powdered ginger, or a 1.25 cm slice of fresh ginger root. Other preparations, including ginger tea, can be used several times a day for similar purposes and for arthritis and pain relief. Ginger tea is available in tea bags, or you can add ½ teaspoon of grated ginger root to a cup of very hot water. On journeys, try crystallised ginger: a 2.5 cm square, about ½ cm thick, contains approximately 500 mg of ginger. *For aching muscles:* Rub several drops of ginger oil, mixed with a tablespoon of almond oil or another neutral oil, on the sore areas. *For relief of colds and flu:* Drink up to four cups of ginger tea a day as needed to reduce symptoms.

⬚ **GUIDELINES FOR USE:** Taking large doses on an empty stomach may lead to indigestion: take with food, and take ginger capsules with fluid. To prevent motion sickness, ginger should be taken three to four hours before your departure, and then every four hours as needed, up to four times a day. For postoperative nausea, begin taking ginger the day before your operation, under medical supervision.

Possible side effects

Ginger is very safe for a broad range of complaints, whether it is taken in a concentrated capsule form, eaten fresh or sipped as a tea or ginger ale. Occasional indigestion seems to be the only documented side effect.

Whether eaten fresh or taken in the form of capsules, ginger is a potent remedy for nausea and dizziness.

Ginkgo biloba

Ginkgo biloba

This popular herbal medicine, derived from one of the oldest species of tree on earth, is widely marketed as a memory booster. Ginkgo biloba does help to combat age-related memory loss, but whether it is a 'smart pill' meant for everyone remains to be seen.

Common uses

- *May slow down the progression of Alzheimer's symptoms; sharpens concentration and memory, particularly in elderly people.*

- *Lessens depression and anxiety in some elderly people.*

- *Alleviates coldness in the extremities (Raynaud's disease) and painful leg cramps (intermittent claudication).*

- *Relieves headaches, tinnitus (ringing in the ears) and dizziness.*

- *May restore erections in men with impotence.*

Forms

- Capsule
- Liquid
- Powder
- Softgel
- Tablet
- Tincture

CAUTION!

■ **Do not use any form of unprocessed ginkgo leaves, including teas; they contain potent chemicals that can trigger allergic reactions. Select standardised extracts (GBE) in which the allergens have been removed during processing.**

REMINDER: *If you have a medical or psychiatric condition, consult your doctor before taking supplements.*

What it is

The medicinal form of the herb is extracted from the fan-shaped leaves of the ancient ginkgo biloba tree, a species that has survived in China for more than 200 million years. A concentrated form of the herb, known as ginkgo biloba extract, or GBE, is used to make the supplement. Commonly called ginkgo, GBE is obtained by drying and milling the leaves and then extracting the active ingredients in a mixture of acetone and water.

What it does

Ginkgo may have beneficial effects on both the circulatory and the central nervous systems. It increases blood flow to the arms and legs and the brain by regulating the tone and elasticity of blood vessels, from the largest arteries to the tiniest capillaries. It also acts like aspirin by helping to reduce the 'stickiness' of the blood, thereby lowering the risk of blood clots. Ginkgo appears to have antioxidant properties as well, mopping up the damaging compounds known as free radicals and aiding in the maintenance of healthy blood cells. Some researchers report that it enhances the nervous system by promoting the delivery of additional oxygen and blood sugar (glucose) to nerve cells.

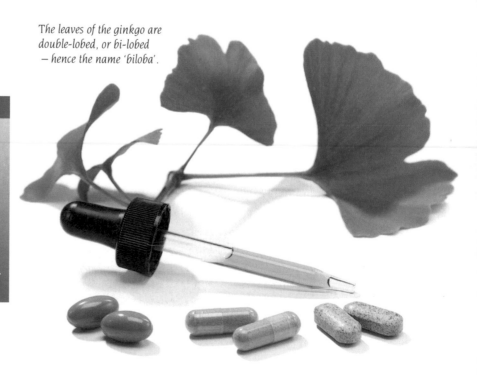

The leaves of the ginkgo are double-lobed, or bi-lobed — hence the name 'biloba'.

PREVENTION: Modern interest in ginkgo centres on the herb's potential as a preventative for age-related memory loss. There is also an indication that ginkgo may make healthy people better able to focus their thoughts or to remember. So far it is those people who are already suffering from diminished blood flow to the brain who have benefited most from taking the herb. Current research is trying to determine whether ginkgo's ability to prevent blood clots may stave off heart attacks or strokes.

MAJOR BENEFITS: The fact that ginkgo aids blood flow to the brain – thereby increasing its oxygen supply – is particularly important to elderly people whose arteries may have narrowed with cholesterol build-up or other conditions. Diminished blood flow has been linked to Alzheimer's disease and memory loss, as well as to anxiety, headaches, depression, confusion, tinnitus and dizziness. All may be helped by ginkgo.

ADDITIONAL BENEFITS: Ginkgo also promotes blood flow to the arms and legs, which makes it useful for reducing the pain, cramping and weakness caused by narrowed arteries in the leg, a disorder called intermittent claudication. There are indications that the herb may improve circulation to the extremities in people with Raynaud's disease, and help victims of scleroderma, a rare autoimmune disorder.

In addition some research suggests that, by increasing blood flow to the nerve fibres of the eyes and ears, ginkgo may be of value in treating macular degeneration or diabetes-related eye disease (both leading causes of blindness) as well as some types of hearing loss.

Other studies are in progress to assess the possible effectiveness of ginkgo in speeding up recovery from certain strokes and head injuries, as well as in treating other conditions that may be related to circulatory or nervous system impairment, including impotence, multiple sclerosis and nerve damage linked to diabetes. Before the introduction of leaf extracts, traditional Chinese healers used ginkgo nuts for treating asthma because they appear to alleviate wheezing and other respiratory complaints.

How to take it

DOSAGE: Use supplements that contain ginkgo biloba extract, or GBE, the concentrated form of the herb. *As a general memory booster and for poor circulation*: Take 120 mg of GBE daily, divided into two or three doses. *For Alzheimer's disease, depression, tinnitus, dizziness, impotence or other conditions caused by insufficient blood flow to the brain*: Take up to 240 mg a day.

GUIDELINES FOR USE: It commonly takes four to six weeks, and in some cases up to 12 weeks, for the herb's effects to be noticed. Generally, it is considered safe for long-term use in recommended dosages. You can take ginkgo with or without food. No adverse effects have been reported in pregnant or breastfeeding women who take the herb.

Possible side effects

In rare cases, ginkgo may cause irritability, restlessness, diarrhoea, nausea or vomiting, but these effects are usually mild and transient. People starting to take the herb may also notice headaches during the first day or two of use. If side effects are troublesome, discontinue ginkgo or reduce the dosage.

Ginseng

Panax ginseng
P. quinquefolius
Eleutherococcus senticosus

Common uses

- *Combats the physical effects of stress.*
- *Boosts vitality and enhances immunity.*
- *Chinese ginseng may treat impotence and infertility in men.*

Forms

- Capsule
- Dried herb/tea
- Powder
- Softgel
- Tablet
- Tincture

There are three main types of ginseng, any of which can exert a variety of protective effects on the body when taken at the correct dosage. Chinese ginseng is frequently added to manufactured beverages, but the amounts used are usually too small to be effective.

What it is

Panax ginseng – also called Asian, Chinese or Korean ginseng – has been used in Chinese medicine for thousands of years to enhance both longevity and the quality of life; it is the most widely available and extensively studied form of the herb. Another species, Panax quinquefolius, or American ginseng, is grown mainly in the American Midwest and exported to China. Siberian ginseng (Eleutherococcus senticosus) comes from Siberia, and is distantly related to the other two.

The medicinal part of the plant is its slow-growing root, which is harvested after four to six years, when its overall ginsenoside content – the main active ingredient in Panax ginsengs – is at its peak; there are 13 different ginsenosides in all. Panax ginsengs also contains panaxans, substances that can lower blood sugar, and polysaccharides, complex sugar molecules that enhance the immune system. 'White' ginseng is simply the dried root; 'red' ginseng (usually from Korea) has been steamed and dried. Most research studies have been done with white Chinese ginseng. Siberian ginseng is characterised by containing eleutherosides, which have similar properties to ginsenosides.

What it does

The primary health benefits of the three ginsengs derive from their antioxidant properties, their power to stimulate the immune system, and their ability to protect the body against the adverse effects of stress.

PREVENTION: All three ginsengs may help the body to combat a range of illnesses. They stimulate the production of specialised immune cells called 'killer T cells', which destroy harmful viruses and bacteria.

Research has also indicated that Chinese ginseng may inhibit the growth of certain cancer cells. A large Korean study found that the risk of cancer developing in people who took Panax ginseng was half that in subjects who did not take it. Although ginseng powders and tinctures

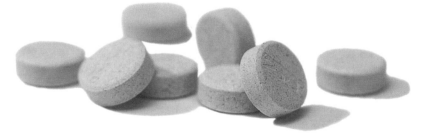

Widely available in capsule and tablet form, ginseng can restore energy and relieve stress.

were shown to lower the risk of cancer, eating fresh ginseng root or drinking ginseng juice or tea did not have the same effect.

✺ **ADDITIONAL BENEFITS:** Ginseng may benefit people who are feeling fatigued and stressed and those recovering from long illnesses. It has been shown to balance the release of stress hormones in the body and to support the organs that produce these hormones: the pituitary gland and hypothalamus at the base of the brain, and the adrenal glands, located on top of the kidneys.

Chinese ginseng may help to correct impotence by improving erectile function through dilating blood vessels. Animal studies indicate that it increases testosterone levels and sperm production, bringing potential benefit to men with fertility problems.

Many long-distance runners and body-builders take ginseng to boost physical endurance. Herbalists believe that the ginsengs can combat fatigue by raising vitality. While Chinese ginseng is more applicable to the male system, Siberian ginseng may be more suitable for women, particularly those with menstrual cycle irregularities. American ginseng is highly regarded for its tonic effects, and has traditionally been used for treating digestive tract disorders. Otherwise the three ginsengs have many similarities in properties and use.

How to take it

⬜ **DOSAGE:** *For general health or to combat fatigue:* Take 100 to 250 mg *Panax ginseng* extract (or 300 to 400 mg Siberian ginseng) once or twice a day. *To support the body in times of stress or during recovery from illness:* Take the above dose twice a day. *For male impotence and infertility:* Take the above dose twice a day.

◉ **GUIDELINES FOR USE:** Start at the lower end of the dosage range and increase your intake gradually. Some experts recommend that you stop taking ginseng for a week every two or three weeks and then resume your regular dose. In some cases, ginseng may be rotated with other herbs which stimulate the immune system, such as astragalus.

Possible side effects

At the recommended doses, ginseng is unlikely to cause any side effects. There have been reports that higher doses cause nervousness, insomnia, headache and stomach upset; if you have any of these problems, reduce your dose. The combination of ginseng and caffeine may intensify these reactions. Some women report increased menstrual bleeding or breast tenderness with high doses of Chinese ginseng. If this occurs, try using Siberian ginseng instead.

RECENT FINDINGS

Men with erectile dysfunction may benefit from ginseng. In one study involving 45 patients, 900 mg of Korean red ginseng, taken three times a day, improved erection in 60% of patients .

DID YOU KNOW?

The name 'ginseng' is derived from the ancient Chinese word *jen shen* (meaning 'man root') because the ginseng root (below) often resembles the shape of the human body.

Glucosamine

This promising arthritis fighter helps to build cartilage – which provides cushioning at the tips of the bones – and protects and strengthens the joints as it relieves pain and stiffness. Although your body produces its own glucosamine, supplements can be helpful.

Common uses

- *Relieves pain, stiffness and swelling of the knees, fingers and other joints caused by osteoarthritis or rheumatoid arthritis.*

- *Helps to reduce arthritic back and neck pain.*

- *May speed up the healing of sprains and strengthen joints, preventing future injury.*

Forms

- Capsule
- Cream and skin patches
- Tablet

CAUTION!

REMINDER: *If you have a medical condition, consult your doctor before taking supplements.*

What it is

Glucosamine (pronounced glue-KOSE-a-mean) is a fairly simple molecule that contains the sugar glucose. It is found in relatively high concentrations in the joints and connective tissues, where the body uses it to form the larger molecules necessary for cartilage repair and maintenance. In recent years glucosamine has become available as a nutritional supplement. Various forms are sold, including glucosamine sulphate and N-acetyl-glucosamine (NAG). Glucosamine sulphate is the preferred form for arthritis: it is readily used by the body (90% to 98% is absorbed through the intestine) and appears to be very effective in relieving this condition.

What it does

Although some doctors hail glucosamine as an arthritis cure, no single supplement or combination of supplements can claim that title. Glucosamine does, however, provide significant relief from pain and inflammation for about half of arthritis sufferers – especially those with the common age-related form known as osteoarthritis. It can also help people with rheumatoid arthritis and other types of joint injuries.

✪ **MAJOR BENEFITS:** Used to treat arthritis in about 70 countries around the world, glucosamine can ease pain and inflammation, increase range of motion, and help to repair ageing and damaged joints in the knees, hips, spine and hands. Recent studies show that it may be even more effective for relieving pain and inflammation than nonsteroidal anti-inflammatory drugs (NSAIDs), such as aspirin and ibuprofen, commonly taken by arthritis sufferers – without their harmful side effects. Moreover, while NSAIDs mask arthritis pain, they do little to combat progression of the disease – and may even make it worse by impairing the body's ability to build cartilage. By contrast, glucosamine helps to make cartilage and may repair damaged joints. Although it cannot do much for people with advanced arthritis, when cartilage has completely worn away, it may benefit the millions of people with mild to moderately severe symptoms.

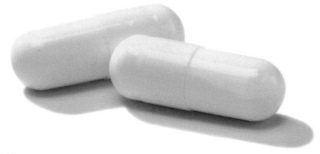

✥ ADDITIONAL BENEFITS: As a general joint strengthener, glucosamine may be useful for the prevention of arthritis and all forms of age-related degenerative joint disease. It may also speed healing of acute joint injuries, such as a sprained ankle or finger. Athletes and sportsmen and women often take glucosamine to help to prevent muscle injuries.

How to take it

◪ DOSAGE: The usual dosage for arthritis and other conditions is 500 mg glucosamine sulphate three times a day, or 1500 mg daily. This amount has been shown to be safe for all individuals and effective for most.

◉ GUIDELINES FOR USE: Glucosamine is typically taken long term and appears to be very safe. It may not bring relief as quickly as conventional pain relievers or anti-inflammatories do (it usually works in two to eight weeks), but its benefits are far greater and longer lasting when it is used over a period of time. Take glucosamine with meals to minimise the chance of digestive upset.

In addition to glucosamine, some supplements contain a related cartilage component called chondroitin sulphate and sometimes other nutrients, such as niacin or S-adenosylmethionine (SAM). These are purported to have enhanced cartilage-building properties, but research-based evidence for such benefits is lacking. Other supplements that are sometimes taken along with glucosamine for the relief of arthritis include boswellia, a tree extract from India; devil's claw from Namibia; celery seed extract; and the topical pain reliever cayenne cream. No adverse reactions have been reported when glucosamine is used with other supplements or with prescription or over-the-counter medications.

Possible side effects

Supplements of glucosamine – a natural substance produced in the body – appear to be virtually free of side effects, although no long-term studies have been done. Gastrointestinal effects, such as indigestion or nausea, are rare in those who take glucosamine supplements. Should any of these symptoms occur, try taking glucosamine with meals.

RECENT FINDINGS

A study at the Beijing Union Medical College Hospital, involving 178 patients with osteoarthritis of the knee, showed that 1500 mg of glucosamine sulphate taken daily was just as effective in reducing symptoms as 1200 mg of ibuprofen – and that it was significantly better tolerated by the patients.

━✧━

An Australian study involving 63 patients with osteoarthritis of the knee found that the direct application to the knee of a cream containing glucosamine and chondroitin was effective in relieving pain. Improvement was evident within four weeks.

DID YOU KNOW?

Older dogs that have trouble moving around may benefit from glucosamine sulphate. It has been shown to be as safe and effective for the canine species as it is for humans.

FACTS & TIPS

■ Supplements are the best source of extra glucosamine because dietary sources of the nutrient are quite obscure. Foods that are relatively rich in glucosamine include crabs, oysters and the shells of prawns.

Goldenseal

Hydrastis canadensis

The Cherokee, Iroquois and other Native American tribes valued goldenseal as a remedy for everything from insect bites and bloating to eye infections and stomach aches. Today the root of this herb is used by medical herbalists in the USA and throughout Europe.

Common uses

- *Soothes inflamed mucous membranes, as in sinusitis.*
- *Promotes healing of mouth ulcers and cold sores and helps to destroy the virus that causes warts.*
- *Bolsters the immune system.*
- *Alleviates digestive disorders.*
- *May help urinary tract infections.*
- *Treats eye infections.*

Forms

- Capsule
- Dried herb/tea
- Liquid
- Ointment/cream
- Softgel
- Tincture

CAUTION!

- Goldenseal should not be used by pregnant women or people with high blood pressure or glaucoma.

REMINDER: *If you have a medical condition, consult your doctor before taking supplements.*

What it is

Related to the buttercup, goldenseal is a perennial herb native to North America. The dried root has long been used to soothe inflamed or infected mucous membranes; today it is appreciated for its ability to help the body to fight infection. The plant was first called goldenseal in the 19th century, acquiring its name from the rich yellow of the root and the small cuplike scars found there. These scars, which appear on the previous year's root growth, resemble the wax seals formerly used to close envelopes – hence the name 'goldenseal'.

The key medicinal compounds in goldenseal are the alkaloids berberine and hydrastine. Berberine is also responsible for the root's rich yellow colour – so vibrant, in fact, that Native Americans and early settlers utilised goldenseal as a dye as well as a medicinal herb. The alkaloids have a bitter taste, so goldenseal tea often includes other herbs or is mixed with a sweetener such as honey.

What it does

The primary benefit of goldenseal is its overall effect on immunity. Not only does it increase the power of the immune system to fight infection, but it can also combat both bacteria and viruses directly.

PREVENTION: Taking goldenseal as soon as you detect symptoms of a cold or flu may prevent the illness from developing fully – or at least minimise the symptoms – by enhancing the activity of virus-fighting white blood cells.

ADDITIONAL BENEFITS: Goldenseal fights bacteria, making it useful for mild urinary tract infections (if you begin taking it early enough) and

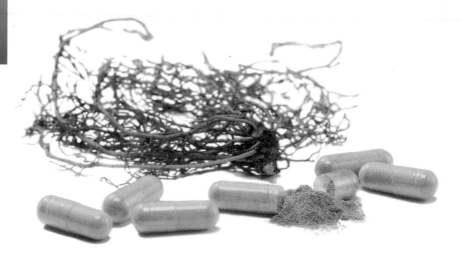

The root of the goldenseal plant is dried and then ground to a powder for use in supplements.

sinus infections. It may also help to soothe nausea and vomiting by stimulating digestive secretions and working to destroy the bacteria that may be causing the symptoms.

As one of several herbs that stimulate the immune system – others include echinacea, pau d'arco and astragalus – goldenseal can play a role in relieving the symptoms of chronic fatigue syndrome, a disabling disorder that may be partly caused by a weakened immune system. It also helps to fight cold sores and shingles (both caused by the herpes virus). Unless advised otherwise by a practitioner, use it for no more than a week or two at a time.

Applied topically, goldenseal tincture is beneficial for mouth ulcers and warts. The tincture promotes the healing of the sores and directly fights the human papilloma virus that causes warts. Once cooled and strained, goldenseal tea can be used as an eyewash to relieve eye infections such as conjunctivitis. Be sure to prepare a fresh batch daily, and store it in a sterile container so the tea does not get contaminated.

How to take it

☑ **DOSAGE:** *For colds, flu and other respiratory infections:* As soon as you begin to feel symptoms, take 125 mg of goldenseal extract (in combination with 200 mg of echinacea extract) up to four times a day for no more than five days. *For urinary tract infections:* Drink several cups of goldenseal tea a day. *For nausea and vomiting:* Take 125 mg extract every four hours as needed. *For chronic fatigue syndrome:* Use 125 mg extract twice a day in rotation with other immune-stimulating herbs. *For cold sores and shingles:* Take 125 mg of goldenseal extract with 200 mg echinacea extract four times a day. *For mouth ulcers and warts:* Apply goldenseal tincture directly to the sores three times a day. *For eye infections:* Use 1 teaspoon dried herb per 600 ml of hot water. Steep, strain through muslin or a fine cloth and cool, then apply as an eyewash three times a day; make a new solution every day.

◉ **GUIDELINES FOR USE:** Take goldenseal supplements with meals. Unlike echinacea and other herbs that stimulate the immune system, goldenseal should be used only when you feel that you are coming down with a cold, flu or some other illness, and only for the duration of the illness. The single exception to this rule is when you are taking goldenseal in rotation with other herbs to strengthen the immune system.

Possible side effects

When taken at recommended doses and for suggested lengths of time, goldenseal is safe to use and has few side effects. Very high doses may irritate the mucous membranes of the mouth and cause them to become excessively dry.

CASE HISTORY
Going for gold

Alexa K. always reacted badly to antibiotics. Although she needed them to combat her sinus infections, the side effects – dizziness, nausea, diarrhoea – often made the drugs worse than the illness.

When a herbalist told her to try goldenseal extract, Alexa was sceptical. But she took the goldenseal, and in a few days her sinus infection was gone – without a single side effect.

Now goldenseal is a part of Alexa's sinus first-aid kit. At the first sign of an infection she starts taking it, along with the immune stimulator echinacea.

Though antibiotics are sometimes necessary, in the past few years Alexa has often been able to avoid them. 'Those miserable side effects are history!' she reports.

Gotu kola

Centella asiatica

Reputed to be a favourite food of elephants, famously long-lived animals, gotu kola is associated by many people with longevity. Though scientific research has not shown that the herb can extend your life, there is little doubt that it provides important health benefits.

Common uses

- *Treats burns and wounds.*
- *Builds connective tissue.*
- *Strengthens veins.*
- *Improves memory.*

Forms

- Capsule
- Dried herb/tea
- Powder
- Tablet
- Tincture

CAUTION!

- **Pregnant women should not use gotu kola.**

REMINDER: If you have a medical condition, consult your doctor before taking supplements.

What it is

The medicinal use of gotu kola has its roots in India, where the herb continues to be part of the ancient healing tradition called Ayurveda. Word of its therapeutic benefits for skin disorders gradually spread throughout Asia and Europe, and in fact gotu kola has been used in France since the 1880s to treat burns and other wounds.

A red-flowered plant that thrives in hot, swampy areas, gotu kola grows naturally in India, Sri Lanka, Madagascar, middle and southern Africa, Australia, China and the southern USA. The appearance of this slender creeping perennial changes according to whether it is growing in water (broad, fan-shaped leaves) or on dry land (small, thin leaves). The plant's leaf is most commonly used medicinally.

What it does

Whether taken internally or applied externally as a compress, gotu kola has many beneficial effects. Components of the herb include chemicals called triterpenes (especially asiaticoside), which appear to enhance the formation of collagen in bones, cartilage and connective tissue. In addition they promote healthy blood vessels and may help to balance the activity of neurotransmitters, the chemical messengers in the brain.

MAJOR BENEFITS: Gotu kola's singular effect on connective tissue – promoting its healthy development and inhibiting the formation of hardened areas – makes it potentially important for treating many skin conditions. It can be therapeutic for burns, keloids (overgrown scar tissue) and wounds (including surgical incisions and skin ulcers). Gotu kola also seems to strengthen cells in the walls of blood vessels, improving blood flow, which makes it valuable in the treatment of varicose veins. Research results are often impressive. In more than a dozen studies observing gotu kola's effect on veins (which are surrounded by supportive connective-tissue sheaths), about 80% of patients with varicose veins and similar problems showed substantial improvement. Other studies indicate that applying gotu kola topically to psoriasis lesions may aid healing in sufferers of this condition as well.

ADDITIONAL BENEFITS: Gotu kola has been used to increase mental acuity for thousands of years. Current research supports a role for the herb in boosting memory, improving learning capabilities and possibly reversing some of the memory loss associated with Alzheimer's disease.

In one study, 30 children with learning difficulties were found to have significantly better concentration and attention levels after taking gotu kola for 12 weeks than they did at the start of the study. Early findings reveal that animals given gotu kola for two weeks were able to learn and remember new behaviours much better than animals not given the herb.

How to take it

✓ **DOSAGE:** *To treat varicose veins*: Take 200 mg of the standardised extract three times a day. *For burns*: Use 200 mg twice a day until they heal. To *improve memory or possibly slow down the progress of Alzheimer's disease*: Take 200 mg three times a day. You can substitute 1 gram of the crude herb for each 200 mg dose of the standardised extract.

◉ **GUIDELINES FOR USE:** In most cases gotu kola is taken internally as a tablet or capsule, with or without meals, but gotu kola tea or tincture can also be applied externally to the skin for psoriasis, burns, wounds, incisions or scars. You can use both oral and topical preparations of the herb over the same period of time.

To apply gotu kola topically, soak a compress in tea or tincture and apply it directly to problem areas. Start with a relatively weak solution and increase the strength as needed. To brew gotu kola tea, steep 1 or 2 teaspoons of dried leaf in a cup of very hot water for 10 to 15 minutes. You can also make a paste to apply to patches of skin affected by psoriasis: break open capsules and mix 2 teaspoons of dried gotu kola powder in a small amount of water.

Possible side effects

Taking gotu kola orally or using a topical preparation generally does not cause problems. Skin rash (dermatitis), sensitivity to sunlight and headaches are rare side effects. If you experience these symptoms, reduce the dosage or stop using the herb.

FACTS & TIPS

■ Gotu kola is also known as *Centella asiatica*, Indian pennywort, Indian water navelwort, talepetrako or hydrocotyle. Marsh pennywort (*Hydrocotyle vulgaris*), a related species native to Europe, has no known therapeutic properties.

■ Though the names sound similar, there is no relationship between gotu kola and the kola (or cola) nut used in cola drinks. The kola nut is a stimulant containing caffeine; gotu kola is a very mild sedative and is caffeine-free.

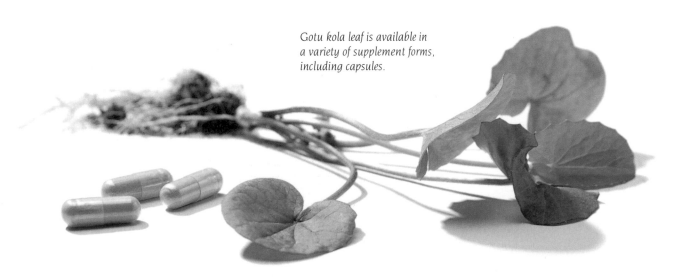

Gotu kola leaf is available in a variety of supplement forms, including capsules.

Grape seed extract

With antioxidant properties many times more powerful than vitamin C or vitamin E, grape seed extract can do much to promote a healthy heart and to reduce the risk of cancer. It also has the power to improve well-being in myriad ways.

Common uses

- Treats blood vessel disorders.
- Protects against damage to vision.
- Lessens the risk of heart disease and cancer.
- Reduces the rate of collagen breakdown in the skin.

Forms

- Capsule
- Liquid
- Tablet

What it is

An extract from the tiny seeds of red grapes has become one of the leading natural medicines in Europe. It belongs to the group of plant substances called flavonoids – antioxidants which protect the body's cells from damage by unstable oxygen molecules called free radicals. Grape seed extract contains oligomeric proanthocyanidin complexes (OPCs), also called proanthocyanidins. Once called pycnogenols (pik-NODGE-en-alls), OPCs are believed to play an important role in preventing heart disease and cancer. 'Pycnogenol' with a capital P is the trademark for a specific OPC derived from maritime pine bark; it can be used in place of grape seed extract, but it is more expensive, and many practitioners do not believe that it is worth the extra cost.

What it does

Grape seed extract exerts a powerful, positive influence on blood vessels. It is no coincidence that the active substances in this extract, OPCs, are key ingredients in one of the drugs most frequently prescribed for blood vessel (vascular) disorders in western Europe.

Grape seed extract contains both oil-soluble and water-soluble components, so it can penetrate all types of cell membranes, delivering antioxidant protection throughout the body. It is also one of the few substances that can cross the blood-brain barrier, which means that it may protect brain cells from free-radical damage.

✪ MAJOR BENEFITS: With its powerful ability to enhance the health of blood vessels, grape seed extract may not only reduce the risk of heart attack and stroke but also strengthen fragile or weak capillaries and increase blood flow, particularly to the extremities. For this reason many practitioners find it a beneficial supplement for almost any type

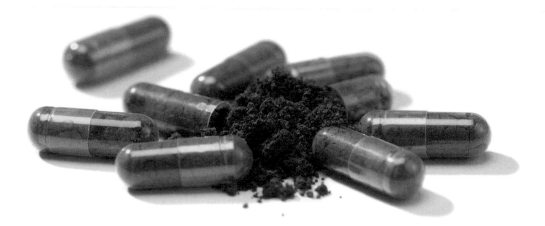

of vascular insufficiency as well as for conditions that are associated with poor vascular function, including diabetes, varicose veins, some cases of impotence, numbness and tingling in the arms and legs, and even painful leg cramps.

Grape seed extract affects even the tiniest blood vessels, so it can have a beneficial impact on circulation in the eye. It is often recommended as a supplement to combat macular degeneration and cataracts – two of the most common causes of blindness in elderly people. Grape seed extract may also be beneficial in people who regularly use computers. At least one study has shown that taking 300 mg of the extract daily for just 60 days reduced eye strain related to computer monitor work and improved contrast vision.

Many practitioners now endorse grape seed extract for its cancer-fighting properties. Working as antioxidants, OPCs correct damage to the genetic material of cells that could possibly cause tumours to form.

✱ **ADDITIONAL BENEFITS:** Grape seed extract helps to preserve and reinforce the collagen in the skin, so it is often included in cosmetic creams to improve skin elasticity.

Relief from allergy symptoms is another benefit of the extract; it inhibits the release of symptom-causing compounds such as histamine, which, in turn, helps to control a variety of allergic reactions, from hay fever to urticaria. The extract also blocks the release of prostaglandins, chemicals involved in allergic reactions and in pain and inflammation, particularly that of the menstrual disorder called endometriosis.

How to take it

⬛ **DOSAGE:** *For antioxidant protection*: Take 100 mg daily. *For therapeutic benefits*: Doses are usually 200 mg daily. Choose supplements that are standardised to contain 92% to 95% proanthocyanidins, or OPCs.

◉ **GUIDELINES FOR USE:** After 24 hours, only about 28% of grape seed extract's active components remain in the body, so it is important to take supplements at the same time every day, particularly when they are used to combat disease.

Possible side effects

No side effects from taking grape seed extract have been reported, and no toxic reactions have been noted.

Green tea

Camellia sinensis

Common uses
- *May help to prevent cancer.*
- *Protects against heart disease.*
- *Inhibits tooth decay.*
- *Promotes longevity.*

Forms
- Capsule
- Liquid
- Powder
- Tablet
- Tea

CAUTION!

- **Pregnant and breastfeeding women should limit their consumption of green tea to two cups a day.**

REMINDER: If you have a medical condition, consult your doctor before taking supplements.

According to Chinese legend, green tea was first drunk about 2700 BC, when an emperor sitting under a tea bush saw a few leaves fall into his cup of hot water – and sipped the brew. This type of tea has now been discovered to contain a highly promising anticancer compound.

What it is

The traditional process that yields green tea is simple: the leaves from the tea plant are first steamed, then rolled and dried. The steaming kills enzymes that would otherwise ferment the leaves. With other types of tea the leaves are allowed to ferment either partially (for oolong tea) or fully (for black tea). The lack of fermentation gives green tea its unique flavour and, more importantly, preserves virtually all the naturally present polyphenols – strong antioxidants that can protect against cell damage. Other substances in green tea that may also be beneficial are fluoride, catechins and tannins.

What it does

Green tea possesses compounds that may provide powerful protection against several cancers and, possibly, heart disease. Studies indicate that it also fights infection and promotes longevity.

PREVENTION: The prevalence of certain types of cancer is lower among people who drink green tea. In one large-scale study researchers found that Chinese men and women who drank green tea as seldom as once a week for six months had lower rates of rectal, pancreatic and possibly colon cancers than those who rarely or never drank it. In women, the risk of rectal or pancreatic cancer was nearly halved. Preliminary research suggests that green tea may also provide protection against breast, stomach and skin cancers.

Studies investigating how green tea might guard against cancer have pointed to the potency of its main antioxidant, the polyphenol EGCG (epigallocatechin-gallate). Some scientists believe that EGCG may be one of the most effective anticancer compounds ever discovered, protecting cells from damage and boosting the body's own production of antioxidant enzymes. One US study found that EGCG prompts cancer cells to stop reproducing by stimulating a natural process of programmed cell death called apoptosis. Remarkably, EGCG does not cause damage to healthy cells. Separate research at the Medical College of Ohio indicates that EGCG inhibits the production of urokinase, an enzyme that cancer cells need in order to grow. In animals, blocking urokinase shrinks tumours and sometimes causes the cancer to go into complete remission.

ADDITIONAL BENEFITS: The antioxidant effect of the polyphenols in green tea may also help to protect the heart. In test-tube studies these compounds appeared to suppress the damage to LDL cholesterol, thought to be an initial step in the build-up of plaque in the arteries. A Japanese study of 1371 men linked daily consumption of green tea to the prevention of heart disease. In addition, green tea contains fluoride, which provides an overall antibacterial effect and may help to guard against tooth decay. Preliminary evidence suggests that green tea may also have a beneficial effect on arthritis and in the healing of wounds.

How to take it

☑ **DOSAGE:** You can get the benefits of green tea either by taking green tea capsules or tablets, or by drinking several cups of the brew each day. Your aim should be to take in 240 to 320 mg of polyphenols.

When using supplements, buy those standardised to contain at least 50% polyphenols. At this concentration two 250 mg supplements would provide 250 mg of polyphenols. Studies show that four cups of freshly brewed green tea also supply a recommended amount of polyphenols.

◈ **GUIDELINES FOR USE:** Take green tea supplements at meals with a full glass of water. Drink freshly brewed green tea either on its own or with meals. To make tea, use 1 teaspoon of green tea leaves per 225 ml of very hot water. Let the brew steep for three to five minutes; then strain and drink it.

Possible side effects

Green tea is very safe both as a supplement and as a beverage, but people who are sensitive to caffeine may not want to drink large amounts of it because each cup contains about 40 mg of caffeine. Green tea supplements, however, have very little caffeine. The recommended dose of green tea supplements provides the same amount of polyphenols as four cups of green tea, but generally contains only 5 to 6 mg of caffeine.

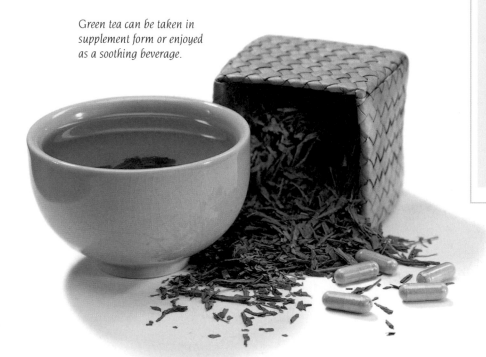

Green tea can be taken in supplement form or enjoyed as a soothing beverage.

Hawthorn

Crataegus oxyacantha

If you are diagnosed with any form of heart disease you will want to know all about hawthorn. This herb, historically used both as a diuretic and as a treatment for kidney and bladder stones, is now one of the most widely prescribed remedies for heart problems.

Common uses

- Relieves the chest pain of angina.
- Lowers high blood pressure.
- Helps the heart to pump more efficiently in people with heart disease.
- Corrects irregular heartbeat (cardiac arrhythmia).

Forms

- Capsule
- Dried herb/tea
- Powder
- Tablet
- Tincture

CAUTION!

REMINDER: *If you have a medical condition, consult your doctor before taking supplements.*

What it is

For centuries hawthorn, a shrub or tree that grows up to 9 metres high, has been trimmed to hedge height and planted along the edges of fields or as a garden boundary. As a divider it both looks attractive and discourages trespassers: it produces pretty white flowers and vibrant red berries, but it also has large thorns. (The crown of thorns worn by Christ at the Crucifixion is believed to have been woven from hawthorn twigs.)

Knowledge of the cardioprotective benefits of hawthorn was widespread among peoples of different eras and locations, from the ancient Greeks to the Native Americans, who considered the herb a potent heart tonic. Modern use of hawthorn originated with the 19th-century Irish physician Dr D. Greene of Ennis, who had great success in treating heart disease. Greene guarded his heart formula closely, and it was not until after his death in the 1890s that his secret remedy was revealed to be tincture of hawthorn berry.

What it does

Hawthorn is a herb that directly benefits the workings of the heart and the arteries. It can dilate blood vessels, increase the heart's energy supply and improve its pumping ability. These gentle but valuable cardiac effects can probably be traced to its abundant supply of plant compounds called flavonoids – especially oligomeric proanthocyanidin complexes (OPCs) – which function as potent antioxidants.

Hawthorn supplements are derived from the plant's leaves and flowers, its red berries (right), or a combination of all three.

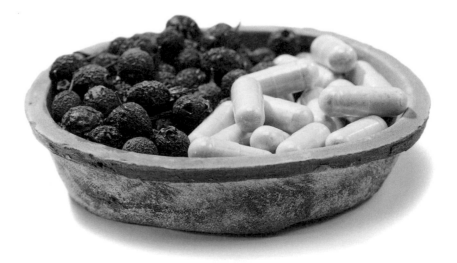

⚫ MAJOR BENEFITS: Hawthorn can have beneficial effects on the heart. It widens the arteries by interfering with an enzyme called ACE (angiotensin-converting enzyme), which constricts blood vessels. This action improves blood flow through the arteries, which makes the herb a good remedy for people with angina. In addition, chronically constricted arteries can lead to high blood pressure (because the heart must work harder to pump blood through inflexible arteries), so hawthorn may reduce blood pressure in those with mild hypertension.

Hawthorn also seems to block enzymes that weaken the heart muscle, thereby strengthening its pumping power. This property makes it especially useful for people with mild heart disease who do not need strong heart medications such as digitalis. Moreover, the antioxidant properties of hawthorn may help to protect against damage associated with the build-up of plaque in the coronary arteries.

⚫ ADDITIONAL BENEFITS: Hawthorn has a long history as a treatment for other conditions as well. It seems to exert a calming effect and functions as a sleeping aid in some people who suffer from insomnia. Several researchers have also noted that hawthorn preserves collagen – the protein that composes connective tissue – which is damaged in such diseases as arthritis.

How to take it

⚫ DOSAGE: The recommended dose of hawthorn extract ranges from 300 to 450 mg a day in capsule or tablet form, and from 1 teaspoon to 1 tablespoon of the tincture, depending on the type of heart condition. People at risk of heart disease may wish to take a 100 to 150 mg supplement or 1 teaspoon of the tincture daily as a heart disease preventative.

⚫ GUIDELINES FOR USE: If you are taking large doses, hawthorn works best when the daily amount is split up and taken at three different times during the day. Hawthorn may take a couple of months to build up in your system and produce noticeable results.

Possible side effects

Hawthorn is widely regarded as one of the safest herbal preparations. Although there have been reports of nausea, sweating, fatigue and skin rashes, these side effects are rare. Hawthorn appears to be safe to use with drugs prescribed for heart disease; you may even need less of some heart medications while you are taking it. But consult your doctor before trying hawthorn, and never stop taking a prescribed drug (or reduce the dose) except on your doctor's advice.

Iodine

Many people associate iodine with the orange-brown topical antiseptic used to clean childhood cuts and grazes, but the real value of this potent trace mineral springs from its role in the manufacture of thyroxine, the hormone responsible for regulating metabolism.

Common uses

- *Corrects an iodine deficiency.*
- *Ensures proper functioning of the thyroid gland.*
- *May help to treat fibrocystic breasts.*

Forms

- Capsule
- Liquid
- Tablet

What it is

Although the body needs only tiny amounts of iodine, this mineral is so crucial to an individual's overall health that in the 1920s US government officials decided that it should be added to a foodstuff common to nearly everyone – table salt. The introduction of iodised salt to the American diet virtually eliminated one severe form of mental retardation called cretinism. In the UK salt is not routinely iodised, although you can buy an iodised brand of salt if you wish to supplement iodine in this way. Apart from iodised salt, fish and seafood are the best dietary sources of iodine, as well as fruit, vegetables and cereals grown in iodine-rich soil.

Despite the recognised importance of this vital mineral, however, about 1.6 billion people in the world, mostly in developing countries, still suffer from iodine deficiency.

What it does

Unique among minerals, iodine has only one known function in the body: it is essential to the thyroid gland for manufacturing thyroxine, a hormone that regulates metabolism in all the body's cells.

PREVENTION: By getting enough iodine, a pregnant woman can prevent certain types of mental retardation in her developing foetus.

ADDITIONAL BENEFITS: Unlike many other minerals, iodine does not seem to help in the treatment of specific diseases, but it plays a crucial role in assuring the health of the thyroid, the butterfly-shaped gland that surrounds the windpipe (trachea). When your iodine intake is adequate your body contains about 40 mg of it, and 75% of that amount is stored in the thyroid. This gland controls the body's overall metabolism, which determines how quickly and efficiently calories are burned. It also regulates growth and development in children, reproduction, nerve and muscle function, the breakdown of proteins and fats, the growth of nails

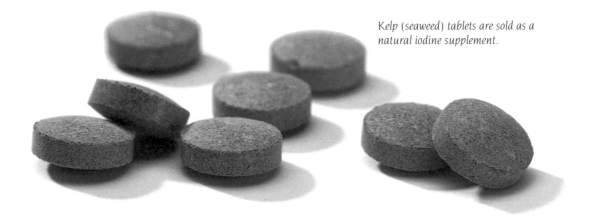

Kelp (seaweed) tablets are sold as a natural iodine supplement.

and hair, and the use of oxygen by every cell in the body. There is some evidence that iodine derived from an organic source may be effective in reducing the pain of fibrocystic breasts, but patients should discuss this type of supplementation with their doctor first.

How much you need

The recommended target for iodine is 140 mcg daily for adult men and women. One teaspoon of iodised salt contains about 300 mcg of iodine, but there is a wide range of other dietary sources (see below).

⊟ **IF YOU GET TOO LITTLE:** Iodine deficiency is extremely rare in developed countries, but the first signs include an enlarged thyroid gland, known as a goitre. Lack of iodine can cause the gland to expand in an attempt to increase its surface area and trap as much of the iodine in the bloodstream as possible. Although a low iodine intake can result in low levels of thyroid hormone (hypothyroidism), the most likely cause is a condition known as myxoedema, which results from autoimmune damage (when the body's immune system turns on itself). Hypothyroidism is characterised by fatigue, dry skin, a rise in blood fats, a hoarse voice, delayed reflexes and reduced mental clarity. Consult your doctor if you have these symptoms.

⊞ **IF YOU GET TOO MUCH:** There is very little risk of iodine overdose, even at levels 10 to 20 times the recommended amount. However, if you ingest 30 times the recommended amount you are likely to experience a metallic taste, mouth sores, swollen salivary glands, diarrhoea, vomiting, headache, a rash and difficulty in breathing. Ironically, a goitre can also develop if you consistently take extremely large amounts of iodine, which is one of the causes of thyrotoxicosis. This condition may be associated with high levels of thyroid hormone, leading to over-activity, rapid reflexes, anxiety and excessive weight loss.

How to take it

⊘ **DOSAGE:** You probably get all the iodine you need from your daily diet, especially if you regularly eat fish. Iodine is also a standard ingredient in many multivitamin and mineral supplements. People on a thyroid hormone should always discuss their condition with their doctor before taking individual iodine supplements.

◉ **GUIDELINES FOR USE:** When prescribed, iodine supplements can be taken at any time of the day, with or without food.

Other sources

The mineral can also be found in saltwater fish and in sea vegetation, such as kelp. Soil in coastal areas also tends to be iodine-rich, as are the dairy products derived from cows grazing there. The same is true for fruits and vegetables grown in soil high in iodine. Commercial baked goods – such as breads and cakes – can also be good sources of iodine.

RECENT FINDINGS

An analysis of ten different studies conducted in countries where iodine deficiency is common found evidence that an iodine deficiency can affect motor skills, decreasing reaction time, manual dexterity, coordination and muscle strength. The analysis, headed by UNICEF researchers, also revealed that the IQ of people who were iodine deficient was some 13 points below that of those with adequate iodine.

FACTS & TIPS

■ Even though health-food shops often promote sea salt as a healthier alternative to table salt, it is not iodised and therefore is not a good source of iodine.

Iron

A surprising number of people have insufficient iron in their diets – and few realise that lack of the mineral can make them weak, unable to concentrate and more susceptible than normal to infection. Too much iron, however, can be dangerous, so be cautious about taking supplements.

Common uses

- *Treats iron-deficiency anaemia.*

- *Often needed during pregnancy; by women with heavy menstrual periods; or in other situations determined by your doctor.*

Forms

- Capsule
- Liquid
- Softgel
- Tablet

CAUTION!

■ Avoid high-dose supplements containing iron alone, unless they have been prescribed by your doctor. Some people suffer from haemochromatosis, an inherited disease which causes them to absorb too much iron, and most don't even know they have it. (Early symptoms include fatigue and aching joints.)

■ A supplement containing iron alone could also mask a cause of anaemia, such as a bleeding ulcer, and prevent your doctor from making an early, life-saving diagnosis.

REMINDER: If you have a medical condition, consult your doctor before taking supplements.

What it is

Needed throughout the body, iron is an essential part of haemoglobin, the oxygen-carrying component of red blood cells. The mineral is also found in myoglobin, which supplies oxygen to the muscles, and is part of many enzymes and immune-system compounds. The body, which gets most of the iron it needs from foods, carefully monitors its iron status, absorbing more of the mineral when demand is high (during periods of rapid growth, such as pregnancy or childhood) and less when stores of it are adequate. Because the body loses iron when bleeding, menstruating women may often have low levels. Vegetarians, people on weight-loss diets and endurance athletes may experience iron shortfalls as well.

What it does

By helping the blood and muscles to deliver oxygen, iron supplies energy to every cell in the body. Yet iron deficiency is surprisingly common in the UK. According to government surveys, the majority of women do not reach their dietary target of 14.8 mg daily. Although for most people it is very difficult to develop an iron deficiency from poor nutrition (iron is found in many foods), women with heavy menstrual periods may be particularly at risk and will benefit from iron supplementation, as will people with medical conditions that give rise to iron-deficiency anaemia.

✪ **MAJOR BENEFITS:** Keeping your body well supplied with iron provides vitality, helps your immune system function at its best and gives your mind an edge. Studies show that even mild iron deficiency – well short of the levels commonly associated with anaemia – can cause adults to have a short attention span and teenagers to do poorly in school.

How much you need

The recommended daily amount for iron is 8.7 mg a day for men and for postmenopausal women. For younger women it is 14.8 mg a day, with no recommendation for an additional requirement during pregnancy. To combat anaemia, additional iron – through either diet or supplements – is typically needed for a period of weeks or months.

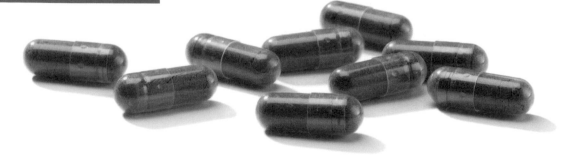

⊖ **IF YOU GET TOO LITTLE:** If you get too little iron in your diet or lose too much through heavy menstrual periods, stomach bleeding (commonly caused by arthritis drugs) or cancer, your body draws on its iron reserve. Initially there are no symptoms, but as your iron supply dwindles, so does your body's ability to produce healthy red blood cells. The result is iron-deficiency anaemia, marked by weakness, fatigue, paleness, breathlessness, palpitations and increased susceptibility to infection.

⊕ **IF YOU GET TOO MUCH:** Some studies link too much iron to an increased risk of chronic diseases, including heart disease and colon cancer. Excess iron can be particularly dangerous in adults with a genetic tendency to overabsorb it (haemochromatosis), and in children, who are especially susceptible to iron overdose.

How to take it

▨ **DOSAGE:** Unless a practitioner advises otherwise, iron should be taken only in the form of a multivitamin or multimineral supplement at no more than the recommended daily amount. Anaemia requires a careful diagnosis, and treatment to correct the underlying cause. When prescribed by a doctor, iron is typically taken in a form called ferrous salts – usually ferrous sulphate, ferrous fumarate or ferrous gluconate. A typical prescribed dose provides about 30 mg of iron one to three times daily. Most men and postmenopausal women do not need iron supplements and should consider taking a multivitamin or multimineral supplement that does not contain this nutrient.

◉ **GUIDELINES FOR USE:** Iron is best absorbed when taken on an empty stomach. However, if iron upsets your stomach, have it with meals, preferably with a small amount of meat and a food or drink rich in vitamin C, such as broccoli or orange juice, to help boost the amount of iron your body absorbs.

Other sources

Iron-rich foods include liver, beef and lamb. Clams, oysters and mussels also contain iron. Vegetarians can get adequate amounts of iron from beans and peas, leafy green vegetables, dried fruits, such as apricots and raisins, and fortified breakfast cereals. Brewer's yeast, kelp, molasses and wheat bran are also good sources.

If you need to increase your iron intake, choose raisins as a snack.

Kelp and spirulina

Health enthusiasts are looking to the seas and lakes for algae and plant proteins that are powerful food supplements. Predominant among the aquatic plants that have been found to contain various beneficial substances are kelp and spirulina.

Common uses

Kelp
- *Treats an underactive thyroid gland.*
- *Provides essential nutrients.*

Spirulina
- *Treats bad breath.*
- *Adds protein, vitamins and minerals to the diet.*

Forms
- Capsule
- Liquid
- Powder
- Tablet
- Tincture

CAUTION!

■ **Kelp may aggravate the condition of patients taking medication for an overactive thyroid.**

REMINDER: If you have a medical condition, consult your doctor before taking supplements.

What they are

Kelp and spirulina are two very different types of aquatic alga. Kelp, a long-stemmed seaweed, is derived from various species of brown algae known as *Fucus* or *Laminaria*. It is a prime source of iodine, a mineral crucial in preventing thyroid problems.

The smaller spirulina (also known as a blue-green alga) is actually a single-celled microorganism, or microalga, that closely resembles a bacterium. Because its spiral-shaped filaments are rich in the plant pigment chlorophyll, spirulina turns the lakes and ponds where it grows a dark blue-green.

What they do

Kelp and spirulina have been used medicinally for thousands of years in China. Devotees make many claims for their powers – ranging from increased libido to reduced hair loss – but most are highly speculative. The algae do, however, have some confirmed medicinal properties.

✪ **MAJOR BENEFITS:** The high iodine content of kelp makes it useful for treating an underactive thyroid caused by a shortage of iodine. This remedy is rarely necessary, however, because iodised salt supplies plenty of this mineral. Kelp is also marketed as a weight-loss aid, but it is probably effective only in the extremely rare cases when weight gain is secondary to an iodine-deficient underactive thyroid. Kelp should be taken only under a doctor's close supervision for the treatment of thyroid disorders.

Spirulina is a prime source of chlorophyll so it is ideal for combating one of life's most troublesome minor complaints: bad breath. It can be an extremely effective remedy, provided that the condition is not due to gum disease or chronic sinusitis. Spirulina is a key ingredient of many commercial chlorophyll breath-fresheners.

Spirulina is the most popular of the blue-green algae supplements.

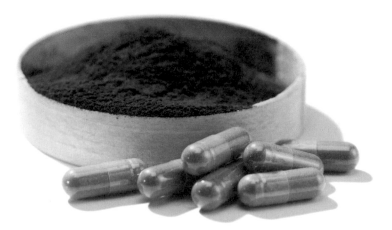

✱ **ADDITIONAL BENEFITS:** Sometimes kelp and spirulina are included in vegetarian and macrobiotic diets. In addition to iodine, kelp provides carotenoids as well as fatty acids, potassium, magnesium, calcium, iron and other nutrients. Spirulina contains protein, vitamins (including B_{12} and folic acid), carotenoids and other nutrients. The concentrations of all these substances appear to be fairly low, however. There are many less expensive – and better tasting – sources of vitamins and minerals than kelp and spirulina, including an array of popular garden vegetables.

Various other claims are made for kelp and spirulina – that they boost energy, relieve arthritis, enhance liver function, prevent heart disease and certain types of cancer, boost immunity, suppress HIV and AIDS, and protect cells against damage from X-rays or heavy metals such as lead. But most studies on these supplements have been done in test tubes or with animals, and more research is needed.

How to take them

⬚ **DOSAGE:** *To use kelp for an underactive thyroid:* Use kelp only when it is recommended by your doctor; if iodine is needed, your doctor can prescribe an appropriate dose. Powder forms dissolve easily in water, though some people do not like the taste. Tablets, capsules and tinctures are equally effective.

To freshen the breath with spirulina: Use a commercial, chlorophyll-rich 'green' drink (the label will often say if the chlorophyll is derived in part from spirulina) or mix a teaspoon of spirulina powder in half a glass of water. Swish the liquid around the mouth, then swallow it. Alternatively, chew a tablet thoroughly and then swallow it. Repeat three or four times a day, or as needed.

◉ **GUIDELINES FOR USE:** Take with food to minimise the chances of digestive upset. Pregnant or breastfeeding women may want to avoid kelp because of its high iodine content, though spirulina seems to be very safe.

Possible side effects

Occasionally nausea or diarrhoea develops in those taking kelp or spirulina; if this side effect occurs, lower or stop the dose. Up to 3% of the population is sensitive to iodine and may experience adverse reactions to long-term ingestion of kelp – including a painful enlargement of the thyroid gland that disappears once the kelp is discontinued. This condition is most common in Japan, where seaweed is a dietary staple.

Kelp is an important source of iodine.

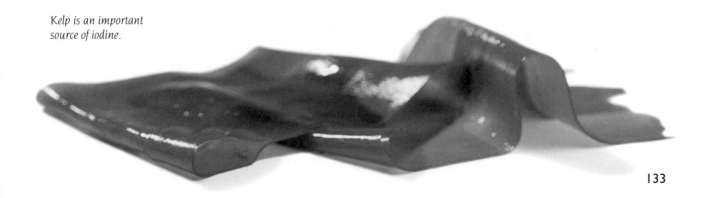

Lecithin and choline

These closely related nutrients with rather daunting scientific names are essential for the proper functioning of every cell in the body. They have particularly important roles to play in maintaining a healthy liver and nervous system.

Common uses

- Aid in the prevention of gallstones.
- Strengthen the liver, which makes them useful in the treatment of hepatitis and cirrhosis.
- Help the liver to eliminate toxins from the bodies of cancer patients undergoing chemotherapy.
- Diminish indigestion symptoms.
- May boost memory and enhance brain function.

Forms

- Capsule
- Liquid
- Powder
- Softgel
- Tablet

What they are

Lecithin (pronounced LESS-i-thin) is a fatty substance found in many animal and plant-based foods, including liver, eggs, soya beans, peanuts and wheat germ. It is often added to processed foods – including ice cream, chocolate, margarine and salad dressings – to help blend, or emulsify, the fats with water. It is also manufactured in the body.

Lecithin is considered an excellent source of choline, one of the B vitamins, primarily in the form called phosphatidylcholine. Once in the body, the phosphatidylcholine breaks down into choline, so that when you take lecithin, or absorb lecithin from foods, your body gets choline. However, only 10% to 20% of the lecithin found in plants and other natural sources consists of phosphatidylcholine.

Although dietary lecithin is a primary source of choline, choline is also found in liver, soya beans, egg yolks, grape juice, peanuts, cabbage and cauliflower. Choline supplements are available in health-food shops, and choline is a common ingredient of B-complex vitamins or other combination formulas.

What they do

Lecithin and choline are needed for a range of bodily functions. They help to build cell membranes and facilitate the movement of fats and nutrients in and out of cells. They aid in reproduction and in foetal and infant development; they are essential to liver and gall bladder health; and they may promote a healthy heart. Choline is also a key component of the brain chemical acetylcholine, which plays a prominent role in memory and muscle control.

As a result of their widely distributed effects, lecithin and choline have been touted for almost everything – from curing cancer and AIDS to lowering cholesterol. Even though the evidence for some of these claims is weak, the nutrients should not be dismissed out of hand.

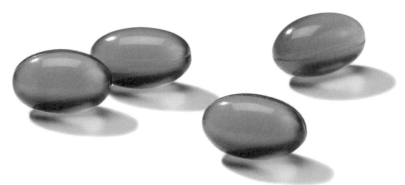

Lecithin supplements come in a variety of forms, including softgels.

✵ MAJOR BENEFITS: Lecithin and choline may be especially helpful in the treatment of gall bladder and liver diseases. Lecithin is a key component of bile, the fat-digesting substance, and low levels of this nutrient are known to precipitate gallstones. Taking supplements with lecithin or phosphatidylcholine, its purified extract, may help to treat or prevent this disorder. Lecithin may also be beneficial for the liver: the results of a ten-year study on baboons showed that it prevented severe liver scarring and cirrhosis caused by alcohol abuse, and other studies have indicated that it helps to relieve liver problems associated with hepatitis.

Choline is often included in liver complex formulas along with other liver-strengthening supplements, such as the amino acid methionine, the B vitamin inositol and the herbs milk thistle and dandelion. These preparations, sometimes called lipotropic combinations or factors, can protect against the build-up of fats within the liver, improve the flow of fats and cholesterol through the liver and gall bladder, and help the liver to rid the body of dangerous toxins. They may be especially effective in treating liver or gall bladder diseases, such as hepatitis, cirrhosis or gallstones, as well as conditions that benefit from good liver function, such as endometriosis (the leading cause of female infertility), and side effects from chemotherapy. Choline, along with the B vitamins pantothenic acid and thiamin, may also relieve indigestion.

✵ ADDITIONAL BENEFITS: These two nerve-building nutrients may be useful for improving memory in people with Alzheimer's disease, as well as for preventing neural tube birth defects (spina bifida), boosting performance in endurance sports and treating twitches and tics (tardive dyskinesia) caused by antipsychotic drugs. Lecithin and choline have also been proposed as possible remedies for high cholesterol and even cancer. However, more studies are needed to define their role in these and other diseases.

How to take them

☑ DOSAGE: Lecithin is usually given in a dosage of two 1200 mg capsules twice a day. It can also be taken in a granular form: 1 teaspoon contains 1200 mg of lecithin. Choline can be obtained from lecithin, although phosphatidylcholine (500 mg three times a day) or plain choline (500 mg three times a day) may be a better source. Choline can also be taken as part of a lipotropic combination product. In the UK no recommended amounts have been set for lecithin and choline, but the US Food and Drug Administration (FDA) has recognised choline as an essential nutrient and has recommended daily intakes of 550 mg for men and 425 mg for women.

◉ GUIDELINES FOR USE: Lecithin and choline should be taken with meals to enhance absorption. Granular lecithin has a nutty taste and can be sprinkled over foods or mixed into drinks.

Possible side effects

In high doses, lecithin and choline may cause sweating, nausea, vomiting, bloating and diarrhoea. Taking very high dosages of choline (10 grams a day) may produce a fishy body odour or a heart rhythm disorder.

Lutein

Lutein is a yellow pigment found in egg yolk, some algae, many plants and in the light sensitive cells at the back of the eye, where it helps to maintain healthy vision. Increased intake of lutein is linked with reduced risk of macular degeneration, the main cause of blindness in older people.

Common uses

- Important for eye health.
- Essential for the development of the macular pigment which protects light sensitive cells in the retina from free radical dmage.
- May lower the risk of macular degeneration.
- May improve vision in people with cataracts.
- May provide protection against some cancers.

Forms

- Capsule
- Softgel
- Sublingual spray
- Tablet

What it is

Lutein (and its chemical isomer zeaxanthin) is a member of the carotenoid family, *see page 64*. It gives the yellow colour to fruits and vegetables, such as mango, papaya, sweetcorn and tomato. However, the highest amounts of lutein are found in dark green vegetables such as kale, spinach and turnip greens. Broccoli, Brussels sprouts, peas, leeks and some types of lettuce, particularly Cos and Romaine lettuce are also good dietary sources. The greener the vegetable, the more lutein it contains, and raw vegetables are better sources than cooked.

The amount of lutein found in the average UK diet is between 1 mg and 3 mg a day. Though official UK recommendations for lutein intake have not been made, results of research suggest that an appropriate intake could be 6 mg a day. Even people who eat large quantities of fruit and vegetables could find that hard to manage.

What it does

Lutein is an antioxidant. This means that it has the ability to neutralise harmful free radicals (substances produced by pollution, radiation, fried and burnt foods, sunlight and combustion) that may have entered the body. These free radicals can damage cells and accelerate ageing. At one time, it was thought that all antioxidants served the same purpose but there is growing evidence that they have specific functions.

Lutein is thought to play an important role in maintaining healthy vision because it is the main pigment found in the central region of the retina, known as the macula. This is the region of maximum visual sensitivity. As we get older, the cells with retinal pigment become less efficient, the retina degenerates and central vision is gradually lost. This process is known as age-related macular degeneration (ARMD).

One of the causes of macular degeneration is damage from the free radicals in sunlight. Lutein may protect the macula by acting as an optical filter for sunlight and as an antioxidant to soak up the free radicals. Lutein may also play a role in maintaining immunity.

MAJOR BENEFITS: Scientific studies have generally found an increased risk of macular degeneration with low levels of lutein in the diet or in the blood; however, conclusive evidence that increased intakes will reduce the incidence of ARMD or help to treat it is not yet available. Small studies have provided encouraging results. A recent US study found that supplementation with lutein and other antioxidants in people with early ARMD had a beneficial effect on macular function. And another trial published in *Optometry* found that a daily dose of 10 mg lutein, alone or with other antioxidant supplements, improved visual function in 90 patients with atrophic ARMD over a period of 12 months.

Research looking at the role of lutein in cataract prevention has so far not been encouraging. But lutein supplements have been found to improve visual acuity and glare sensitivity in people with cataracts.

Pending the results of further research, it is important to consume a diet rich in leafy green vegetables, which should supply high amounts of lutein. If you do not like fresh vegetables, your diet may be lacking in this nutrient.

✳ **ADDITIONAL BENEFITS:** High dietary intake of lutein has been linked with reduced risk of some cancers, most notably endometrial, ovarian and breast cancer. A US study found an intake of more than 7,300 mcg (7.3 mg) a day of lutein was associated with a 70 per cent reduced risk of endometrial cancer. The risk of ovarian cancer has been shown to be reduced by 40 per cent in women with a weekly intake of lutein of more than 24,000 mcg (24 mg) compared with a weekly intake of less than 3,800 mcg (3.8 mg). In another study, lutein intake of more than 7,162 mcg (7.162 mg) daily was associated with a 53 per cent reduction in the risk of developing breast cancer compared with consumption of less than 3652 mcg (3.652 mg) daily.

How to take it

⬛ **DOSAGE:** *For general good eye health*: Take 6 mg daily (if your diet does not contain dark leafy green vegetables.) Supplements containing these amounts are available. *For prevention*: To reduce the risk of eye disorders such as cataracts and macular degeneration, take 6-15 mg lutein daily.

◉ **GUIDELINES FOR USE:** Take with food in a single daily dose. Benefits develop slowly and may not fully develop for six months to two years.

Possible side effects

There are no known side effects from either short-term or long-term use of lutein. No interactions with drugs have been found.

RECENT FINDINGS

A randomised controlled trial published in *Nutrition* investigated 17 people with age-related cataracts. Supplementation with 15 mg lutein three times a week for up to two years resulted in improved visual performance (visual acuity and glare sensitivity) compared with placebo.

—〰—

A short-term study published in *Ophthalmology* found that supplementation with lutein, vitamin E and nicotinamide daily for 180 days in 30 patients with early ARMD and visual acuity of 6/9 or better found that treatment had a beneficial effect on macular function.

FACTS & TIPS

These foods can supply your daily lutein needs :

■ A serving of kale or turnip tops three times a week

■ A daily serving of spinach

■ A daily serving of broccoli and a leafy green salad

■ A daily serving of sprouts, peas and sweetcorn.

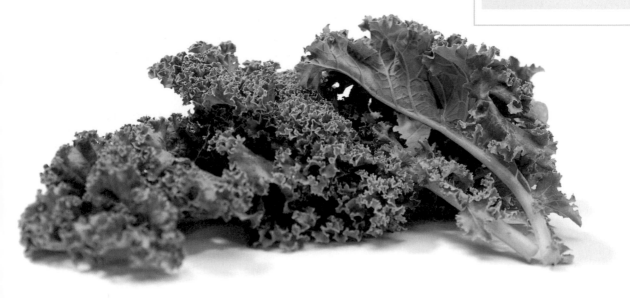

Magnesium

Although little heralded, magnesium may be one of the most important health-promoting minerals. Studies suggest that, as well as enhancing some 300 enzyme-related processes in the body, magnesium may help to prevent or combat many chronic diseases.

Common uses

- Helps to protect against heart disease and arrhythmia.
- Eases symptoms of chronic fatigue and fibromyalgia.
- Lowers high blood pressure.
- May reduce the severity of asthma attacks.
- Improves symptoms of premenstrual syndrome (PMS).
- Aids in preventing the complications of diabetes.

Forms

- Capsule
- Powder
- Tablet

What it is

The average person's body contains just under 30 grams of magnesium, but this small amount is vital to a number of bodily functions. Many people do not have adequate stores of magnesium, often because they rely too heavily on processed foods, which contain very little of this mineral. In addition, magnesium levels are easily depleted by stress, certain diseases or medications and intense physical activity. For this reason, nutritional supplements may be needed for the maintenance of optimal health. Supplements come in many forms, including magnesium acetate, magnesium carbonate, magnesium citrate, magnesium gluconate, magnesium oxide and magnesium sulphate.

What it does

One of the most versatile minerals, magnesium is involved in energy production, nerve function, muscle relaxation and bone and tooth formation. In conjunction with calcium and potassium, magnesium regulates heart rhythm and clots blood; it also aids in the production and use of insulin.

PREVENTION: Recent research indicates that magnesium is beneficial for the prevention and treatment of heart disease. Studies show that the risk of dying of a heart attack is lower in areas with 'hard' water, which contains high levels of magnesium. Some researchers speculate that if everyone drank hard water the number of deaths from heart attacks might decline by 19%. Magnesium appears to lower blood pressure, and has also been found to aid recovery after a heart attack by inhibiting blood clots, widening arteries and normalising dangerous arrhythmias.

Preliminary studies suggest that an adequate intake of magnesium may help to prevent non-insulin-dependent (type 2) diabetes. American researchers at Johns Hopkins University measured magnesium levels in more than 12,000 people who did not have diabetes, then tracked them for six years to see who developed the disease. Individuals with the lowest magnesium levels had a 94% greater chance of developing the disease than those with the highest levels. Further studies are needed to see if magnesium supplements can prevent the disease.

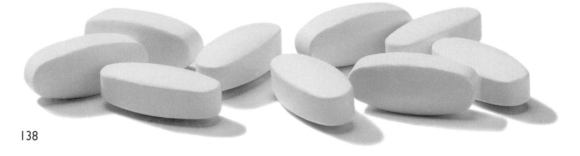

✥ **ADDITIONAL BENEFITS:** Magnesium relaxes muscles, so it is useful for sports injuries, chronic fatigue and fibromyalgia. It also seems to ease PMS and menstrual cramps, and may increase bone density in postmenopausal women, helping to stem the onset of osteoporosis. In addition, magnesium expands airways, which aids in the treatment of asthma and bronchitis. Studies are inconclusive about magnesium's role in preventing or treating migraines, but one study says it may improve the effect of sumatriptan, a prescription drug used for migraines.

How much you need

The recommended daily amount for magnesium is 300 mg for men and 270 mg for women. Higher doses are required for teenage girls (300 mg) and for disease prevention or treatment.

⊟ **IF YOU GET TOO LITTLE:** Even moderate deficiencies can increase the risk of heart disease and diabetes. Severe deficiencies can result in irregular heartbeat, fatigue, muscle spasms, irritability, nervousness and confusion.

✥ **IF YOU GET TOO MUCH:** Magnesium may cause diarrhoea and nausea. More serious side effects – including muscle weakness, lethargy, confusion and difficulty in breathing – can develop if the body is unable to process high doses properly. Large amounts lower blood pressure. and may therefore cause dizziness. But overdoses of magnesium are rare because absorption decreases as intake increases, and because the kidneys are usually efficient at eliminating excess amounts.

How to take it

🖉 **DOSAGE:** *For heart disease prevention*: Take 300 mg a day. *For arrythmias, asthma and recovery from heart failure*: Use 300 mg a day. *For chronic fatigue*: Take 150 mg of magnesium, preferably as magnesium citrate, twice a day. *For diabetes and high blood pressure*: Take 300 mg a day.

◉ **GUIDELINES FOR USE:** Magnesium is best absorbed when taken with each meal. If supplements cause diarrhoea, lower the dose or try magnesium glucomate, which has a gentler effect on the digestive tract.

Other sources

Good food sources of magnesium are whole grains, nuts, legumes, dark green leafy vegetables and shellfish.

One generous serving of wild rice supplies a third of an adult's daily magnesium needs.

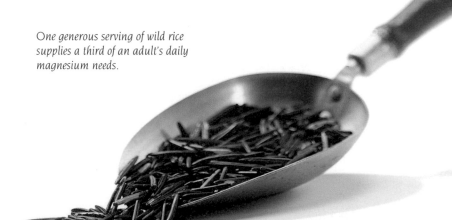

Milk thistle

Silybum marianum

The medicinal use of milk thistle can be traced back to ancient Greece and Rome. Today researchers around the world have completed more than 300 scientific studies that attest to the benefits of this herb, particularly in the treatment of liver ailments.

Common uses

- *Protects liver from toxins, including drugs, poisons and chemicals.*
- *Treats liver disorders such as cirrhosis and hepatitis.*
- *Reduces liver damage from excessive alcohol.*
- *Aids in the treatment and prevention of gallstones.*
- *Helps to clear psoriasis.*

Forms

- Capsule
- Softgel
- Tablet
- Tincture

CAUTION!

- Any liver disease requires careful evaluation and treatment by a doctor.

REMINDER: If you have a medical condition, consult your doctor before taking supplements.

What it is

Known by its botanical name, *Silybum marianum*, as well as by its main active ingredient, silymarin, milk thistle is a member of the sunflower family, with purple flowers and milky white leaf veins. The herb blooms from June to August, and the shiny black seeds used for medicinal purposes are collected at the end of summer.

What it does

Milk thistle is one of the most extensively studied and documented herbs in use today. Scientific research continues to validate its healing powers, particularly for the treatment of liver-related disorders. Most of its effectiveness stems from a complex of three liver-protecting compounds, collectively known as silymarin, which constitutes 4% to 6% of the ripe seeds.

⭐ **MAJOR BENEFITS:** Among the benefits of milk thistle is its ability to fortify the liver, one of the body's most important organs. The liver processes nutrients, including fats and other foods. In addition it neutralises, or detoxifies, many drugs, chemical pollutants and alcohol. Milk thistle helps to enhance and strengthen the liver by preventing the depletion of glutathione, an amino acid-like compound that is essential to the detoxifying process. Moreover, studies have shown that it can increase glutathione concentration by up to 35%. Milk thistle is an effective gatekeeper, limiting the number of toxins which the liver processes at any given time. The herb is also a powerful antioxidant. Even more potent than vitamins C and E, it helps to prevent damage

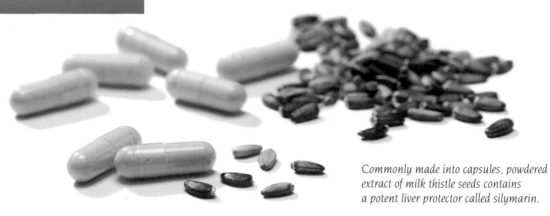

Commonly made into capsules, powdered extract of milk thistle seeds contains a potent liver protector called silymarin.

from highly reactive free-radical molecules. It promotes the regeneration of healthy new liver cells which replace old and damaged ones. Milk thistle eases a range of serious liver ailments, including viral infections (hepatitis) and scarring of the liver (cirrhosis). The herb is so potent that it is sometimes given in an injectable form in hospitable resuscitation rooms to combat the life-threatening, liver-obliterating effects of poisonous mushrooms. In addition, because excessive alcohol depletes glutathione, milk thistle can aid in protecting the livers of alcoholics or those recovering from alcohol abuse.

✳ **ADDITIONAL BENEFITS:** In cancer patients, milk thistle limits the potential for drug-induced damage to the liver after chemotherapy, and it speeds recovery by hastening the removal of toxic substances that can accumulate in the body. The herb also reduces the inflammation and may slow the skin-cell proliferation associated with psoriasis. It may be useful for endometriosis (the most common cause of infertility in women) because it helps the liver to process the hormone oestrogen, which at high levels can make pain and other symptoms worse. Finally, milk thistle can be beneficial in preventing or treating gallstones by improving the flow of bile, the cholesterol-laden digestive juice that travels from the liver through the gall bladder and into the intestine, where it helps to digest fats.

How to take it

▢ **DOSAGE:** The recommended dose for milk thistle is up to 200 mg of standardised extract (containing 70% to 80% silymarin) three times a day; lower doses are often very effective. It is often combined with other herbs and nutrients, such as dandelion, choline, methionine and inositol. This combination may be labelled 'liver complex' or 'lipotropic factors' ('lipotropic' refers to the formula's fat-metabolising properties; it prevents the build-up of fatty substances in the liver). For proper dosage follow the instructions on the packet.

◉ **GUIDELINES FOR USE:** Milk thistle extract seems most effective when taken between meals. However, if you want to take the herb itself, a tablespoon of ground milk thistle can be sprinkled over breakfast cereal, once daily. Milk thistle's benefits may be noticeable within a week or two, though long-term treatment is often needed for chronic conditions. The herb appears to be safe, even for pregnant and breastfeeding women. No interactions with other medications have been noted.

Possible side effects

Virtually no side effects have been attributed to the use of milk thistle, which is considered one of the safest herbs on the market. However, in some people it may have a slight laxative effect for a day or two.

Nettle

Urtica dioica

The healing powers of this herb were recognised by the ancient Greeks. One of its early uses was to remove venom from snakebites. Modern research shows that nettle leaf has a valuable role to play in treating eczema and hay fever, as well as in easing the pain and inflammation of gout.

Common uses

- Helps to reduce inflammation caused by eczema and skin rashes, and to relieve inflamed joints.
- Helps the body to eliminate excess fluid, and alleviates urinary tract infections.
- Relieves allergy symptoms, particularly hay fever.
- May ease prostate symptoms.

Forms

- Capsule
- Dried herb/tea
- Liquid
- Tincture

CAUTION!

REMINDER: If you have a medical condition, consult your doctor before taking supplements.

What it is

Strange as it may seem, the original interest in using nettle for medicinal purposes was probably inspired by the plant's ability to irritate exposed skin. Nettle leaves are covered with tiny hairs – hollow needles actually – that sting and burn upon contact. This effect was believed to be beneficial for joint pain (stinging oneself with nettle is an old folk remedy for arthritis), and for centuries nettle leaf poultices were applied to draw toxins from the skin.

Nettle leaves are also considered a nutritious food, and taste like spinach. They are particularly high in iron and other minerals and are rich in carotenoids and vitamin C. (Select young shoots, which have no stingers.) Found in parts of Europe, the USA and Canada, the plant often grows up to 1½ metres high.

What it does

Nettle leaf has valuable cleansing, detoxifying and diuretic properties, possibly owing to its high content of flavonoids and potassium. It is therefore helpful for alleviating many skin conditions, including childhood eczema, and the arthritic problems of later life. Stinging yourself with nettle leaves probably won't help your joint pain, but nettle tea applied as a compress or nettle supplements taken orally may relieve inflamed joints, especially in people with gout.

⚝ **MAJOR BENEFITS:** As a diuretic, nettle helps the body rid itself of excess fluid, and it may be useful as an auxiliary treatment for many disorders. People suffering from urinary tract infections, for example,

Supplements are a convenient way to obtain the diuretic and antihistamine benefits of nettle leaves.

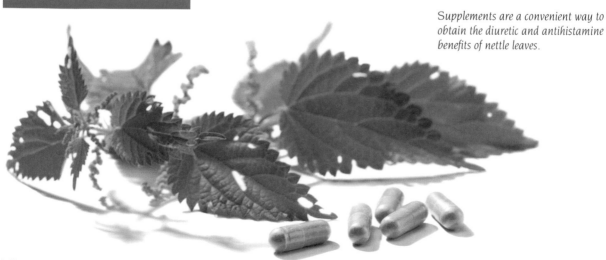

may find that it promotes urination, which flushes infection-causing bacteria out of the body. Women who become bloated just before their periods may experience some relief after taking nettle supplements.

One of the tried-and-tested benefits of nettle leaf is its ability to control hay fever symptoms. Nasal congestion and watery eyes result when the body produces an inflammatory compound called histamine in response to pollen and other allergens. Nettle is a good source of quercetin, a flavonoid that has been shown to inhibit the release of histamine. In one study of allergy sufferers, more than half of the participants rated nettle moderately to highly effective in reducing allergy symptoms when compared with a placebo.

✳ **ADDITIONAL BENEFITS:** Nettle leaf, taken internally, has an astringent action, and so helps to stop bleeding; it is used to treat nosebleeds and heavy menstrual bleeding.

Nettle root – rather than leaf – may be useful for men with enlarged prostate glands, when this is not caused by cancer. This condition, called benign prostatic hyperplasia (BPH), occurs when the prostate enlarges and narrows the urethra (the tube that transports urine out of the bladder), making urination difficult; diagnosis should be established by a doctor. Nettle root may aid in slowing prostate growth.

How to take it

📄 **DOSAGE:** *For fluid retention, allergies, eczema, excessive bleeding and gout:* Drink one cup of nettle tea three times a day; use 1 teaspoon of the dried herb per 250 ml of very hot water. Alternatively, take 250 mg extract three times a day, or one teaspoon of tincture three times a day. You can also apply a compress of nettle tea to painful joints. *For slowing prostate growth in* BPH: Take 250 mg nettle root (not leaf) extract twice a day, in combination with 160 mg of saw palmetto extract.

⊙ **GUIDELINES FOR USE:** Take nettle leaf (leaves, extract or tincture) with food to minimise the risk of stomach upset. If you want to try the fresh leaves as a vegetable, keep in mind that the young shoots can be eaten raw, but older leaves (with mature, stinging hairs) must be cooked to deactivate the stingers.

Possible side effects

Generally, nettle is considered safe, with only a minimal risk of causing an allergic reaction. There have been some reports, however, that it may irritate the stomach, causing indigestion and diarrhoea.

RECENT FINDINGS

In a preliminary study, nettle helped arthritis patients to cut down on painkillers and reduced the side effects of the drugs. No difference was found in pain, stiffness or the level of physical impairment between patients on 200 mg of the anti-inflammatory drug diclofenac (the brand name is Voltaren) and those taking 50 mg of the drug who also ate 50 grams of nettle leaves each day. In previous studies, lowering the diclofenac dose by just 25% lessened the drug's effectiveness in controlling the symptoms of arthritis.

Niacin

Severe deficiency of this B vitamin, also called nicotinamide and vitamin B_3, results in the debilitating disease pellagra, still found in some developing countries. In the western world niacin is used in the prevention and treatment of depression, arthritis and a host of other ailments.

Common uses

- May *improve circulation.*
- May *ease symptoms of arthritis.*
- May *relieve depression.*
- May *prevent progression of type II diabetes.*

Forms

- Capsule
- Tablet

What it is

The chemical structure of niacin is similar to that of the amino acid tryptophan – found in eggs, meat and poultry – and the body is able to obtain about half its niacin requirements by converting it from the chemical ingredients of tryptophan. The remainder has to come directly from the diet; many protein-rich foods are good sources. In addition, niacin can be obtained from dietary supplements and also from the many cereal products that have been fortified with this and other vitamins.

What it does

Niacin is needed to release energy from carbohydrate foods. It is also involved in controlling blood sugar, keeping skin healthy and maintaining the proper functioning of the nervous and digestive systems. The form of niacin usually sold in the UK is nicotinamide.

PREVENTION: In the 1940s and 1950s there were reports of very good clinical results when high doses of nicotinamide were used to treat people with rheumatoid arthritis and osteoarthritis. Within a few months there were improvements in joint function, range of motion, muscle strength and endurance. These findings have been confirmed by more recent studies. It appears that nicotinamide has an anti-inflammatory effect on these conditions and may help to heal damaged cartilage.

ADDITIONAL BENEFITS: Niacin helps to foster healthy brain and nerve cells, and there is some evidence to indicate that nicotinamide can ease depression, anxiety and insomnia. High doses of nicotinamide may reverse the development of type I diabetes – the form that typically appears before the age of 30 – if it is given early enough. However, this therapy should be tried only under medical supervision.

How much you need

The recommended daily amount of niacin intake is 13 mg for women and 17 mg for men. Far higher doses are required for the effective treatment of various disorders, when niacin is being used as a medication rather than a nutrient.

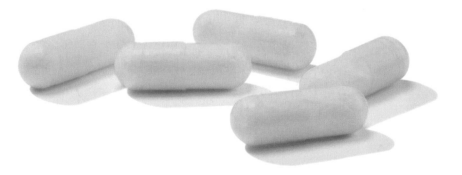

⊟ IF YOU GET TOO LITTLE: A slight niacin deficiency results in patches of irritated skin, appetite loss, indigestion and weakness. Severe deficiencies – which are practically nonexistent in industrialised countries – result in pellagra, a debilitating disease. Symptoms include a rash in areas exposed to sunlight, vomiting, a bright red tongue, fatigue and memory loss.

⊞ IF YOU GET TOO MUCH: Niacin in the form of nicotinamide presents no danger when taken at the levels normally recommended for dietary supplementation. The upper safe limit is 500 mg daily, When high intakes are regularly prescribed by a doctor, it is necessary for a check to be kept on liver function because too much niacin over a long period of time can damage this organ.

How to take it

▨ DOSAGE: *For anxiety and depression*: Take 50 mg of niacin a day; this dose can usually be found as part of a B-complex vitamin. *For insomnia*: Take 500 mg nicotinamide one hour before bedtime. *For arthritis*: Take 500 mg nicotinamide three times a day, but ensure that this treatment is administered only under the supervision of a doctor.

◉ GUIDELINES FOR USE: It is best to take niacin with meals to decrease the likelihood of stomach upset, especially at high doses. Do not take therapeutic doses of any form of niacin if you take cholesterol-lowering prescription drugs.

Other sources

Niacin is found in foods that are high in protein, such as chicken, beef, fish and nuts. Breads, cereals and some pasta are also enriched with niacin. Although they are low in niacin, eggs, milk and other dairy products are good alternative sources of the vitamin because they are high in tryptophan.

Many people obtain their daily requirement of niacin from fortified breakfast cereals.

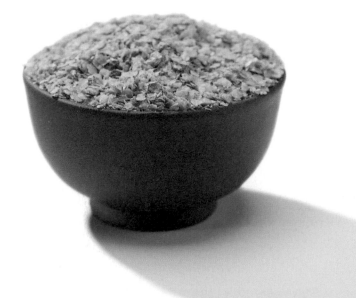

Pau d'arco

Tabebuia impetiginosa

Rumoured to have been prescribed by the Incas to treat serious ailments, the herb pau d'arco has been investigated as a remedy for infectious diseases and cancer. Although its anticancer properties have not yet been confirmed, it may indeed combat a variety of infections.

Common uses

- *Treats thrush.*
- *Helps to get rid of warts.*
- *Reduces inflammation of the airways in bronchitis.*
- *May be useful in treating such immune-related disorders as asthma, eczema, psoriasis and bacterial and viral infections.*

Forms

- Capsule
- Dried herb/tea
- Powder
- Softgel
- Tablet
- Tincture

CAUTION!

- **Pregnant or breastfeeding women should avoid pau d'arco.**
- **Pau d'arco may duplicate the effect of anticoagulant drugs.**

REMINDER: If you have a medical condition, consult your doctor before taking supplements.

What it is

Pau d'arco is obtained from the inner bark of a tree – *Tabebuia impetiginosa* – indigenous to the rain forests of South America. Native tribes have taken advantage of its healing powers for centuries. Pau d'arco is also known as *lapacho*, taheebo or *ipe roxo*. In the UK, however, it is always sold as pau d'arco.

The therapeutic ingredients in pau d'arco include a host of potent plant chemicals called naphthoquinones. Of these, lapachol has been the most intensely studied.

What it does

Lapachol and other compounds in pau d'arco help to destroy the microorganisms that cause diseases and infections, from malaria and flu to thrush. Most people, however, are interested in the potential cancer-fighting properties of the herb.

MAJOR BENEFITS: Pau d'arco appears to combat bacteria, viruses and fungi, reduce inflammation and support the immune system. One of its best-documented uses is for the treatment of thrush; herbalists often recommend a pau d'arco tea douche to restore the normal environment of the vagina. In capsule, tablet, tincture or tea form pau d'arco may be effective in strengthening immunity in cases of chronic fatigue syndrome, chronic bronchitis, or HIV and AIDS. The herb's anti-inflammatory properties likewise may help to treat acute bronchitis, which involves inflammation of the respiratory passages, as well as muscle pain. A directly applied tincture of pau d'arco can eradicate warts.

ADDITIONAL BENEFITS: Pau d'arco's anticancer activity is subject to continuing debate. Because of the herb's traditional reputation as a cancer fighter the US National Cancer Institute (NCI) investigated it, identifying lapachol as its most active ingredient. In animal studies pau

Pau d'arco can be taken as a supplement or brewed as a tea.

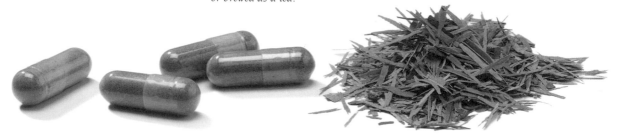

d'arco showed promise in shrinking tumours, and so in the 1970s the NCI began human trials using high doses of lapachol. Again there was some evidence that lapachol was active in destroying cancer cells, but participants taking a therapeutic dose suffered serious side effects, including nausea, vomiting and blood-clotting problems. As a result, research into lapachol and its source, pau d'arco, was abandoned.

Critics of this investigation believe that using therapeutic doses of pau d'arco – and not simply the isolated compound lapachol – would have produced similar benefits without the potentially dangerous blood-thinning effects. It's likely that lapachol interferes with the action of vitamin K, needed for the blood to clot properly. Some researchers suggest that other compounds in pau d'arco supply some vitamin K, so that use of the whole herb would not interfere with blood clotting. Others think that combining lapachol with vitamin K supplements might make it possible for people to take doses of lapachol high enough to permit its potential anti-tumour action to be studied further without provoking a reaction. Despite the controversy many practitioners rely on the historical evidence of pau d'arco's anticancer action and often recommend it as a complement to conventional cancer treatment.

How to take it

☑ **DOSAGE:** When pau d'arco is used in capsule or tablet form the typical dosage is 250 mg of the powered herb twice a day. This dose of pau d'arco is often recommended for chronic fatigue syndrome, or HIV and AIDS, in alternation with other immune-boosting herbs such as echinacea or goldenseal. Pau d'arco is also commonly taken as a tea in dried herb form. To make it, steep 2 or 3 teaspoons of pau d'arco in 500 ml of very hot water; drink the tea over the course of a day.

◉ **GUIDELINES FOR USE:** Herbalists recommend using whole-bark products (not only those that contain just lapachol) because they suspect that the herb's healing properties come from the full range of plant chemicals in the bark. For vaginal yeast infections: Let pau d'arco tea cool to lukewarm before using it as a douche. For warts: Apply a tincture-soaked compress to the affected area at bedtime and leave it on all night. Repeat until the wart disappears. Seek advice from your doctor if you suffer from genital warts.

Possible side effects

Whole-bark products are generally safe; they do not produce the side effects of high doses of lapachol. If pau d'arco tea or supplements cause stomach upset, take them with food.

Peppermint

Mentha piperita

For centuries this powerfully aromatic herb has provided relief for indigestion, colds and headaches. Today medicinal peppermint is most highly prized for its ability to soothe the digestive tract, easing indigestion, irritable bowel syndrome and other abdominal complaints.

Common uses

- *Relieves nausea and indigestion.*
- *Eases symptoms of diverticulitis and irritable bowel syndrome.*
- *Helps to dissolve gallstones.*
- *Sweetens the breath.*
- *Soothes muscle aches.*
- *Eases coughs and congestion caused by allergies or colds.*

Forms

- Capsule
- Dried or fresh herb/tea
- Oil
- Ointment/cream
- Tincture

What it is

Peppermint is cultivated worldwide for use as a flavouring and a herbal medicine. A natural hybrid of spearmint and water mint, peppermint has square stems, pointed dark green or purple oval leaves and lilac-coloured flowers. For medicinal purposes, the leaves and stems of the plant are harvested just before the flowers bloom in summer. The major active ingredient of peppermint is its volatile oil, which is made up of more than 40 different compounds. The oil's therapeutic effect comes mainly from menthol (35% to 55% of the oil), menthone (15% to 30%) and menthyl acetate (3% to 10%). Medicinal peppermint oil is made by steam-distilling the parts of the plant that grow above the ground.

What it does

Particularly effective in treating digestive disorders, peppermint relieves cramps and relaxes intestinal muscles. It freshens the breath and may clear up nasal congestion as well.

⚡ **MAJOR BENEFITS:** Peppermint oil relaxes the muscles of the digestive tract, helping to relieve intestinal cramping and gas. Its antispasmodic effect also makes it useful for alleviating the symptoms of irritable bowel syndrome, a common disorder characterised by abdominal pain, alternating bouts of diarrhoea and constipation, and indigestion. The menthol in peppermint aids digestion because it stimulates the flow of natural digestive juices and bile. This action explains why peppermint oil

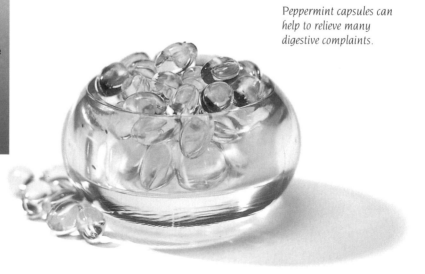

Peppermint capsules can help to relieve many digestive complaints.

is commonly included in over-the-counter antacids. Several studies show that the menthol in peppermint oil also assists in dissolving gallstones, providing a possible alternative to surgery. Consult your doctor before trying the oil for this purpose. You can also put the oil directly on your tongue; it provides a minty antidote to bad breath.

As a tea or an oil, peppermint serves as a mild anaesthetic to the stomach's mucous lining, which helps to reduce nausea and motion sickness. The tea may ease symptoms of diverticulitis as well, including flatulence and bloating.

✱ **ADDITIONAL BENEFITS:** When rubbed on the skin, peppermint oil relieves pain by stimulating the nerves that perceive cold while muting those that sense pain, which makes it a good remedy for aching muscles.

Results of studies into peppermint's traditional use in the treatment of colds and coughs are contradictory. Some tests show that the plant has no effect, but Commission E, a German health board recognised as an authority on the scientific investigation of herbs, found that it was an effective decongestant that reduced inflammation of the nasal passageways. Many people with colds report that inhaling peppermint's menthol enables them to breathe more easily. Peppermint tea also may offer relief from the bronchial constriction of asthma.

How to take it

📋 **DOSAGE:** *For the treatment of irritable bowel syndrome, nausea and gallstones:* Do not ingest peppermint oil itself; enteric-coated capsules release peppermint oil where it's most needed – in the small and large intestine rather than in the stomach. Take one or two capsules (containing 0.2 ml of oil per capsule) two or three times a day, between meals. *To freshen the breath:* Place a few drops of peppermint oil on the tongue. *To relieve flatulence and calm the stomach:* Make a tea by steeping 1 or 2 teaspoons of dried peppermint leaves in 250 ml of very hot water for between 5 and 10 minutes; be sure to cover the cup to prevent the volatile oil from escaping. *For congestion:* Drink up to four cups of peppermint tea a day. *For pain relief:* Add a few drops of peppermint oil to 45 ml (3 tablespoons) of a neutral oil. Apply to the affected areas up to four times daily.

◉ **GUIDELINES FOR USE:** Take enteric-coated capsules between meals. If you prefer peppermint tea, drink a cup three or four times a day, after or between meals. Apply peppermint oil or ointments containing menthol no more than three or four times daily. To take peppermint tincture, put 10 to 20 drops in a glass of water. Peppermint oil should not be used if you are taking homoeopathic treatment, and avoid it during pregnancy.

Possible side effects

Peppermint in the recommended doses generally has no side effects, even when taken for long periods. There have been rare instances of skin rashes and indigestion caused by enteric-coated peppermint oil capsules. Topical peppermint oil can produce allergic skin rashes, especially if heat is being applied as well. If side effects occur, stop using the herb.

Phosphorus

The main function of phosphorus is to interact with calcium to build and maintain strong bones and teeth, but the mineral also plays an essential role in the process of supplying energy to every cell in the body. Fortunately, the likelihood of deficiency is very small.

Common uses

- Builds strong bones and maintains skeletal integrity.
- Helps to form tooth enamel and strengthens teeth.

Forms

- Capsule
- Liquid
- Powder
- Tablet

What it is

Phosphorus is the second most abundant mineral in the body after calcium, and up to 650 grams of it are found in the average person. Although 85% of this mineral is concentrated in the bones and teeth, the rest is distributed in the blood and in various organs, including the heart, kidneys, brain and muscles. Phosphorus interacts with a variety of other nutrients, but its most constant companion is calcium. In the bones the ratio of calcium to phosphorus is around 2:1. In other tissues, however, the ratio of phosphorus to calcium is much higher.

What it does

There is hardly a biological or cellular process that does not, directly or indirectly, involve phosphorus. In some instances the mineral works to protect cells, strengthening the membranes that surround them; in other cases it acts as a kind of biological escort, assisting a variety of nutrients, hormones and chemicals in doing their jobs. There is also evidence that phosphorus helps to activate the B vitamins and enables them to provide all their benefits.

✪ MAJOR BENEFITS: One of phosphorus's most important functions is to team up with calcium to build bones and aid in maintaining a healthy, strong skeleton. The phosphorus-calcium partnership is also crucial for strengthening the teeth and keeping them strong. In addition phosphorus joins with fats in the blood to make compounds called phospholipids which, in turn, play structural and metabolic roles in cell membranes throughout the body. Furthermore, without phosphorus the body could not convert the proteins, carbohydrates and fats from food into energy. The mineral is needed to create the molecule known as adenosine triphosphate, or ATP, which acts like a tiny battery charger, supplying vital energy to every cell in the body.

✪ ADDITIONAL BENEFITS: Phosphorus serves as a cell-to-cell messenger. In this capacity it contributes to the coordination of such body processes as muscle contraction, the transmission of nerve impulses from the brain

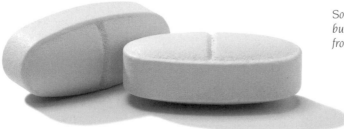

Some multivitamin pills contain phosphorus, but most people get enough of this mineral from their daily diet.

to the body and the secretion of hormones. An adequate phosphorus supply may therefore enhance physical performance and be effective in fighting fatigue. The mineral is necessary for maintaining the pH (the acid-base balance) of the blood and for manufacturing DNA and RNA, the basic components of our genetic makeup.

How much you need

Phosphorus is found in so many foods that the need for supplements is virtually nonexistent. The recommended target for phosphorus in men and women is the same, 550 mg daily. In the past many nutritionists recommended that phosphorus and calcium be taken in a 1:1 ratio, but most recently practitioners have advised that this ratio has little practical benefit. Most people today consume more phosphorus than calcium in their diets.

⊟ **IF YOU GET TOO LITTLE:** Although rare, a deficiency of phosphorus can lead to fragile bones and teeth, fatigue, weakness, a loss of appetite, joint pain and stiffness, and an increased susceptibility to infection. A mild deficiency may produce a modest decrease in energy.

⊞ **IF YOU GET TOO MUCH:** There are no immediate adverse effects from getting too much phosphorus. In the long term, excessive intake of phosphorus may inhibit calcium absorption, though it is uncertain whether this can result in a calcium deficiency that threatens bone health.

How to take it

⊘ **DOSAGE:** Most people get all the phosphorus they require in their everyday diets. In addition a small amount of phosphorus may be included in daily multivitamin and mineral supplements. If you have a medical condition that depletes this mineral, such as a bowel ailment or failing kidneys, your doctor will prescribe an appropriate dose.

◉ **GUIDELINES FOR USE:** Never take individual phosphorus supplements except on medical advice.

Other sources

High-protein foods, such as meat, fish, poultry and dairy products, contain a lot of phosphorus. It is also used as an additive in many processed foods. Soft drinks, particularly colas, often have large amounts. Phosphorus is present in grain products as well, although wholegrain breads and cereals may include ingredients that partially reduce its absorption.

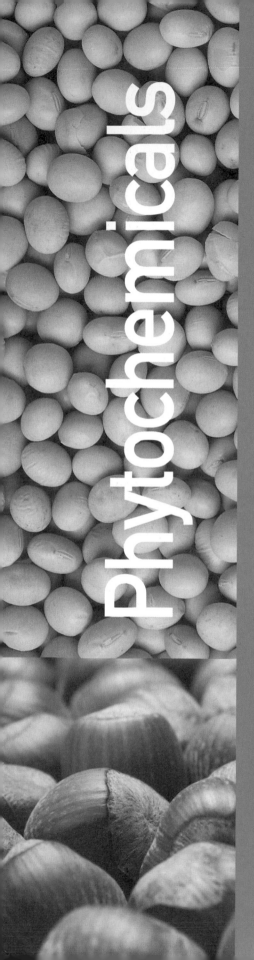

Phytochemicals

Phytochemicals are compounds naturally present in plants. They are neither vitamins, trace minerals nor dietary fibre, but are nevertheless biologically active in the human body. In recent years they have generated particular interest as a result of their potential benefits to health. While most research has focused on fruit and vegetables as sources of phytochemicals, similar substances are found in culinary and medicinal herbs.

Phytochemicals have been shown to have complementary and overlapping effects on the human body. As well as a host of antioxidant, antibacterial and antiviral actions, these include:

- Stimulating liver enzymes that deal with and help to get rid of toxins.
- Stimulating the functioning of the immune system.
- Reducing the danger of blood clots.
- Regulating cholesterol levels and hormone metabolism.
- Reducing blood pressure.

ANTIOXIDANT EFFECTS
Most phytochemicals have powerful antioxidant properties, good examples being flavonoids and carotenoids. This means they are able to neutralise free radicals, the unstable molecules that can cause cell damage.

The antioxidant action of phytochemicals is believed to reduce the risk of heart disease and to limit the development of inflammation in tissues that are being damaged by free radicals. For example, quercetin (found in onions and apples) has an anti-inflammatory action that may help to alleviate allergic respiratory reactions such as hay fever and asthma, skin conditions such as eczema, and inflammatory disorders of the joints and muscles.

FLAVONOIDS
Flavonoids (or bioflavonoids) are a large group of phyto-chemicals, examples of which are found in all plants. Most are colourless, but some are responsible for the bright colours of many fruits and vegetables. The human diet usually includes at least 1 gram per day of flavonoids, and tea and wines (especially red) contain large quantities.

More than 4000 flavonoids have been identified so far, and many of them have been intensively investigated by laboratory and animal studies. Except for one major flavonoid – quercetin – few have been the subject of human studies.

Rutin and hesperidin – found in buckwheat and citrus fruit, respectively – are among the most potent antioxidant flavonoids. Chemical subgroups of flavonoids include OPCs (oligomeric proanthocyanidins, which are abundant in grape seed extract), isoflavones (in soya) and anthocyanosides (the red pigment in, for example, red wines and blackberries).

Other pigments found in plants are the carotenoids, which give red, orange and yellow colours. Unlike the flavonoid pigments they are fat soluble, so the yellow colour of butter is due to beta-carotene from grass eaten by cows.

CABBAGES AND ONIONS

There are two important groups of sulphur-containing phytochemicals. Glucosinolates, believed to provide protection against cancer, are found in all members of the cabbage family, including broccoli, cauliflower and Brussels sprouts.

The onion family contains several closely related sulphur compounds with health benefits – garlic is an especially rich source.

HERBS THAT CONTAIN PHYTOCHEMICALS

As well as being rich sources of flavonoids, most herbs – and particularly herbal medicines – contain phytochemicals that are either protective or have curative properties. For example, liquorice and ginseng (and also soya) contain saponins that are chemically similar to the body's steroids.

Other herbs contain active constituents that are unique to the plant, and are often named accordingly: ginkgolides from ginkgo, echinoside from echinacea, valerenic acid from valerian, and so on.

THE POWER OF PHYTOESTROGENS

The principal phytoestrogens in the human diet are the isoflavones and a group of compounds called lignans, found in rye bran, flaxseed, sesame seeds and nuts.

Most research has been undertaken into isoflavones, which occur almost exclusively in legumes – soya beans are the most important dietary source. The main isoflavones found in soya proteins and soya foods are daidzein, genistein and glycitein.

Although not chemically related, phytoestrogens have some similarities to the female sex hormone oestrodiol, produced by women's bodies, which allows them to bind to oestrogen 'receptors' in cells.

Phytoestrogens will have no effect on the level of blood oestrogen, but by binding to these receptors they have an oestrogenic (oestrogen-like) effect when the hormone is lacking and an anti-oestrogenic effect when it is in excess.

Oestrogen also circulates in men's blood and high levels are associated with increased risk of cancer of the prostate gland. Soya phytoestrogens are believed to have a protective effect against prostate cancer.

The level of oestrogen in a woman's body falls after the menopause. At this time phytoestrogens are thought to provide a substitute for the body's own oestrogen, and may help to relieve symptoms such as hot flushes and dry skin. Phytoestrogens may also help to reduce the loss of bone mineral density that normally occurs after the menopause and is associated with osteoporosis.

THE ASIAN DIET

In Asian countries such as Japan, where the diet is rich in soya foods, menopausal symptoms such as hot flushes are reported much less than in Western countries. For example, in Europe 70-80% of menopausal women experience hot flushes, compared with 57% in Malaysia and 18% in China. One of the

A THERAPEUTIC DOSE OF ISOFLAVONES

Not enough is known about isoflavones to be able to recommend a daily amount, but consumption of isoflavones in Asia is between 25 and 200 mg a day. An intake of 50 to 120 mg isoflavones a day may be needed for therapeutic effects. On average this can be provided by one or two portions of soya products a day, but the isoflavone content is very variable.

The following foods yield approximately 50 mg isoflavones:
- 100 grams firm tofu or 200 grams soft tofu
- 100 grams miso
- 250 ml soya milk or soya yoghurt
- 50 grams soya flour, cooked soya beans or textured vegetable protein (TVP)

Most soya proteins used by the food industry contain 10-300 mg isoflavones per 100 grams. Soy sauce, soya bean oil and lecithin contain virtually no isoflavones.

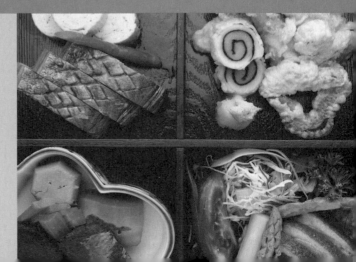

THE MAIN GROUPS OF PHYTOCHEMICALS: WHERE THEY COME FROM AND WHAT THEY DO

PHYTOCHEMICAL GROUPS	EXAMPLES OF COMPOUNDS	MAIN FOOD SOURCES	ACTION
Flavonoids	Kaempferol, quercetin Hesperitin, naringenin, rutin, tangeritin	Artichoke, apples, lettuce, onions, peppers, tea, tomatoes, wine; citrus fruits: grapefruit, oranges, tangerines	Antioxidants; enzyme regulators May prevent cancer and cardiovascular disease; may regulate immunity
Glucosinolates/ Isothiocyanates	Allylisothiocyanates, glucobrassicin, indoles	Cabbage family (broccoli, Brussels sprouts, cauliflower), mustard, watercress	Liver enzyme inducers; may prevent cancer
Hydroxycinnamic acids	Caffeic, chlorogenic and ferulic acids, curcumin	Apples, coffee, curry powder, mustard, pears	Antioxidants; may prevent cancer
Isoflavones	Daidzein, genistein	Soya bean products (soya flour, soya milk, soya protein)	Lower serum lipids; anti-oestrogenic; may prevent breast and prostate cancers
Lignans	Matairesinoll, secoisolaciresinol	Berries, flaxseed, nuts, rye bran	Antioxidant and antioestrogenic effects; may prevent colon and prostate cancers
Monoterpenes	D-carvone, D-limonene, perrillyl alcohol	Cherries, citrus fruits, herbs (dill, mint, caraway)	Liver enzyme inducers; anti-tumour agents (especially in respect of breast, prostate and pancreas), antimicrobial
Organosulphides	Allyl methyl sulphide, diallyl sulphide	Cabbage, garlic, leeks, onions, etc	Reduce blood clotting; lowers blood lipids; liver enzyme inducers; may prevent cancer
Phenols	Ellagic acid, gallic acid, hydroquinone, ρ-cresol	Widespread, including black tea, cocoa beans, green tea, raspberries, strawberries	Antioxidants; anti-inflammatory agents
Phytosterols	B-sitosterol, campesterol, stigmasterol	Vegetable oils (corn, rapeseed, soya bean, sunflower); specialist margarines (such as Benecol) contain ten times as much	Lower total cholesterol and LDL ('bad') cholesterol
Tannins	Theaflavins, thearubigens	Black tea, red wine, roasted coffee	Antioxidants; antimicrobial and anti-inflammatory agents

A POWERFUL WEAPON IN THE BATTLE AGAINST CANCER
Death rates for breast cancer in women are around 27.7 per 100,000 women in the UK compared with 6.6 in Japan. Prostate cancer deaths are similarly around four times greater in the UK than in Japan – and these figures are associated with significantly lower intakes of isoflavones.

most striking dietary differences among women in these areas is their intake of dietary soya protein and the phytoestrogens it contains. Japanese women excrete 100-1000 times more oestrogens in their urine than Western women.

In 1998 a study found that menopausal women who added 40 grams of isolated soya protein with naturally occurring isoflavones to their diet experienced a 45% reduction in hot flushes after 12 weeks.

LOWERING THE INCIDENCE OF OSTEOPOROSIS

Osteoporosis is the main underlying cause of most of the 60,000 hip fractures in England and Wales each year. It is incurable, but – along with increased prescribing of hormone replacement therapy (HRT) to help to prevent loss of bone mineral density – there is growing interest in dietary isoflavones as an alternative means of preventing it.

In Asian women the incidence of fractures due to osteoporosis is lower than in the West, despite the fact that Asian women have smaller frames, consume fewer dairy products and have lower calcium intakes.

A recent study of post-menopausal women found a small but significant increase in bone density with a diet containing 90 mg of total isoflavones that came from soya protein. It is thought that the isoflavones in soya may inhibit

the breakdown of bone. Synthetic isoflavones with the same structure as those in soya protein are also effective in reducing bone loss.

REDUCING THE LIKELIHOOD OF CANCER

A low consumption of fruit and vegetables is now considered by many scientists to be an important factor in increasing the risk of cancer. A reduced risk of cancer appears to be more strongly linked with the intake of certain foods – fruit, vegetables and legumes – than with intake of the antioxidant vitamins C, E and A, or fibre.

This suggests that other, non-essential substances – such as phytochemicals – play a key role in lowering risk. Drinking tea can help too. Animal studies have shown that green tea

PHYTOCHEMICALS AS SUPPLEMENTS

Scientific studies have confirmed the centuries-old wisdom that plant foods are highly protective against many different diseases. The health benefits of plants have been mainly attributed to the vitamins and phytochemicals they contain. Phytochemicals from vegetables, fruit and herbs are now readily available as tablets and tinctures. In addition to being used to complement the diet, many of these preparations can be just as effective as their traditional counterparts in restoring an ailing body to good health.

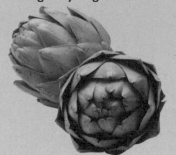

inhibits carcinogenesis (formation of tumours) in the lung and liver, as well as in the intestine and large bowel.

Death rates for breast cancer and prostate cancer are four times higher in the UK than in Japan, and these differences are linked with significantly lower intakes of isoflavones.

PROTECTION AGAINST HEART DISEASE

The commonest cause of heart disease is atherosclerosis, or hardening of the arteries by a fatty substance called plaque.

Flavonoids such as OPCs and quercetin can inhibit the process of atherosclerosis and help to strengthen blood vessels; in this way they may protect against heart disease and circulatory disorders. Equally, differences in the consumption of flavonoids may account for about 25% of the variations in heart disease between different countries.

Risk of atherosclerosis may also be reduced by isoflavones. A recent trial found that a daily dose of 62 mg isoflavones, taken as soya protein, reduced LDL 'bad' cholesterol by 10%.

Isoflavones, especially genistein, are also thought to reduce the risk of heart attacks as a result of their anticoagulant properties, which may impede the formation of clots in the blood and so prevent arterial blockages. However, most of the evidence is derived from laboratory and animal studies, and these need to be confirmed with further study on humans.

Potassium

You are probably careful not to eat too much salt, especially if you are monitoring your blood pressure levels, but you might also want to increase your consumption of potassium. In some people this mineral may do as much to control blood pressure as reducing sodium intake.

Common uses

- *Helps to lower blood pressure.*
- *May prevent high blood pressure, heart disease and stroke.*

Forms

- Liquid
- Powder
- Tablet

CAUTION!

If you suffer from a kidney disease or are taking medication for high blood pressure or heart disease, do not take potassium supplements without consulting your doctor.

REMINDER: If you have a medical condition, consult your doctor before taking supplements.

What it is

The third most abundant mineral in the body after calcium and phosphorus, potassium is an electrolyte – a substance that takes on a positive or negative charge when dissolved in the watery medium of the bloodstream. Sodium and chloride are electrolytes too, and the body needs a balance of these minerals to perform a host of essential functions. Almost all the potassium in the body is found inside the cells.

What it does

Along with the other electrolytes, potassium is used to conduct nerve impulses, initiate muscle contractions and regulate heartbeat and blood pressure. It controls the amount of fluid inside the cells, and sodium regulates the amount outside, so the two minerals work to balance fluid levels in the body. Potassium also enables the body to convert blood sugar (glucose) – its primary fuel – into a stored form of energy (glycogen) that is held in reserve by the muscles and liver. It is a natural diuretic, so helps to remove toxic metabolites, or toxins, from the body.

PREVENTION: Study after study has shown that people who get plenty of potassium in their diets have lower blood pressure than those who get very little. This effect holds true even when sodium intake remains high (though reducing sodium produces better results). In one study 54 people on medication for high blood pressure were divided into two groups. Half followed their regular diet; the other half added three to six servings of potassium-rich foods a day. After a year 81% of those getting extra potassium were able to reduce their drug dosages significantly, compared with only 29% of the individuals following their regular diets.

ADDITIONAL BENEFITS: Through its effects on blood pressure, potassium may also decrease the risk of heart disease and stroke. In one study a group of people with hypertension who ate one serving of a food high in potassium every day reduced their risk of fatal stroke by 40%. A 12-year investigation found that men who got the least amount of

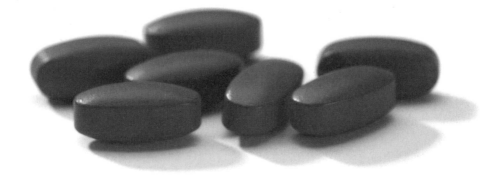

potassium were two and a half times more likely to die from a stroke than men who consumed the most; for women with a low potassium intake, the risk of fatal stroke was nearly five times greater.

How much you need

The recommended target for potassium is 3500 mg a day for both men and women. The mineral is found in a wide variety of foods, fruit and vegetables being particularly rich sources. However, many people do not eat enough of this vital food group, and a third of the UK population has a potassium intake of 2500 mg or less.

⊟ **IF YOU GET TOO LITTLE:** In otherwise healthy people a low intake of potassium is unlikely to produce adverse symptoms. At even lower intakes the first sign of deficiency would be muscle weakness and nausea. A serious deficiency can occur if an individual is taking a potent diuretic (a drug that reduces fluid levels in the body) or is suffering from an extreme case of diarrhoea or vomiting. If potassium is not replaced, such low levels could lead to heart failure.

⊕ **IF YOU GET TOO MUCH:** Potassium toxicity is highly unlikely because most people can safely consume up to 18 grams a day. Toxicity usually occurs only if an individual has a kidney disorder or takes too many potassium supplements. Signs of potassium overload include muscle fatigue and an irregular heartbeat. Even in small doses, potassium supplements may cause stomach irritation and nausea.

How to take it

☑ **DOSAGE:** Most people don't need potassium supplements unless they are taking certain diuretic medications. Try to get sufficient potassium in your daily diet. People who use ACE inhibitors (such as captopril or enalapril) for high blood pressure or angina, and those who have kidney disease, should not take potassium supplements at all.

◉ **GUIDELINES FOR USE:** If you do need to take potassium supplements, take them with food to decrease stomach irritation.

Other sources

Fresh vegetables and fruit – such as potatoes, bananas, oranges and orange juice – are very high in potassium. Meats, poultry, milk and yoghurt are also good sources.

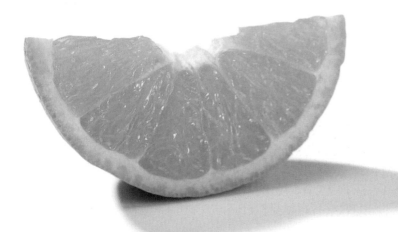

The results of 33 studies show that potassium has a positive impact on blood pressure. People with normal blood pressure who added 2340 mg of potassium a day – from foods, supplements or a combination of both – to their normal diets had an average drop of two points in systolic blood pressure (the upper reading) and one point in diastolic pressure (the lower reading). These small changes reduce by 25% the chance of developing hypertension. The extra potassium offered even greater benefits – a 4.4 point drop in systolic pressure and a 2.5 point drop in diastolic – in people who already had high blood pressure.

DID YOU KNOW?
Sustained exercise depletes the level of potassium in muscles, so athletes must repeatedly replenish their stores of the mineral.

FACTS&TIPS

■ Microwave or steam vegetables whenever you can; boiling them decreases their potassium content. Boiled potatoes lose 50% of their potassium; steamed potatoes lose less than 6%.

■ Potassium supplements should not contain more than 99 mg per tablet (this includes multivitamin and mineral preparations). If you think you need potassium supplements, talk to your doctor about higher-dose pills available on prescription.

Riboflavin

Exciting new research suggests that riboflavin, also known as vitamin B_2, may possess a range of previously unsuspected medicinal powers. It has been credited with counteracting migraines, preventing sight-robbing cataracts, healing skin blemishes – and much more.

Common uses

- Prevents or delays the onset of cataracts.
- Reduces the frequency and severity of migraines.
- Improves skin blemishes caused by rosacea.

Forms

- Capsule
- Tablet

CAUTION!

REMINDER: If you have a medical or psychiatric condition, consult your doctor before taking supplements.

What it is

In 1879 scientists looking through a microscope discovered a fluorescent yellow-green substance in milk, but not until 1933 was it identified as riboflavin. This water-soluble vitamin is part of the B-complex family, which is involved in transforming protein, fats and carbohydrates into fuel for the body. Found naturally in many foods, riboflavin is also added to fortified breads and cereals. It is easily destroyed when exposed to sunlight. Inadequate riboflavin intake often accompanies other B-vitamin deficiencies, which are a common problem in the elderly and alcoholics. Riboflavin is available as a single supplement, in combination with other B vitamins (vitamin B complex), or as part of a multivitamin.

What it does

The body depends on riboflavin for a wide range of functions. It plays a vital role in the production of thyroid hormone, which speeds up metabolism and helps to ensure a steady supply of energy. Riboflavin also aids the body in producing infection-fighting immune cells; it works in conjunction with iron to manufacture red blood cells, which transport oxygen to all the cells in the body. In addition it converts vitamins B_6 and niacin into active forms so that they can do their work.

Riboflavin produces substances that assist antioxidants, such as vitamin E, in protecting cells against damage from the naturally occurring, highly reactive molecules known as free radicals. It is essential for tissue maintenance and repair – the body uses extra amounts to speed the healing of wounds after surgery, burns and other injuries. The vitamin is also necessary to maintain the function of the eyes, and may be important for healthy nerves as well.

◉ **PREVENTION:** By boosting antioxidant activity riboflavin protects many body tissues – particularly the lens of the eye. It may therefore help to prevent the formation of cataracts, the milky opacities in the lenses that impair the vision of so many elderly people. Ophthalmologists urge everyone, especially those with a family history of this eye disorder, to get an adequate, steady supply of riboflavin throughout their lives. The

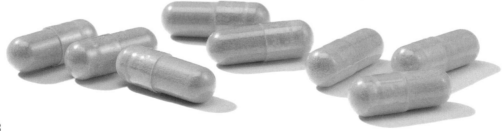

vitamin has also been shown to be highly effective in reducing the frequency and severity of migraine headaches. Migraine sufferers are believed to have reduced energy reserves in the brain, and riboflavin may prevent attacks by increasing the energy supply to brain cells.

ADDITIONAL BENEFITS: Riboflavin has proved valuable in treating skin disorders including rosacea, which causes facial flushing and skin pustules in many adults. In combination with other B vitamins, including vitamin B_6 and niacin, it may help against a broad range of nerve and other ailments, including numbness and tingling, Alzheimer's disease, epilepsy and multiple sclerosis, as well as anxiety, stress and even fatigue. Some doctors prescribe riboflavin supplementation to treat sickle-cell anaemia because many people with the disease have a riboflavin deficiency.

How much you need

The daily recommended target for riboflavin is 1.3 mg a day for men and 1.1 mg for women. These amounts simply prevent general deficiencies; larger doses are usually prescribed for specific conditions.

IF YOU GET TOO LITTLE: Classic deficiency symptoms include cracking and sores in the corner of the mouth and increased sensitivity to sunlight, with watering, burning and itchy eyes. The skin round the nose, eyebrows and ear lobes may peel, and there may be a skin rash in the groin area. A low red blood cell count (anaemia), resulting in fatigue, can also occur.

IF YOU GET TOO MUCH: Excess riboflavin isn't dangerous because the body excretes any extra in the urine. However, high intakes of this vitamin can turn the urine bright yellow – a harmless but unsettling side effect.

How to take it

DOSAGE: *For cataract prevention:* The usual dosage is 25 mg a day. *For rosacea:* Dosages of 40 mg a day are recommended. *For migraines:* Up to 40 mg a day. Many one-a-day vitamins meet the RDA for riboflavin; high-potency multivitamins may contain much higher amounts – 30 mg or more.

GUIDELINES FOR USE: Consult your doctor if you are taking oral contraceptives, antibiotics or psychiatric drugs, which can affect riboflavin needs. Don't take it with alcohol, which reduces absorption of riboflavin in the digestive tract.

Other sources

Good sources of riboflavin include milk, cheese, yoghurt, liver, beef, fish, wholegrain breads and cereals, eggs, avocados and mushrooms.

St John's wort

The ancient Greeks and Romans believed that St John's wort could deter evil spirits. Today the herb has found new and widespread popularity as a natural antidepressant. It is a gentler alternative to conventional medications, with far fewer side effects.

Hypericum perforatum

Common uses

- Treats depression.
- Helps to fight off viral and bacterial infections.
- May help to treat PMS, chronic fatigue syndrome and fibromyalgia.
- Helps to relieve chronic pain.
- Soothes haemorrhoids.
- May aid in weight loss.

Forms

- Capsule
- Cream/ointment
- Softgel
- Tablet
- Tincture

What it is

A shrubby perennial bearing bright yellow flowers, St John's wort is cultivated worldwide. It was named after St John the Baptist because it blooms around 24 June, the day celebrated as his birthday; 'wort' is an old English word for plant. For centuries St John's wort was used to soothe the nerves and to heal wounds and burns. Supplements are made from the dried flowers, which contain a number of therapeutic substances including a healing pigment called hypericin and the chemical hyperforin.

What it does

St John's wort is most frequently used to treat mild depression. Scientists are not sure exactly how the herb works, although it is believed to improve mood and emotions by enhancing brain levels of at least four neurotransmitters, including serotonin.

MAJOR BENEFITS: A recent analysis of 23 different studies of St John's wort concluded that the herb was as effective as antidepressant drugs – and more effective than a placebo – in the treatment of mild to moderate depression. (Few studies have examined its usefulness for more serious depression, though it may prove beneficial for this as well.)

St John's wort may be helpful for many conditions associated with depression too, such as anxiety, stress, premenstrual syndrome (PMS), chronic fatigue syndrome, fibromyalgia or chronic pain; it may even have some direct pain-relieving effects. This herb promotes sound sleep and may be especially valuable when depression is marked by fatigue, sleepiness and low energy levels. It may also aid in treating 'wintertime blues' (seasonal affective disorder, or SAD), a type of depression that develops in the autumn and winter and dissipates in the bright sunlight of spring and summer. Some people are wary of

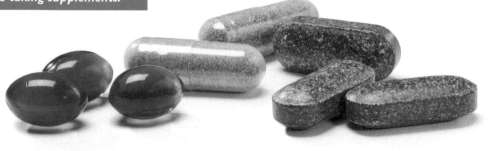

Whether you take softgels, capsules or tablets, St John's wort offers an effective natural remedy for depression.

conventional antidepressants because of their potential for causing undesirable side effects, especially reduced sexual function. St John's wort has far fewer bothersome side effects than these drugs. In addition St John's wort doesn't appear to interact with most other conventional drugs, making it useful for older people taking multiple medications. The herb seems so promising that the US National Institute of Health (NIH) is conducting a major study of its effectiveness.

✳ **ADDITIONAL BENEFITS:** St John's wort fights bacteria and viruses as well. Research indicates that it may play a key part in combating herpes simplex, influenza and Epstein-Barr virus (the cause of glandular fever), and preliminary laboratory studies reveal a possible role for the herb in the fight against AIDS. It also improves liver function. When an ointment made from St John's wort is applied to haemorrhoids it relieves burning and itching. St John's wort may also be useful as a weight-loss aid.

How to take it

✐ **DOSAGE:** The recommended dose is 300 mg of an extract standardised to contain 0.3% hypericin, three times a day. Supplements containing 900 mcg hypericin are also available and can be taken once a day.

◉ **GUIDELINES FOR USE:** Take St John's wort close to mealtime to reduce stomach irritation. In the past, people using the herb were advised not to eat certain foods, including matured cheese and red wine – the same foods best avoided by those taking MAO inhibitors (a treatment for depression). But recent studies suggest that these foods do not present a problem for those on St John's wort.

Like a prescription antidepressant, the herb must build up in your body's tissues before it becomes effective, so be sure to allow at least four weeks to determine whether it works for you. It can be used long term, as needed. Always consult your doctor before taking prescribed antidepressants and St John's wort together. Although adverse reactions are extremely unlikely, it is difficult to evaluate your progress unless the doctor is aware of all the medicines you are taking.

Though no adverse effects have been reported in pregnant or breast-feeding women using the herb, there have been few studies in this group of patients, so caution is advised.

Possible side effects

While uncommon, side effects can include constipation, upset stomach, fatigue, dry mouth and dizziness. People with fair skins are advised to avoid prolonged exposure to sunlight while taking St John's wort. High doses of St John's wort (more than 900 mcg hypericin daily) reduce blood levels of several drugs. If you are taking prescribed medicines, consult your doctor before using this herb. In the Republic of Ireland, St John's wort is now classified as a prescribed medicine.

RECENT FINDINGS

In one recent study 50 people with depression were given either St John's wort or a placebo. After eight weeks 70% of those on St John's wort extract showed marked improvement, as against 45% of those receiving a placebo. No adverse reactions to the herb were noted.

Several recent trials have compared St John's wort with conventional antidepressants in mild to moderate depression. In one study, 240 people were given either St John's wort or Prozac, and two studies tested St John's wort against imipramine. All three trials found that St John's wort was as effective as conventional antidepressants.

DID YOU KNOW?

In Germany, where doctors routinely prescribe herbal remedies, St John's wort is the most common form of antidepressant – and much more popular than conventional drugs such as Prozac and Zoloft.

Saw palmetto

Native Americans regularly consumed the leaf of this small palm tree as a food, so they were probably not plagued by prostate problems. Now frequently prescribed by doctors in Europe, saw palmetto is a herb with men's troubles in mind.

Serenoa repens

Common uses

- *Eases frequent night-time urination and other symptoms of an enlarged prostate.*
- *Relieves prostate inflammation.*
- *May boost immunity and treat urinary tract infections.*

Forms

- Capsule
- Dried herb/tea
- Softgel
- Tablet
- Tincture

CAUTION!

- Anyone finding blood in the urine or having trouble urinating should see their doctor before taking saw palmetto. These symptoms could be related to prostate cancer.

- Saw palmetto affects hormone levels, so men with prostate cancer and anyone taking hormones should discuss use of the herb with their doctor.

REMINDER: If you have a medical condition, consult your doctor before taking supplements.

What it is

The saw palmetto, a small palm tree that grows wild in the southern USA, gets its name from the spiny saw-toothed stems that lie at the base of each leaf. With a life span of 700 years the plant seems almost indestructible, resisting drought, insect infestation and fire. Its medicinal properties are derived from the blue-black berries, which are usually harvested in August and September. This process is sometimes hazardous: harvesters can easily be cut by the razor-sharp leaf stems, and they risk being bitten by the diamondback rattlesnakes that make their homes in the shade of this scrubby palm.

What it does

Saw palmetto has a long history of folk use. Native Americans valued it for treating disorders of the urinary tract. Early colonists, noting the vitality of animals who fed on the berries, gave the fruits to frail people as a general tonic. Through the years it has also been employed to relieve persistent coughs and improve digestion. Today saw palmetto's claim to fame rests mainly on its ability to relieve the symptoms of an enlarged prostate gland – a use verified by a number of scientific studies.

⭐ **MAJOR BENEFITS:** In Italy, Germany, France and other countries, doctors routinely prescribe saw palmetto for the benign (noncancerous) enlargement of the prostate known medically as BPH, which stands for 'benign prostatic hyperplasia', or 'hypertrophy'. When the walnut-sized prostate gland becomes enlarged, a common condition that affects more than half of men over age 50, it can press on the urethra, the tube that carries urine from the bladder through the prostate and out through the penis. The resulting symptoms include frequent urination (especially at

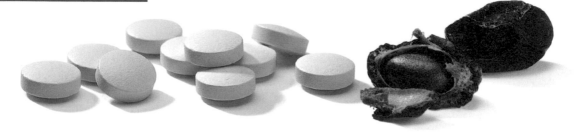

The dried fruit of the saw palmetto tree, often processed into tablets, provides a potent remedy for prostate complaints.

night), weak urine flow, painful urination and difficulty emptying the bladder completely. Researchers believe that saw palmetto relieves the symptoms of BPH in various ways. Most importantly, it appears to alter levels of various hormones that cause prostate cells to multiply. In addition the herb may curb inflammation and reduce tissue swelling.

Studies have found that saw palmetto produces fewer side effects (such as impotence) and quicker results than the conventional prostate drug finasteride (Proscar); it takes only about 30 days to be effective, compared with at least six months for the prescription medication.

✸ **ADDITIONAL BENEFITS:** Although there is strong evidence that saw palmetto relieves the symptoms of BPH, other potential benefits of this herb are more speculative. Saw palmetto has been used to treat certain inflammations of the prostate (prostatitis). In the laboratory it boosts the immune system's ability to kill bacteria, which suggests that it may be a potential treatment for prostate or urinary tract infections. Saw palmetto affects levels of cancer-promoting hormones, so scientists are also investigating its possible role in preventing prostate cancer.

How to take it

⊘ **DOSAGE:** The usual dosage is 160 mg twice a day. Be careful about taking higher amounts: scientific studies have not examined the effects of daily doses above 320 mg. Choose supplements made from extracts standardised to contain 85% to 95% fatty acids and sterols – the active ingredients in the berries that are responsible for its therapeutic effects.

◐ **GUIDELINES FOR USE:** Since prostatic enlargement could be a result of cancer, you must obtain a correct diagnosis before taking this herb to treat BPH. Also consult your doctor before taking saw palmetto for prostatitis. Saw palmetto has a bitter taste, so those using the liquid form may want to dilute it in a small amount of water. The herb can be taken with or without food. Although some healers recommend sipping tea made from saw palmetto, it may not contain therapeutic amounts of the active ingredients – and so provide few benefits for the treatment of BPH.

Possible side effects

Side effects are relatively uncommon, but include mild abdominal pain, nausea, dizziness and headache. If side effects occur, lower the dose or stop taking the herb.

Selenium

Although the significance of this trace mineral was not widely acknowledged until 1979, selenium has now gained prominence as a potentially powerful weapon against cancer. Many researchers believe that it could prove to be one of the most important disease-fighting nutrients.

Common uses

- *Works with vitamin E to help to prevent cancer and heart disease.*
- *Protects against cataracts and macular degeneration.*
- *Fights viral infections; reduces the severity of cold sores and shingles; may slow down the development of HIV/AIDS.*
- *Helps to relieve lupus symptoms.*

Forms

- Capsule
- Tablet

What it is

A trace mineral essential for many body processes, selenium is found in soil. The mineral is present throughout the body but is most abundant in the kidneys, liver, spleen, pancreas and testes.

What it does

Selenium acts as an antioxidant, blocking the rogue molecules known as free radicals that damage DNA. It is part of an antioxidant enzyme (called glutathione peroxidase) that protects cells against environmental and dietary toxins, and is often included with vitamins C and E in antioxidant 'cocktails'. This combination may guard against a range of disorders thought to be caused by free-radical damage – from cancer, heart disease and strokes to cataracts and macular degeneration.

✪ **MAJOR BENEFITS:** Selenium has received a great deal of attention for its role in combating cancer. A five-year US study, conducted at Cornell University and the University of Arizona, showed that taking 200 mcg of selenium daily resulted in 63% fewer prostate tumours, 58% fewer colo-rectal cancers, 46% fewer lung malignancies and a 39% overall decrease cancer. deaths. In other studies, selenium showed promise in preventing cancers of the ovaries, cervix, rectum, bladder, oesophagus, pancreas and liver, as well as leukaemia. Studies of cancer patients reveal that people with the lowest blood levels of selenium developed more tumours and had a higher rate of disease recurrence, a greater risk of cancer spreading and a shorter overall survival rate than those with high selenium levels.

In addition, selenium can protect the heart, primarily by reducing the 'stickiness' of the blood and decreasing the risk of clotting, which in turn lowers the risk of heart attack and stroke. Selenium increases the ratio of HDL ('good') cholesterol to LDL ('bad') cholesterol, which is critical for a healthy heart. Smokers and anyone who has already had a heart attack or stroke may gain the greatest cardiovascular benefits from selenium supplements, though everyone may profit from taking selenium in a daily vitamin and mineral supplement.

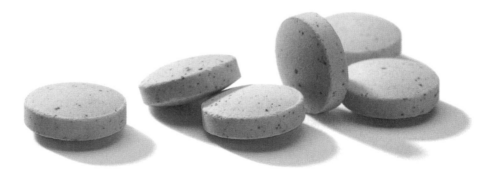

✳ **ADDITIONAL BENEFITS:** Selenium may be useful in preventing cataracts and macular degeneration, the leading causes of impaired vision or blindness in the elderly. It is also vital for converting thyroid hormone, which is needed for the proper functioning of every cell in the body, from a less active form (called T4) to its active form (known as T3). In addition, selenium is essential for a healthy immune system, assisting the body in defending itself against harmful bacteria and viruses as well as cancer cells. Its immunity-boosting effects may play a role in fighting the herpes virus that is responsible for cold sores and shingles, and it is also being studied for possible effectiveness against HIV, the virus that causes AIDS.

When combined with vitamin E, selenium appears to have some anti-inflammatory benefits as well. These two nutrients may improve chronic conditions such as rheumatoid arthritis, psoriasis, lupus and eczema.

How much you need

The recommended target intake for selenium is 75 mcg for men and 60 mcg for women daily. However, a therapeutic dose of up to 200 mcg a day may be needed to produce major benefits.

⊟ **IF YOU GET TOO LITTLE:** Soil with low levels of selenium, such as in the UK, produces food containing relatively low levels of the nutrient. Consistent intakes below the recommended amount could lead to higher incidences of cancer, heart disease, immune problems and inflammatory conditions of all kinds, particularly those affecting the skin. Insufficient amounts of selenium during pregnancy could increase the risk of birth defects (especially those involving the heart) or, possibly, sudden infant death syndrome (SIDS). Early symptoms of selenium deficiency include muscular weakness and fatigue.

⊞ **IF YOU GET TOO MUCH:** It is hard to get too much selenium from your diet, but if you are taking this mineral in supplement form it is important to remember that the margin of safety between a therapeutic dose of selenium (up to 350 mcg a day) and a toxic dose (as little as 900 mcg) is small compared with that of other nutrients. Symptoms of toxicity include nervousness, depression, nausea and vomiting, a garlicky odour to the breath and perspiration, and a loss of hair and fingernails.

How to take it

⊘ **DOSAGE:** Most nutritionists agree that the optimum dose for long-term use of selenium should be between 100 and 200 mcg daily.

◉ **GUIDELINES FOR USE:** Vitamin E greatly enhances the effectiveness of selenium; people at risk of heart disease may wish to add foods rich in this vitamin to their diet.

Other sources

The most abundant sources of selenium include Brazil nuts, seafood, poultry and meats. Grains, particularly oats and brown rice, may also have significant amounts, depending on the selenium content of the soil in which they were grown.

RECENT FINDINGS

Recent studies show that in the test tube selenium works relatively quickly, helping cells to grow and die at normal rates and protecting them from becoming cancerous. Researchers believe that selenium's cancer-fighting benefits may be fast-acting in the body as well.

Studies in mice show that a deficiency in either selenium or vitamin E – both antioxidants – can convert a latent, inactive virus into its active, disease-causing form. This may help to explain why selenium is effective against cold sores and shingles, which are both caused by reactivation of a dormant herpes virus.

DID YOU KNOW?

Brazil nuts are very rich in selenium; one nut may contain about 75 mcg, the recommended daily target for a man. Kidneys are also an excellent source of selenium; a single lamb's kidney contains about 50 mcg.

Tea tree oil

Melaleuca alternifolia

For centuries aboriginal Australians relied on the leaves of the tea tree to fight infections. Today tea tree oil is valued throughout the world as a potent antiseptic, and scientists have confirmed its powerful ability to combat harmful bacteria and fungal infections.

Common uses

- *Disinfects and promotes the healing of cuts and scrapes.*
- *Minimises scarring.*
- *Speeds recovery from insect bites and stings, including bee stings.*
- *Fights athlete's foot, fungal nail infections and yeast infections.*

Forms

- Cream
- Gel
- Oil
- Vaginal suppository

CAUTION!

- Tea tree oil is for topical use only. Do not ingest; it can be toxic. Keep it away from eyes.

- Consult your doctor before applying to deep open wounds.

REMINDER: If you have a medical condition, consult your doctor before taking supplements.

What it is

A champion infection fighter, tea tree oil has a pleasant nutmeg-like scent. It comes from the leaves of *Melaleuca alternifolia*, or the tea tree, a species that grows only in Australia (and is completely different from the species of *Camellia* used to make black, oolong and green drinking teas). Extracted through a steam-distillation process, quality tea tree oil contains at least 40% terpinen-4-ol – the active ingredient responsible for its healing effects – and less than 5% cineole, a substance that causes skin irritation if too much is present. With the rise of antibiotics after the Second World War, tea tree oil fell out of favour. Recently interest in it has revived, and more than 700 tonnes are now produced annually.

What it does

Tea tree oil is used topically to treat a variety of common infections. Once applied to the skin, the oil makes it impossible for many disease-causing fungi to survive. Studies have shown that it also fights various bacteria, including some that are resistant to powerful antibiotics. Doctors think that one reason why tea tree oil is so effective is that it readily mixes with skin oils, allowing it to attack the infective agent quickly and actively.

✪ **MAJOR BENEFITS:** Tea tree oil's antiseptic properties are especially useful for treating cuts and scrapes, as well as insect bites and stings. The oil promotes the healing of minor wounds, helps to prevent infection and minimises any future scarring. As an antifungal agent, tea tree oil fights the fungus *Trichophyton*, the culprit in athlete's foot, a similar infection of the groin and some nail infections. It may also be effective against *Candida albicans* and *Tricho-monas vaginalis*, two of the organisms that cause vaginal infections. Some fungal infections can be stubborn to treat, however, and your doctor may need to prescribe a more potent conventional antifungal medication.

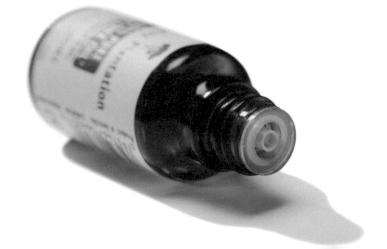

✳ **ADDITIONAL BENEFITS:** Tea tree oil may be beneficial in the treatment of acne. In one study, a gel containing 5% tea tree oil was shown to be as effective against acne as a lotion with 5% benzoyl peroxide, the active ingredient in most over-the-counter acne medications. But there were fewer side effects with tea tree oil: it caused less scaling, dryness and itching than the benzoyl peroxide formula. Another study found that a solution containing 0.5% tea tree oil offered protection against *Pityrosporum ovale*, a common dandruff-causing fungus. Sometimes tea tree oil is suggested as a treatment for warts, which are caused by viruses, though studies have not confirmed its efficacy in this respect.

How to take it

🖉 **DOSAGE:** *To treat athlete's foot, skin wounds or nail infections*: Apply a drop or two of pure, undiluted tea tree oil to affected areas of the skin or nails two or three times a day. Tea tree oil creams and lotions can also be used. *To treat vaginal yeast infections*: Insert a commercially available tea tree oil vaginal suppository every 12 hours, for up to five days.

◉ **GUIDELINES FOR USE:** Tea tree oil is for topical use only. Never take tea tree oil orally. If you ingest it, or a child does, phone your doctor or get to a hospital casualty department immediately. Rarely, tea tree oil can cause an allergic skin rash in some people. Before using the oil for the first time, dab a small amount on your inner arm with a cotton swab. If you are allergic, your arm will quickly become red or inflamed. If this response occurs, dilute the oil by adding a few drops to a tablespoon of bland oil, such as vegetable oil or almond oil, and try the arm test again. If you have no skin reaction it is safe to apply the diluted oil elsewhere.

Possible side effects

Although tea tree oil can cause minor skin irritation, it otherwise appears to be safe for topical use. Like many herbal oils in pure, undiluted form, it can irritate the eyes and mucous membranes.

Tea tree oil is often added to soaps and skin-care products because of its ability to destroy bacteria.

Thiamin

Most of us get enough thiamin in our diets to meet our basic needs, but many nutritionists believe that some people, especially older adults, are mildly deficient in this B vitamin, which makes a vital contribution to a healthy metabolism and a properly functioning nervous system.

Common uses

- Aids energy production.
- Promotes healthy nerves.
- May improve mood.
- Strengthens the heart.
- Soothes indigestion.

Forms

- Capsule
- Tablet

CAUTION!

REMINDER: If you have a medical or psychiatric condition, consult your doctor before taking supplements.

What it is

Thiamin, an often overlooked but key member of the B-complex vitamin family, is known as vitamin B_1 because it was the first B vitamin to be discovered. Although severe thiamin deficiency is a thing of the past, even a moderate deficit has health consequences. Thiamin is available as an individual supplement, but it is advisable to get it from a B-complex supplement because it works closely with the other B vitamins.

What it does

Thiamin is essential for converting the carbohydrates in foods into energy. It also promotes healthy nerves and may be useful in treating certain types of heart disease.

✪ **MAJOR BENEFITS:** In people with heart disease, thiamin can improve the pumping power of the heart. Thiamin levels in the body are depleted by long-term treatment with diuretic drugs, which are often prescribed for heart patients to reduce the fluid build-up associated with the disease. In one study, patients with heart disease who took furosemide (a diuretic) were given either 200 mg a day of thiamin or a placebo. After six weeks, the thiamin group showed a 22% improvement.

By helping to maintain healthy nerves, thiamin may minimise tingling and numbness in the hands and feet, a problem that frequently plagues people with diabetes or other diseases that cause nerve damage.

✪ **ADDITIONAL BENEFITS:** In combination with choline and pantothenic acid (also B vitamins), thiamin can enhance the digestive process and provide relief from indigestion. Some researchers think that a thiamin deficiency is linked to mental illnesses, including depression, and that high-dose thiamin supplementation may be beneficial.

Thiamin may also help to boost memory in people with Alzheimer's disease – but evidence is far from conclusive. However, the confusion that is common in older adults after surgery may be prevented by

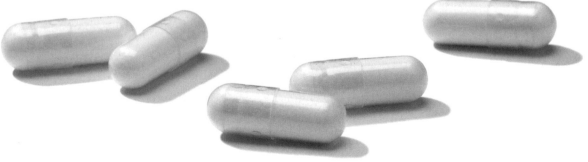

additional doses of thiamin in the weeks before an operation. Doctors also use thiamin to treat the psychosis related to alcohol withdrawal. Antiseizure medications interfere with the vitamin's absorption, so people taking them may need extra thiamin; this may also reduce the fuzzy thinking that such drugs can cause.

How much you need

The recommended amount of 1 mg a day for men and 0.8 mg a day for women is enough to maintain good health and to prevent a thiamin deficiency. However, higher doses are recommended for therapeutic use.

⊟ **IF YOU GET TOO LITTLE:** A mild thiamin deficiency may go unnoticed. Its symptoms are irritability, depression, muscle weakness and weight loss. A severe thiamin deficiency causes beriberi, a disease that leads to mental impairment, the wasting away of muscle, paralysis, nerve damage and eventually death. Once rampant in many countries, beriberi is rare today. It is seen only in parts of Asia where the diet consists mainly of white rice, which is stripped of thiamin and other nutrients during milling. In the UK, thiamin is added to white flour and many breakfast cereals.

⊞ **IF YOU GET TOO MUCH:** There are no adverse effects associated with high doses of thiamin, because the body is efficient at eliminating excess amounts through the urine.

How to take it

▨ **DOSAGE:** Specific disorders can benefit from supplemental thiamin. *For heart disease*: Take 50 mg of thiamin daily. *For numbness and tingling*: Take 50 mg of thiamin a day, preferably as part of a B-complex supplement. *For depression*: Take 50 mg daily as part of a B-complex supplement. *For indigestion*: Take 50 mg a day in the morning. *For alcoholism*: Take 50 mg daily, preferably as part of a B-complex supplement.

◉ **GUIDELINES FOR USE:** Thiamin is best absorbed in an acidic environment. Take it with meals, when stomach acid is produced to digest food. Divide your dose in half and take the halves at different times of the day; high doses are readily flushed out of the body in urine.

Other sources

Lean pork is probably the best dietary source of thiamin, followed by whole grains, dried beans and nuts and seeds. Enriched grain products also contain thiamin.

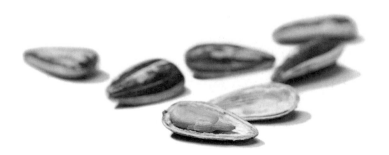

Turmeric

Curcuma longa

A main ingredient of curry powder, turmeric has been used in Indian and Chinese medicine for thousands of years to relieve conditions ranging from flatulence to menstrual irregularities. It is now recognised in the West as a powerful antioxidant and anti-inflammatory agent.

Common uses

- *Reduces inflammation, especially in shoulder, knee and elbow joints.*
- *Can relieve the inflammation and pain of rheumatoid arthritis.*
- *May lower cholesterol levels and reduce tendency to thrombosis.*
- *May help to prevent cancer, particularly of the colon and mouth.*

Forms

- Capsule
- Powder
- Tablet

CAUTION!

- Do not exceed the recommended dose. Although generally safe, turmeric in large doses may cause gastrointestinal problems or even ulcers.

REMINDER: If you have a medical condition, consult your doctor before taking supplements.

What it is

The yellow-flowered turmeric plant is a member of the ginger family. It is grown in Indonesia, China, India and other parts of the tropics, where the dried aromatic root-like stem is ground to form a powder. It contains yellow-coloured curcumin, the key active component, and also an orange-coloured volatile oil. The herb has been shown to have a positive effect on a variety of medical conditions.

Apart from its culinary uses, turmeric is used as a preservative, colorant and flavouring agent in many food products including baked foods, pickles and meat products.

What it does

Turmeric has an antioxidant effect approximately equivalent to that of Vitamins C and E, meaning that it provides powerful protection against the damage that can be done to the cells of the body by unstable oxygen molecules called free radicals. Turmeric, and especially its component curcumin, acts as an anti-inflammatory agent both when applied topically as a poultice and when used orally. Laboratory studies suggest that turmeric may have significant anticarcinogenic properties, and animal studies indicate that it may lower blood cholesterol levels. Its anti-inflammatory and antioxidant properties, combined with its ability to increase the secretion of bile and the production of liver enzymes, explains its liver-protective effects against toxins.

⊕ **MAJOR BENEFITS:** If turmeric is taken internally its principal effects are associated with the ability of curcumin to suppress the release of

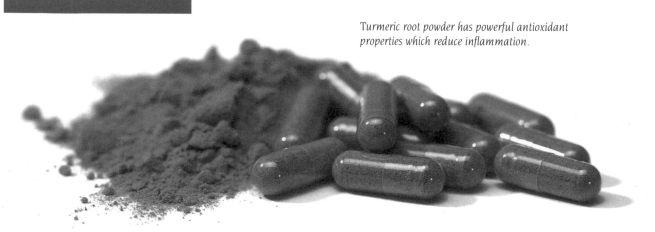

Turmeric root powder has powerful antioxidant properties which reduce inflammation.

inflammatory agents within the body's tissues. It is also thought to stimulate the production of cortisone from the adrenal glands, which indirectly assists the healing process.

Curcumin has been shown in animal studies to have therapeutic properties equivalent to those of cortisone and phenylbutazone in cases of acute inflammation (although it is only half as effective in chronic cases), with the advantage that it has no toxic results. If turmeric is applied to the skin, as is common in India, it can ease pain and inflammation in muscles and joints. Laboratory research has shown that turmeric can not only inhibit the early development of cancer cells but may also stop the progression of the disease as well as boosting the body's own antioxidant system. By lowering cholesterol levels and preventing the coagulation of blood platelets, turmeric has a role to play in combating atherosclerosis, even when taken in small doses.

Its combination of antioxidant and anti-inflammatory properties, together with its ability to increase bile acid output, provides evidence to support the traditional use of turmeric for protecting the liver. A preliminary study has shown the herb to be helpful for people with indigestion. By both hindering the formation of wind and releasing it if it does form, turmeric has a positive effect on the gastrointestinal system and can also inhibit intestinal spasm.

⊛ **ADDITIONAL BENEFITS:** In a clinical trial, patients suffering from rheumatoid arthritis were given 1200 mg of curcumin a day and the results were compared with those of a group given the traditional treatment of 300 mg of phenylbutazone. Both groups reported similar improvements in walking time, stiffness and joint swelling, and, unlike phenylbutazone, curcumin has no adverse side effects when taken in the correct amounts.

How to take it

⊘ **DOSAGE:** The recommended dose for turmeric is between 500 mg and 1000 mg of the dried standardised root extract (containing 95% curcuminoids) per day. *As an anti-inflammatory:* Take 300 mg up to three times a day with meals.

◉ **GUIDELINES FOR USE:** If turmeric is combined with the enzyme bromelain to improve absorption, it should be taken between meals for best results.

Possible side effects

Turmeric appears to be very safe in recommended doses. However, there is some evidence to suggest that – because turmeric enhances the release of bile in the liver – high doses should not be taken by people with gallstones, since gallstones can hinder the flow of bile.

BUYING GUIDE

■ When you are buying a turmeric supplement ensure that it is a standardised root extract containing 95% curcuminoids.

RECENT FINDINGS

In one trial 62 patients with ulcerating mouth or skin tumours which had not responded to traditional treatments such as chemotherapy, radiotherapy or surgery were treated with an external application of turmeric extract or curcumin three times a day for 18 months. At the end of the study it was found that itching had been reduced by 70%, pain by 50% and the size of the lesion by 10%.

DID YOU KNOW?

Turmeric's name comes from the Latin *terra merita*, meaning 'meritorious earth'. This may have been an early reference to the plant's many beneficial properties.

FACTS & TIPS

■ Increasing the turmeric intake in your diet may be beneficial in some cases, but it would be necessary to consume large quantities to obtain the amount required for a specific medical effect.

■ There is no evidence that turmeric has irritant effects when taken in recommended amounts. Indeed, it may provide protection against the formation of ulcers.

Valerian

Valeriana officinalis

It is three o'clock in the morning and you are wide awake – again. You wish there was something that you could safely take to induce temporary oblivion. Valerian may be the answer: this herb gently encourages sleep without the unpleasant side effects of conventional drugs.

Common uses
- *Promotes restful sleep.*
- *Soothes stress and anxiety.*
- *Improves the symptoms of some digestive disorders.*

Forms
- Capsule
- Dried herb/tea
- Softgel
- Tablet
- Tincture

CAUTION!

■ If taken during the day after a poor night's sleep, valerian may cause drowsiness.

■ If you are pregnant or breast-feeding, do not use valerian.

REMINDER: If you have a medical or psychiatric condition, consult your doctor before taking supplements.

What it is

In the UK, Germany and other European countries, valerian is officially approved as a sleep aid by medical authorities. A perennial plant native to North America and Europe, valerian has pinkish-coloured flowers that grow from a tuberous rootstock, or rhizome. Harvested when the plant is two years old, the rootstock contains a number of important compounds – valepotriates, valeric acid and volatile oils among them – that at one time or another were each thought to be responsible for the herb's sedative powers. Many herbalists believe that valerian's effectiveness may be the result of synergy among the various compounds.

What it does

Taken for centuries as an aid to sleep, valerian can also act as a calming agent in stressful daytime situations. It is used in treating anxiety disorders and conditions worsened by stress, such as diverticular disorders and irritable bowel syndrome.

✪ **MAJOR BENEFITS:** Compounds in valerian are able to raise levels in the brain of a nerve chemical (neurotransmitter) called gamma-aminobutyric acid, or GABA. It is through this interaction that valerian promotes sleep and eases anxiety. Unlike benzodiazepines – drugs such as diazepam (Valium) or alprazolam (Xanax), commonly prescribed for these disorders – valerian is not addictive and does not make you feel drugged. Rather than inducing sleep directly, valerian calms the brain and body so sleep

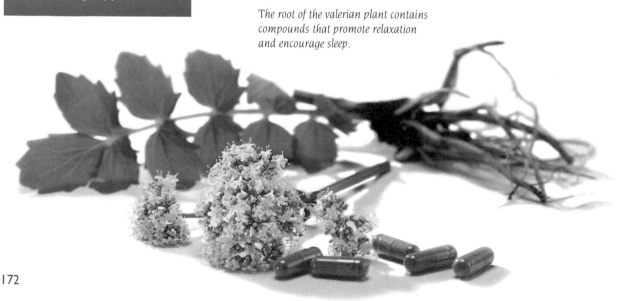

The root of the valerian plant contains compounds that promote relaxation and encourage sleep.

can occur naturally. One of the benefits of valerian for insomniacs is that, when taken at recommended doses, it doesn't make you feel groggy in the morning as some prescription drugs do.

According to various studies, valerian works as well as prescription drugs for many individuals, and when compared with a placebo, appears to lull a person to sleep. In one study, 128 people were given one of two valerian preparations or a placebo. It was found that the herb improved sleep quality: those taking valerian fell asleep more quickly and woke up less often than those receiving a placebo. In another study involving insomniacs, nearly all reported improved sleep when taking valerian, and 44% classified their sleep quality as perfect.

Although modern interest in valerian as an aid against anxiety is relatively recent, the herb is increasingly recommended by herbalists for this purpose.

✪ **ADDITIONAL BENEFITS:** Valerian helps to relax the smooth muscle of the gastrointestinal tract, making it valuable for the treatment of irritable bowel syndrome and diverticular disorders, which often involve painful spasms of the intestine. In addition, because flare-ups of these disorders are sometimes triggered by stress, valerian's calming action may also account for its effectiveness.

How to take it

▨ **DOSAGE:** *For insomnia*: Take 250 to 500 mg of the powdered extract in capsule or tablet form or 1 teaspoon of the tincture 30 to 45 minutes before bedtime. Studies show that, for most people, higher doses bring no additional benefit. However, if the low dose does not work for you, you can safely use as much as 900 mg (2 teaspoons of the tincture). *For anxiety*: Consume 250 mg twice a day and 250 to 500 mg prior to bedtime.

◉ **GUIDELINES FOR USE:** Valerian has a slightly unpleasant taste, so if you choose the tincture try blending it with a little honey or sugar to make it more palatable. Although valerian is not addictive, it is inadvisable to rely on any substance, herbal or otherwise, to help you to fall asleep each night. Therefore, avoid taking valerian nightly for more than two weeks in a row, and ensure that you do not combine it with prescription sleeping drugs or tranquillisers. It is safe to take valerian with other herbs, such as chamomile, melissa (also known as lemon balm) or passionflower, which may increase its effectiveness as a sleeping aid. Valerian can also be used with St John's wort if you are feeling depressed.

Possible side effects

Studies have shown that, even in amounts 20 times higher than normally recommended, valerian has no dangerous side effects. However, extremely large doses can cause dizziness, restlessness, blurred vision, nausea, headache, giddiness and grogginess in the morning.

BUYING GUIDE

■ When buying valerian, it is advisable to look for a product which contains a 5:1 herb extract ratio.

RECENT FINDINGS

Prescription sleeping drugs often cause grogginess the morning after they are taken and can impair a person's ability to drive or to perform other tasks that require concentration. Valerian does not, according to a German study. Researchers compared the effects of valerian, valerian and hops, a benzodiazepine drug and a placebo. The herbal preparations and the drug all improved sleep quality. The benzodiazepine drug reduced performance the following morning, but the herbs did not.

DID YOU KNOW?

Valerian preparations have a very disagreeable odour – so much so that inexperienced users may think they have a bad batch. Don't be put off by the smell; it's quite normal.

Vitamin A

This essential nutrient keeps the eyesight keen, the skin healthy and the immune system strong. Consequently the body needs adequate levels of vitamin A to ensure the prevention of various eye problems, a number of skin disorders and a wide range of infections.

Common uses

- *Helps the body to fight colds, flu and other types of infections.*
- *Promotes skin health and healing of wounds, burns and ulcers.*
- *Maintains healthy eyes.*
- *Benefits the lining of the digestive tract.*

Forms

- Capsule
- Liquid
- Softgel
- Tablet

CAUTION!

■ Vitamin A can build up to toxic levels, so be careful not to get too much, and remember that the beta-carotene form of the vitamin is safer.

■ Women who are pregnant or considering pregnancy should not take more than 1500 mcg of vitamin A daily; higher doses may cause birth defects. It is important to practise effective birth control when taking doses higher than 1500 mcg and for at least a month afterwards.

REMINDER: If you have a medical condition, consult your doctor before taking supplements.

What it is

Vitamin A, a fat-soluble nutrient, is stored in the liver. The body gets part of its vitamin A from animal fats and makes part in the intestine from beta-carotene and other carotenoids in fruit and vegetables. Vitamin A is present in the body in various chemical forms called retinoids – so named because the vitamin is essential to the health of the retina.

What it does

This vitamin prevents night blindness, maintains the skin and cells that line the respiratory and gastrointestinal tracts and helps to build teeth and bones. It is vital for normal reproduction, growth and development. In addition, vitamin A is crucial to the immune system, including the plentiful supply of immune cells that line the airways and digestive tract and form an important line of defence against disease.

MAJOR BENEFITS: Vitamin A is perhaps best known for its ability to maintain vision, especially night vision, assisting the eye in adjusting from bright light to darkness. It can also alleviate 'dry eye', a complaint which is common in many developing countries and is specifically associated with severe vitamin A deficiency.

By boosting immunity, vitamin A greatly strengthens resistance to infections, including sore throat, colds, flu and bronchitis. It may also combat cold sores and shingles (caused by a herpes virus), warts (a viral skin infection), eye infections and vaginal yeast infections – and perhaps even help to control allergies. The vitamin may help the immune system to battle against breast and lung cancers and improve survival rates in those with leukaemia; in addition, animal studies suggest it inhibits melanoma, a deadly form of skin cancer. Another benefit for cancer patients is that the effectiveness of chemotherapy may be enhanced when the body has good levels of vitamin A.

ADDITIONAL BENEFITS: Vitamin A was first used in the 1940s to treat skin disorders, including acne and psoriasis, but the doses were high and toxic. Scientists later developed safer vitamin A derivatives (notably retinoic acid); now sold as prescription drugs, these include the acne and antiwrinkle cream Retin-A. Lower doses of vitamin A (7500 mcg a day)

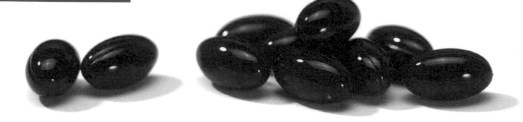

can be used, but only under the supervision of a doctor, to treat a range of skin conditions, including acne, dry skin, eczema, rosacea and psoriasis. When vitamin A levels in the body are good, the healing of skin wounds is promoted, and even recovery from sprains and strains may be hastened. The value of good vitamin A levels even extends to the lining of the digestive tract, where it helps to treat inflammatory bowel disease and ulcers. In addition, getting enough of this vitamin will speed up recovery in people who have had strokes. Women with heavy or prolonged menstrual periods are sometimes deficient in this vitamin.

How much you need

The recommended target for vitamin A is 600 mcg a day for women and 700 mcg a day for men.

⊟ **IF YOU GET TOO LITTLE:** Although quite rare in the UK, a vitamin A deficiency can cause night blindness (even total blindness) and a greatly lowered resistance to infection. Milder cases of deficiency do occur, especially in the elderly, who often have vitamin-poor diets. Infections such as pneumonia can deplete vitamin A stores.

⊞ **IF YOU GET TOO MUCH:** Although levels of up to 1500 mcg a day are safe, supplementation with vitamin A should not be undertaken unless prescribed by a doctor. This advice is particularly important for women who are pregnant or are likely to become pregnant, because of risk of damage to the developing foetus. Above these levels, an overabundance of vitamin A can be a real problem. A single dose of 150,000 mcg may induce weakness and vomiting; and as little as 7500 mcg a day for six years has been reported to cause serious liver disease (cirrhosis). Signs of toxicity include dry, cracking skin and brittle nails, hair that falls out easily, bleeding gums, weight loss, irritability, fatigue and nausea.

How to take it

▣ **DOSAGE:** To avoid an excessive intake of vitamin A it is advisable to take supplements containing no more than the recommended daily allowance of 800 mcg a day. Alternatively, take vitamin A in the form of mixed carotenoids.

◉ **GUIDELINES FOR USE:** Take supplements with food; a little fat in the diet aids absorption. Vitamin E and zinc help the body to use vitamin A, which in turn boosts absorption of iron from foods.

Other sources

Vitamin A is richly represented in fish, egg yolks, butter, offal such as liver (90 grams provide more than 2500 mcg), and fortified milk (check the label to be sure). Yellow, orange, red and dark green fruits and vegetables have large amounts of beta-carotene and many other carotenoids, which the body makes into vitamin A when needed.

Vitamin B$_6$

The 'workhorse' of nutrients, vitamin B$_6$ is probably involved in more bodily processes than any other vitamin. Surveys indicate, however, that a fifth of women and the same proportion of elderly people are not obtaining enough of this critically important nutrient from their daily diets.

Common uses

- Helps to prevent cardiovascular disease and strokes.
- Helps to lift depression.
- Eases insomnia.
- Treats carpal tunnel syndrome.
- May lessen PMS symptoms.
- Helps to relieve asthma attacks.

Forms

- Capsule
- Liquid
- Tablet

What it is

Vitamin B$_6$ performs more than 100 jobs innumerable times a day. It functions primarily as a coenzyme, a substance that acts in concert with enzymes to speed up chemical reactions in the cells.

Another name for vitamin B$_6$ is pyridoxine. In supplement form it is available as pyridoxine hydrochloride or pyridoxal-5-phosphate (P-5-P). Either form satisfies most needs, but some nutritionally aware doctors prefer P-5-P because it may be more easily absorbed.

What it does

Forming red blood cells, helping cells to make proteins, manufacturing brain chemicals (neurotransmitters) such as serotonin and releasing stored forms of energy are just a few of the functions of vitamin B$_6$. There is also evidence to suggest that it plays a role in preventing and treating many diseases.

PREVENTION: Getting enough B$_6$ through diet or supplements may help to prevent heart disease. Working with folic acid and vitamin B$_{12}$, this vitamin assists the body in processing homocysteine, an amino acid-like compound that has been linked to an increased risk of heart disease and other vascular disorders when large amounts are present in the blood.

ADDITIONAL BENEFITS: Some women suffering from premenstrual syndrome (PMS) report that vitamin B$_6$ provides relief from many of the symptoms. This beneficial effect probably occurs as a result of the vitamin's involvement in clearing excess oestrogen from the body. In its role as a building block for neurotransmitters, vitamin B$_6$ may be useful in reducing the likelihood of epileptic seizures as well as improving the moods of people suffering from depression. In fact, up to 25% of people with depression may be deficient in vitamin B$_6$.

The vitamin also maintains nerve health. People with diabetes, who are at risk of nerve damage, can also benefit from supplements of vitamin B$_6$. In addition, it is effective in easing the symptoms of carpal tunnel syndrome, which involves nerve inflammation in the wrist. And for people with asthma, vitamin B$_6$ may reduce the intensity and frequency of attacks; it is especially important for those taking the asthma drug theophylline.

How much you need

The recommended target for vitamin B_6 is 1.2 mg a day for women and 1.4 mg a day for men. Therapeutic doses are higher.

⊟ **IF YOU GET TOO LITTLE:** A recent survey found that a fifth of all women fail to meet the recommended target for vitamin B_6. Women taking oral contraceptives may have especially low levels of this vitamin. Mild deficiencies of B_6 can raise homocysteine levels, increasing the risk of heart and vascular diseases. Symptoms of severe deficiency, which is rare, are skin disorders such as dermatitis, sores around the mouth and acne. Neurological signs include insomnia, depression and, in extreme cases, seizures and brain wave abnormalities.

⊞ **IF YOU GET TOO MUCH:** High doses of vitamin B_6 (more than 2000 mg a day) can cause nerve damage when taken for long periods. In rare cases, prolonged use at lower doses (more than 200 mg a day) can have the same consequence. Fortunately, nerve damage is completely reversible once you discontinue the vitamin. If you are using vitamin B_6 for nerve pain, contact your doctor if you experience any new numbness or tingling and stop taking the vitamin. Doses up to 10 mg a day are safe for long-term use, but doses of up to 200 mg may be taken for short periods of time.

How to take it

▨ **DOSAGE:** You can keep homocysteine levels in check with just 3 mg of B_6 a day, but a daily dose of 50 mg is often recommended. Higher doses are needed for therapeutic uses. *For PMS:* Take 100 mg of B_6 a day. *For acute carpal tunnel syndrome:* Try 50 mg of B_6 or P-5-P three times a day. *For asthma:* Take 50 mg of B_6 twice a day.

◉ **GUIDELINES FOR USE:** Vitamin B_6 is best absorbed in amounts of no more than 100 mg at one time. When you are taking higher doses this more gradual intake will also decrease your chances of nerve damage.

Other sources

Fish, poultry, meats, chickpeas, potatoes, avocados and bananas are all good sources of vitamin B_6.

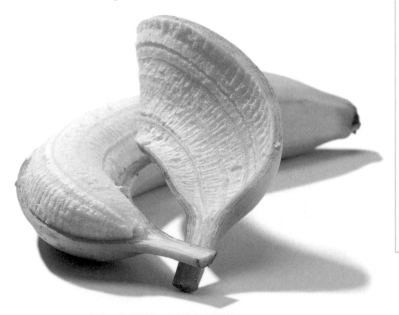

Vitamin B$_{12}$

Although this vitamin is plentiful in most people's diets, after the age of 50 some people have a limited ability to absorb it from food. Supplements may be useful, because even mild deficiencies may increase the risk of heart disease, depression and possibly Alzheimer's disease.

Common uses

- *Prevents a form of anaemia.*
- *Helps to reduce depression.*
- *Thwarts nerve pain, numbness and tingling.*
- *Lowers the risk of heart disease.*
- *May improve multiple sclerosis and tinnitus.*

Forms

- Capsule
- Tablet

CAUTION!

- If you take a vitamin B$_{12}$ supplement you must also have a folic acid supplement: a high intake of one can mask a deficiency of the other.

- Diagnosis of pernicious anaemia should be made by a doctor, and regular follow-up blood tests may be necessary.

REMINDER: *If you have a medical or psychiatric condition, consult your doctor before taking supplements.*

What it is

Vitamin B$_{12}$, also known as cobalamin, was the most recent vitamin to be discovered. In the late 1940s it was identified as the substance in calves' liver that cured pernicious anaemia, a potentially fatal disease primarily affecting older adults. Vitamin B$_{12}$ is the only B vitamin the body stores in large amounts, mostly in the liver. The body absorbs B$_{12}$ through a very complicated process: digestive enzymes in the presence of enough stomach acid separate B$_{12}$ from the protein in foods. The vitamin then binds with a substance called intrinsic factor (a protein produced by cells in the stomach lining) before being carried to the small intestine, where it is absorbed. Low levels of stomach acid or an inadequate amount of intrinsic factor – both of which occur with age – can lead to deficiencies. However, because the body has good reserves of B$_{12}$, it can take several years for a shortfall to develop.

What it does

Vitamin B$_{12}$ is essential for cell replication and is particularly important for red blood-cell production. It maintains the protective sheath around nerves (myelin), assists in converting food to energy and plays a critical role in the production of DNA and RNA, the genetic material in cells.

PREVENTION: Moderately high blood levels of homocysteine, an amino acid-like substance, have been linked to an increased risk of heart disease. Working with folic acid, vitamin B$_{12}$ helps the body to process homocysteine and so may lower that risk. Vitamin B$_{12}$ has beneficial effects on the nerves, and therefore may help to prevent a number of neurological disorders as well as the numbness and tingling often associated with diabetes. It may also play a part in treating depression.

ADDITIONAL BENEFITS: Research shows that low levels of vitamin B$_{12}$ are common in people with Alzheimer's disease. Whether the deficiency is a contributing factor to the disease or simply a result of it is unknown. The nutrient does, however, keep the immune system healthy. Some studies suggest that it lengthens the period of time between infection

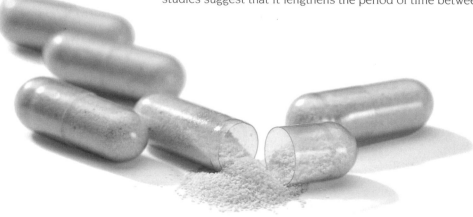

with the HIV virus and the development of AIDS. Other research indicates that adequate B_{12} intake improves immune responses in older people. With its beneficial effect on nerves, vitamin B_{12} may ease tinnitus (ringing in the ears). As a component of myelin it is valuable in treating multiple sclerosis, a disease that involves the destruction of this nerve covering.

How much you need

The recommended amount for vitamin B_{12} is 1.5 mcg a day for adults. Supplements of vitamin B_{12} may be important for older people and vegans (who eat no meat or dairy products).

⊟ **IF YOU GET TOO LITTLE:** Symptoms of a vitamin B_{12} deficiency include fatigue, depression, numbness and tingling in the extremities caused by nerve damage, muscle weakness, confusion and memory loss. Dementia and pernicious anaemia can develop; both are reversible if caught early.

The level of B_{12} in the blood decreases with age. People with ulcers, Crohn's disease or other gastrointestinal disorders are at risk, as are those taking prescription medication for epilepsy (seizures), chronic indigestion or gout. Excessive alcohol also hinders absorption of vitamin B_{12}.

⊞ **IF YOU GET TOO MUCH:** Excess vitamin B_{12} is readily excreted in urine, and there are no known adverse effects from a high intake of it.

How to take it

▨ **DOSAGE:** A general dose of 1000 mcg of vitamin B_{12} a day may be useful for heart disease prevention, pernicious anaemia, numbness and tingling, tinnitus and multiple sclerosis. If you are deficient in B_{12}, higher doses may be needed. Or if you do not produce enough intrinsic factor, B_{12} injections or a prescription nasal spray may be necessary; ask your doctor for further information and guidance.

◉ **GUIDELINES FOR USE:** Take vitamin B_{12} once a day, preferably in the morning, along with 400 mcg of folic acid. Most multivitamins contain at least the recommended amount of vitamin B_{12} and folic acid; B-complex supplements have higher amounts. For larger therapeutic amounts look for a supplement with just vitamin B_{12} or B_{12} with folic acid. Using a sublingual (under-the-tongue) form enhances absorption.

Other sources

Animal foods are the primary source of B_{12}. These include offal, brewer's yeast, oysters, sardines and other fish, eggs, meat and cheese. Many breakfast cereals are fortified with this vitamin as well.

Boost your vitamin B_{12} intake with cheese.

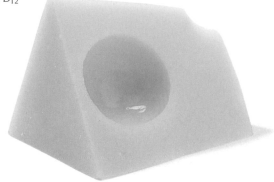

Vitamin C

Vitamin C is probably better known and more widely used than any other nutritional supplement, but even people who are particularly familiar with the uses of this versatile nutrient may be surprised to discover the extent of the health benefits it can provide.

Common uses

- *Enhances immunity.*
- *Minimises cold symptoms; shortens duration of illness.*
- *Speeds wound healing.*
- *Promotes healthy gums.*
- *Treats asthma.*
- *Helps to prevent cataracts.*
- *Protects against some forms of cancer and heart disease.*

Forms

- Capsule
- Liquid
- Powder
- Tablet

CAUTION!

- If you suffer from kidney stones, kidney disease or haemochromatosis, a genetic tendency to store excess iron, limit your daily intake to 500 mg (vitamin C enhances iron absorption).

- Vitamin C can distort the accuracy of medical tests for diabetes, colon cancer and haemoglobin levels. Let your doctor know if you're taking it.

REMINDER: If you have a medical condition, consult your doctor before taking supplements.

What it is

As early as 1742 lemon juice was known to prevent scurvy, a debilitating disease that often plagued long-distance sailors, but not until 1928 was the healthful component in lemon juice identified as vitamin C. Its anti-scurvy, or antiscorbutic, effect is the root of this vitamin's scientific name: ascorbic acid. Today, interest in vitamin C is based less on its ability to cure scurvy than on its potential to protect cells. As the body's primary water-soluble antioxidant, vitamin C helps to fight damage caused by unstable oxygen molecules called free radicals – especially in those areas that are mostly water, such as the interiors of cells.

What it does

Vitamin C is active throughout the body. It helps to strengthen the capillaries (the tiniest blood vessels) and cell walls and is crucial for the formation of collagen (a protein found in connective tissue). In these ways vitamin C prevents bruising, promotes healing and keeps ligaments (which connect muscle to bone), tendons (which connect bone to bone) and gums strong and healthy. It also aids the production of haemoglobin in red blood cells and helps the body to absorb iron from foods.

PREVENTION: As an antioxidant, vitamin C offers protection against cancer and heart disease; several studies have shown that low levels of this vitamin are linked to heart attacks. In addition, vitamin C may actually lengthen life. In one study, men who consumed more than 300 mg of vitamin C a day (from food and supplements) lived longer than men who consumed less than 50 mg a day.

Another study found that, over the long term, vitamin C supplements protect against cataracts, a clouding of the lens of the eye that interferes with vision. Women who took vitamin C for ten years or more had a 77% lower rate of early 'lens opacities', the first stage of cataracts, than women who did not take supplements.

ADDITIONAL BENEFITS: Does vitamin C prevent colds? Probably not, but it can help to lessen their symptoms and may shorten their duration. In a 1995 analysis of studies exploring the connection between vitamin C

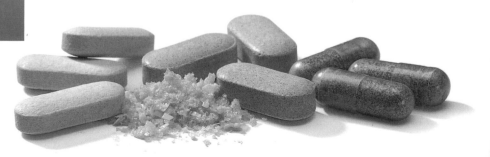

and colds, the researchers concluded that taking 1000 to 6000 mg a day at the onset of cold symptoms reduces the cold's duration by 21% – about one day. Other studies have shown that vitamin C helps elderly patients to fight severe respiratory infections. Vitamin C also appears to be a natural antihistamine. High doses of the vitamin can block the effect of inflammatory substances produced by the body in response to pollen, pet hair or other allergens.

The vitamin is an effective asthma remedy as well. Numerous studies have found that vitamin C supplements helped to prevent or improve asthmatic symptoms. For people with type 1 diabetes, which interferes with the transport of vitamin C into cells, supplementing with 1000 to 3000 mg a day may prevent complications of the disease, such as eye problems and high cholesterol levels.

How much you need

The recommended target for vitamin C for men and women is 40 mg a day (80 mg for smokers). However, even conservative nutritionists think an optimal intake is at least 200 mg a day, and they recommend higher doses for the treatment of specific diseases.

▣ **IF YOU GET TOO LITTLE:** You would have to consume less than 10 mg of vitamin C a day to get scurvy, but receiving less than 50 mg a day has been linked with a higher risk of heart attack, cataracts and a shorter life.

⊞ **IF YOU GET TOO MUCH:** Large doses of vitamin C – more than 1000 mg a day – can cause loose stools, diarrhoea, flatulence and bloating; all can be corrected by reducing your daily dose. At this level the vitamin may interfere with the absorption of copper and selenium, so make sure you consume enough of these minerals in food or supplements. Continued high doses of vitamin C may lead to the development of kidney stones in susceptible individuals.

How to take it

☑ **DOSAGE:** For *general health*: 200 mg of vitamin C a day through foods and supplements. For *the treatment of various diseases*: Depending on the condition, 1000 mg a day may be appropriate.

◉ **GUIDELINES FOR USE:** Large amounts are most easily absorbed in 200 mg doses, taken with meals throughout the day. The vitamin works very well when combined with other antioxidants, such as vitamin E.

Other sources

Citrus fruits and juices, broccoli, dark-green leafy vegetables, red peppers, strawberries and kiwi fruits are all good sources of vitamin C.

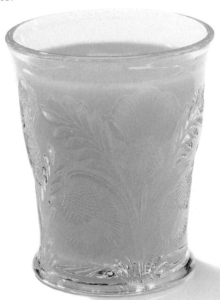

RECENT FINDINGS

Vitamin C may help to prevent reblockage (restenosis) of arteries after angioplasty (an alternative to bypass surgery). A study of 119 angioplasty patients found that restenosis occurred in just 24% of those who took 500 mg of vitamin C a day for four months, but in 43% of those who did not take the vitamin.

———

In addition to being an antioxidant, vitamin C helps the body to recycle other antioxidants. In one study, vitamin E concentrations were 18% higher in those who got more than 220 mg of vitamin C a day than in people who got 120 mg or less.

———

Vitamin C may help to prevent arthritis. A large study, involving 25,000 people, found that the risk of arthritis was significantly higher in those whose diet was low in vitamin C and fruit and vegetables.

DID YOU KNOW?

A 225 ml glass of freshly squeezed orange juice supplies 124 mg of vitamin C – well over half the daily target thought to be desirable for optimal health.

Vitamin D

Called the sunshine vitamin – because your body makes all it needs with enough sunlight – vitamin D is essential for healthy bones and may slow the progression of osteoporosis. It is also believed to strengthen the immune system and possibly prevent some cancers.

Common uses

- Aids in the body's absorption of calcium.

- Promotes healthy bones.

- Strengthens teeth.

- May protect against some types of cancer.

Forms

- Capsule
- Liquid
- Softgel
- Tablet

CAUTION!

■ Overuse of vitamin D supplements can result in elevated blood levels of calcium, leading to weight loss, nausea and heart and kidney damage.

REMINDER: If you have a medical condition, consult your doctor before taking supplements.

What it is

Technically a hormone, vitamin D is produced within the body when the skin is exposed to the ultraviolet B (UVB) rays in sunlight. Theoretically, spending a few minutes in the sun each day supplies all the vitamin D your body needs, but many people do not get enough sun to generate adequate vitamin D, especially in winter.

What is more, the body's ability to manufacture vitamin D declines with age, so vitamin D deficiencies are common in older people. But even young adults may not have sufficient vitamin D stores. One study of nearly 300 patients (of all ages) hospitalised for a variety of causes found that 57% of them did not have high enough levels of vitamin D. Of particular concern was the observation that a vitamin D deficiency was present in a third of the people who obtained the recommended amount of vitamin D through diet or supplements. This finding suggests that current recommendations for vitamin D may not be high enough.

What it does

The basic function of vitamin D is to regulate blood levels of calcium and phosphorus, helping to build strong bones and healthy teeth.

🔻 **PREVENTION:** Studies have shown that vitamin D is important in the prevention of osteoporosis, a disease that causes porous bones and thus an increased risk of fractures. Without sufficient vitamin D, the body cannot absorb calcium from food or supplements, no matter how much calcium you consume. When blood calcium levels are low, the body will move calcium from the bones to the blood to supply the muscles – especially those of the heart – and the nerves with the amount they need. Over time, this reallocation of calcium leads to a loss of bone mass.

Often combined with calcium or added to multivitamin preparations, vitamin D is also available as a separate supplement – in the form of softgels, for example.

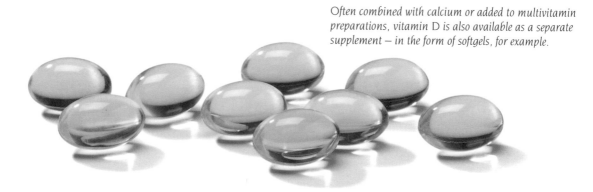

✱ **ADDITIONAL BENEFITS:** Scientists are continuing to discover more about the functions of vitamin D in the body. Some studies suggest that it is important for a healthy immune system; others indicate that it may help to prevent prostate, colon or breast cancer. One study found that adequate vitamin D slowed the progression of osteoarthritis in the knees, although it did not prevent the disease from developing in the first place.

How much you need

A recommended daily target for vitamin D has not been set for adults because it is assumed that sufficient will be made through the action of sunlight on the skin. However, for people over 65, and for pregnant or breastfeeding women, the recommended target is 10 mcg a day.

⊟ **IF YOU GET TOO LITTLE:** A vitamin D deficiency can harm the bones, causing a bone-weakening disease in children (rickets) and increase the risk of osteoporosis in adults. A deficiency can also cause diarrhoea, insomnia, nervousness and muscle twitches. The likelihood of a child developing rickets today is remote, however, since children typically spend enough time in the sun to generate ample vitamin D.

⊞ **IF YOU GET TOO MUCH:** Although your body effectively rids itself of any extra vitamin D it makes from sunlight, too many supplements may create problems. Daily doses of 25 to 50 mcg over six months can cause constipation or diarrhoea, headache, loss of appetite, nausea and vomiting, heartbeat irregularities and extreme fatigue. Continued high doses can disrupt the balance of calcium and phosphate, weaken the bones and allow calcium to accumulate in soft tissues, such as muscles.

How to take it

☑ **DOSAGE:** As little as 10 to 15 minutes of midday sunlight on your face, hands and arms two or three times a week can supply all the vitamin D you need. But if you are over 50, or you do not get outdoors much between the hours of 8am and 3pm or you always wear sunscreen, you might want to consider vitamin D supplements. Many practitioners recommend 10 to 15 mcg a day for people over 50, while 5 to 10 mcg a day is probably sufficient for younger adults.

◉ **GUIDELINES FOR USE:** Supplements can be taken at any time of day, with or without food. Most daily multivitamins contain up to 10 mcg of vitamin D. It is also often found in calcium supplements.

Other sources

Many breakfast cereals are fortified with 1 to 2.5 mcg of vitamin D in each serving. Fatty fish, such as herring, salmon and tuna, are naturally rich in this vitamin.

Vitamin E

A crucially important nutrient with antioxidant capability, vitamin E offers a multitude of benefits, including protection against heart disease, cancer and a range of other disorders. As it works at the body's cellular level, vitamin E may even slow down the ageing process.

Common uses

- Helps to protect against heart disease, certain cancers and various other chronic ailments.
- May delay or prevent cataracts.
- Enhances the immune system.
- Protects against toxins from cigarette smoke and other pollutants.
- Aids in skin healing.

Forms

- Capsule
- Cream
- Liquid
- Oil
- Softgel
- Tablet

CAUTION!

- People on prescription blood-thinning drugs (anticoagulants) or aspirin should consult their doctor before using vitamin E.

- Do not take vitamin E two days before or after surgery.

REMINDER: If you have a medical condition, consult your doctor before taking supplements.

What it is

Vitamin E is a generic term for a group of related compounds called tocopherols, which occur in four major forms: alpha, beta, gamma and delta-tocopherols. Alpha-tocopherol is the most common and most potent form of the vitamin. Vitamin E is fat-soluble, and so is stored for relatively long periods in the body, mainly in fat tissue and the liver. It is found in only a few foods, and many of these are high in fat, which makes it difficult to get the amount of vitamin E you require while on a low-fat diet. Supplements can therefore be very useful in obtaining optimal amounts of this nutrient.

What it does

One of vitamin E's basic functions is to protect cell membranes. It also helps the body to use selenium and vitamin K. But vitamin E's current reputation comes from its disease-fighting potential as an antioxidant – meaning that it assists in destroying or neutralising free radicals, the unstable oxygen molecules that cause damage to cells.

PREVENTION: By safeguarding cell membranes and acting as an antioxidant, vitamin E may play a role in preventing cancer. Some compelling research indicates that vitamin E can help to protect against cardiovascular disease, including heart attacks and strokes, by reducing the harmful effects of LDL ('bad') cholesterol and by preventing blood clots. In addition, vitamin E may offer protection because it works to reduce inflammatory processes that have been linked to heart disease. Findings from two large studies suggest that vitamin E may reduce the risk of heart disease by 25% to 50% – and it may prevent chest pain (angina) as well. Recent findings suggest that taking vitamin E with vitamin C may help to block some of the harmful effects of a fatty meal.

ADDITIONAL BENEFITS: Vitamin E protects cells from free-radical damage, which leads some clinicians to think that vitamin E may retard the ageing process. There is also evidence to suggest that it improves

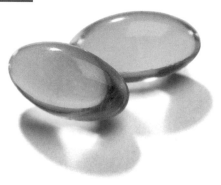
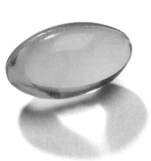

The vitamin E oil contained in softgels can be used to heal minor skin wounds.

immune function in the elderly, combats toxins from cigarette smoke and other pollutants, postpones the development of cataracts and slows the progression of Alzheimer's disease – and perhaps of Parkinson's disease.

Other research found that vitamin E can relieve the severe leg pain caused by a circulatory problem called intermittent claudication. It may alleviate premenstrual breast pain and tenderness as well. In addition, many people report that applying creams or oils containing vitamin E to skin wounds helps to promote healing.

How much you need

Although a recommended daily amount for vitamin E has not been set, recommended safe intakes are 4 mg a day for men and 3 mg a day for women. Safe intake levels may be enough to prevent deficiency, but higher doses are needed to provide the full antioxidant effect.

⊟ **IF YOU GET TOO LITTLE:** When the levels of vitamin E consumed are below the recommended safe intakes, neurological damage may occur and the life of red blood cells may be shortened. However, people who eat a balanced diet are unlikely to be at risk.

⊞ **IF YOU GET TOO MUCH:** No toxic effects from large doses of vitamin E have been discovered. Minor effects, such as headaches and diarrhoea, have rarely been reported. But large doses of vitamin E can interfere with the absorption of vitamin A.

How to take it

▨ **DOSAGE:** Many nutritionists recommend that, to benefit from the disease-fighting potential of vitamin E, you should take 250 to 500 mg daily in capsule or tablet form. (This total includes amounts obtained from a multivitamin.) Doses of up to 800 mg have been recommended for those at high risk of heart disease and certain cancers. It may be particularly effective when taken with vitamin C.

◉ **GUIDELINES FOR USE:** Try to take vitamin E supplements at the same time each day. Combining it with a meal decreases stomach irritation and increases the absorption of this fat-soluble vitamin. For topical use, break open a capsule and apply the oil directly to your skin, or use a commercial cream containing vitamin E as needed.

Other sources

Wheat germ is an outstanding dietary source of vitamin E: 2 tablespoons contain the equivalent of 40 mg. Beneficial amounts of vitamin E are also found in vegetable oils, nuts and seeds (such as almonds and sunflower seeds), green leafy vegetables and whole grains.

Hazelnuts are one of the foods that offer a good source of vitamin E.

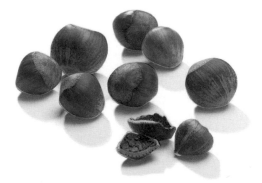

Vitamin K

Doctors have long used vitamin K, which promotes blood clotting, to help to reduce blood loss after surgery and to prevent bleeding problems in newborn babies. This vitamin also aids in building strong bones and may be useful for combating the threat of osteoporosis.

Common uses

- Reduces the risk of internal haemorrhaging.

- Protects against bleeding problems after surgery.

- Helps to build strong bones, and to ward off or treat osteoporosis.

Forms

- Liquid
- Tablet

CAUTION!

■ Supplemental vitamin K (more than is found in a multivitamin) should be taken only with your doctor's supervision.

REMINDER: If you have a medical condition, consult your doctor before taking supplements.

What it is

In the 1930s Danish researchers noticed that baby chickens fed a fat-free diet developed bleeding problems. They eventually solved the problem with an alfalfa-based compound that they named vitamin K, for *Koagulation*. Scientists now know that most of the body's vitamin K needs are met by the beneficial activity of bacteria in the intestines that produce this vitamin, and only about 20% comes from foods. Deficiencies are rare in healthy people, even though the body does not store vitamin K in high amounts. Synthetic supplements are available by prescription. Other names for vitamin K are phytonadione and menadiol.

What it does

This single nutrient sets in motion the entire blood-clotting process as soon as a wound occurs. Without it, we might bleed to death. Researchers have discovered that vitamin K plays a protective role in bone health as well.

PREVENTION: Doctors may recommend preventative doses of vitamin K if bleeding or haemorrhaging is a concern. Even when no deficiency exists, surgeons frequently order vitamin K before an operation to reduce the risk of postoperative bleeding. Under medical supervision it can also be prescribed for excessive menstrual bleeding. Though it is not yet a widely accepted treatment, vitamin K may provide benefits for those suffering from osteoporosis. Some studies show that it helps the body to make use of calcium and decreases the risk of fractures. Vitamin K may be especially important for bone health in older women. Not surprisingly, it is included among the ingredients in many bone-building formulas.

ADDITIONAL BENEFITS: Vitamin K may play a role in cancer prevention and help those undergoing radiation therapy. Recent findings also put vitamin K in the arsenal of heart-supporting nutrients: some evidence suggests it may halt the build-up of disease-causing plaque in arteries and reduce the blood level of LDL ('bad') cholesterol. But more research is needed to define the role of vitamin K in these and other disorders.

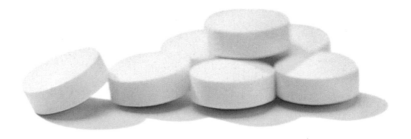

How much you need

Although a recommended daily amount for vitamin K has not been set, the recommended safe intake for adults is 1 mcg a day per 1 kilogram of body weight.

⊟ **IF YOU GET TOO LITTLE:** In healthy people, a vitamin K deficiency is rare because the body manufactures most of what it requires. In fact, deficiencies are found only in those with liver disease or intestinal illnesses that interfere with fat absorption. However, vitamin K levels can drop as a result of long-term use of antibiotics. One of the first signs of a deficiency is a tendency to bruise easily. Those at risk need careful medical monitoring because they could bleed to death in the event of a serious injury.

⊞ **IF YOU GET TOO MUCH:** It is hard to get too much vitamin K because it is not abundant in any one food (except leafy greens). Although even megadoses are not toxic, high doses can be dangerous if you are taking anticoagulants. Large doses also may cause flushing and sweating.

How to take it

⊘ **DOSAGE:** Multivitamins often contain between 25 and 60 mcg of vitamin K. Bone-building formulas provide around 300 mcg a day, the equivalent of adding a large leafy salad to your daily diet. Higher doses (such as those in prenatal multivitamins) may be prescribed under medical supervision for those with specific medical needs.

◉ **GUIDELINES FOR USE:** When prescribed, vitamin K should be taken with meals to enhance absorption.

Other sources

Leafy green vegetables, including – per serving – kale (550 mcg) and Swiss chard (300 mcg), are richest in vitamin K. Broccoli, spring onions and brussels sprouts are also good sources. Other foods with some vitamin K are pistachio nuts, vegetable oils, meats and dairy products.

RECENT FINDINGS

Green tea is sometimes erroneously considered the leading source of vitamin K; it has 1700 mcg in 225 grams. Many doctors consequently advise their patients on anti-coagulants (blood thinners) to skip the tea. In fact, that's the amount of vitamin K in 225 grams of tea leaves – which would make hundreds of cups of brewed tea. According to an American study, a cup of green tea contains virtually no vitamin K.

FACTS & TIPS

■ If you take blood-thinning medications and eat lots of leafy green vegetables, which are rich in vitamin K, let your doctor know. Your dose of medication may need to be adjusted.

■ Vitamin E helps the body to use vitamin K, but too much vitamin E – more than 700 mg a day – taken long term may impair vitamin K function and increase your risk of bleeding.

A serving of kale provides the equivalent of more than five 100 mcg tablets of vitamin K.

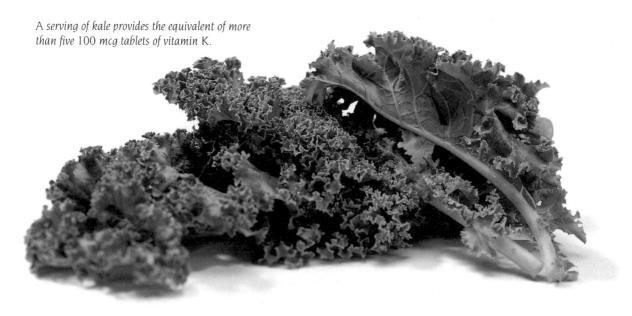

White willow bark

Used for thousands of years to treat fevers and headaches, white willow bark contains a chemical forerunner of today's most popular painkiller – aspirin. The herb is sometimes called 'herbal aspirin' but has few of that drug's side effects.

Salix alba

Common uses

- *Relieves acute and chronic pains, including back and neck pain, headaches and muscle aches.*
- *Reduces arthritis inflammation.*
- *May lower fevers.*

Forms

- Capsule
- Dried herb/tea
- Powder
- Tablet
- Tincture

CAUTION!

■ Avoid white willow bark if you are allergic to aspirin. When subject to fever, children and teenagers should also avoid the herb.

■ Pregnant or breastfeeding women should consult their doctors before taking white willow bark, because its safety has not been established in these situations.

REMINDER: If you have a medical condition, consult your doctor before taking supplements.

What it is

White willow bark comes from the stately white willow tree, which can grow up to 23 metres tall. In China its medicinal properties have been appreciated for centuries, but not until the 18th century was the herb recognised as a pain reliever and fever reducer in the West. European settlers brought the white willow tree to North America, where they discovered that local tribes were already using native willow species to alleviate pain and fight fevers.

In 1828 the plant's active ingredient, salicin, was isolated by German and French scientists. Ten years later, European chemists manufactured from it salicylic acid, a chemical cousin to aspirin. Aspirin, or acetyl-salicylic acid, was later created from a different salicin-containing herb called meadowsweet. By the end of the 19th century the Bayer Company had begun commercially producing aspirin, which was marketed as a new and safer pain reliever than wintergreen and black birch oil, the herbs commonly employed at that time for reducing pain.

All parts of the white willow contain salicin, but concentrations of this chemical are highest in the bark, which is collected in early spring from trees that are two to five years old. *Salix alba*, or white willow, is the most popular species for medicinal use, but other types of willow are also rich in salicin, including *Salix fragilis* (crack willow), *Salix purpurea* (purple willow) and *Salix daphnoides* (violet willow). These species are often sold simply as willow bark in health-food shops.

What it does

In the body, the salicin from white willow bark is metabolised to form salicylic acid, which reduces pain, fever and inflammation. Though the

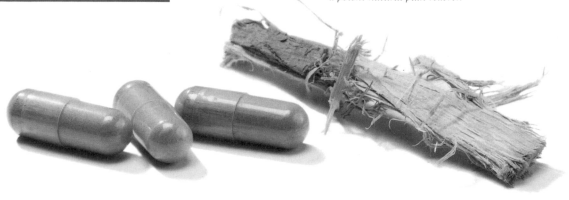

Bark from the white willow tree – dried, concentrated, and packaged into capsules or tablets – is the source of a potent natural pain reliever.

herb is slower acting than aspirin, its beneficial effects last longer, and it causes fewer adverse reactions. Most notably, it does not produce stomach bleeding – one of aspirin's most potentially serious side effects.

✤ **MAJOR BENEFITS:** White willow bark can be very effective for relieving headaches as well as acute muscle aches and pains. It can also alleviate all sorts of chronic pain, including back and neck pain. When recommended for arthritis, especially if there is pain in the back, knees, and hips, it can reduce swelling and inflammation and increase joint mobility. In addition it may help to ease the pain of menstrual cramps – the salicin interferes with the action of hormone-like chemicals called prostaglandins that can contribute to inflammation and cause pain.

✤ **ADDITIONAL BENEFITS:** White willow bark, like aspirin, may be useful for alleviating fevers.

How to take it

✐ **DOSAGE:** Take one or two capsules or tablets three times a day, or as needed to relieve pain, calm a fever or reduce inflammation (follow the instructions on the packet). Look for preparations that are standardised to contain 15% salicin. This dosage provides between 60 and 120 mg a day of salicin. Standardised extracts can also be taken in tincture or powder form. White willow bark teas are likely to be less effective than standardised extracts because they supply only a small amount of pain-relieving salicin.

◉ **GUIDELINES FOR USE:** White willow bark is safe to use long term. It has a bitter, astringent taste, so the most convenient way to take it is probably in capsule or tablet form. Do not consume white willow bark with aspirin because it can amplify the side effects of aspirin.

As a precaution, do not give the herb to a child or teenager under 16 who has a cold, flu or chicken pox. Taking aspirin can put these young people at risk of a potentially fatal brain and liver condition called Reye's syndrome. Salicin, the therapeutic ingredient in white willow bark, is unlikely to cause this problem because it is metabolised differently from aspirin, but its similarities to the painkiller warrant a cautious approach. Paracetamol is a better choice than white willow bark or aspirin for children and teenagers.

Possible side effects

This herb rarely causes side effects at recommended doses. However, higher doses can lead to an upset stomach, nausea or tinnitus. If any of these occur, lower the dosage or stop taking the herb. Consult your doctor if side effects persist.

Wild yam

Dioscorea villosa

Common uses

- *Relieves menstrual cramps.*
- *May ease the pain of endometriosis.*
- *Reduces inflammation.*

Forms

- Capsule
- Cream
- Dried herb/tea
- Softgel
- Tablet
- Tincture

CAUTION!

- **Pregnant women should not use wild yam.**

REMINDER: If you have a medical condition, consult your doctor before taking supplements.

Misconceptions about the active ingredients in wild yam have led to exaggerated claims. The herb has been hailed as a natural alternative to hormone replacement therapy following the menopause. Wild yam has not been proved effective for this purpose, but it does have other benefits.

What it is

In some countries 'yam' describes a type of sweet potato with reddish flesh. This vegetable is not related, even distantly, to wild yam, a native plant of North and Central America that was first used medicinally by the Aztecs and Mayas for its pain-relieving qualities. Later, European settlers took advantage of the wild yam's therapeutic properties and utilised it for treating joint pain and colic. The root is the part of the plant that has medicinal value. Sold as a dried herb for use in tea, it is also available in several other forms.

What it does

In recent years wild yam has been extolled for its ability to mimic certain hormones – especially progesterone – and said to relieve menopausal or PMS symptoms. Most of these claims remain scientifically unproven, however. It is true that wild yam contains a substance called diosgenin that can be converted to progesterone in the laboratory, but the human body is unable to make this conversion.

Some holistic practitioners have reported that patients suffering from premenstrual syndrome (PMS) and menopausal symptoms experienced good results with wild yam cream, which is applied to the soft areas of

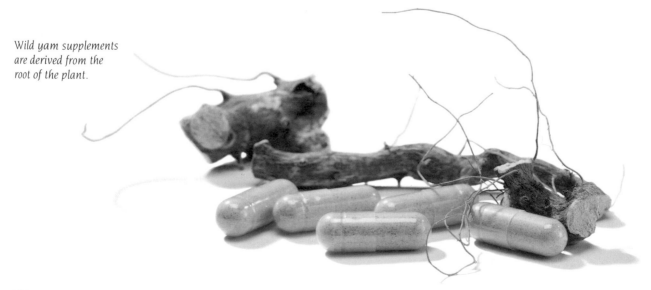

Wild yam supplements are derived from the root of the plant.

the body (abdomen and thighs). How the cream helps is unclear. Sometimes manufacturers of the creams add laboratory-synthesised progesterone, which could well account for some of the therapeutic effects. Despite positive reports from patients, the value of pure wild yam creams has yet to be scientifically proven.

When taken in any of the available forms, wild yam does have other medicinal effects. Some herbalists believe that crude forms of it may help to rectify hormonal imbalances associated with PMS and the menopause because it contains oestrogen-like substances. In addition, wild yam acts as a muscle relaxant, antispasmodic and anti-inflammatory, which may explain why it alleviates menstrual complaints in some women.

✷ **MAJOR BENEFITS:** Wild yam contains substances called alkaloids, which are muscle relaxants that especially target muscles in the abdomen and pelvis. This action suggests that wild yam may be of value in treating digestive disorders such as Crohn's disease and irritable bowel syndrome. It can also ease menstrual cramps and the pain associated with endometriosis, a disorder of the uterine lining.

Some women find that wild yam combined with another herb, such as chasteberry, is particularly effective in relieving the symptoms of PMS; this is the result of both normalisation of hormone balance and anti-inflammatory action.

✷ **ADDITIONAL BENEFITS:** Other active ingredients found in wild yam, known as steroidal saponins, play a role in alleviating muscle strains, chronic muscle pain and arthritis.

How to take it

☑ **DOSAGE:** In order to receive the therapeutic benefits of wild yam, take a ½ teaspoon of tincture three or four times a day, or 500 mg of wild yam in capsule, tablet or softgel form twice a day. If you prefer, drink a cup of wild yam tea three times a day.

✷ **GUIDELINES FOR USE:** Take wild yam supplements or tincture with food to minimise the risk of stomach upsets. To make wild yam tea, pour a cup of very hot water over 1 or 2 teaspoons of the dried herb and let it steep for 15 minutes. You can add other soothing herbs to the tea – valerian or peppermint, for example – when using it for digestive disorders.

Possible side effects

In extremely large amounts wild yam supplements and tinctures can cause nausea and diarrhoea.

DID YOU KNOW?
The first contraceptive pill to be produced was derived from diosgenin, the hormone-like compound found in wild yam.

Zinc

Every cell in the body needs zinc, but many of us do not get enough of this vital mineral. Zinc is contained in enzymes – chemicals that do everything from digesting food to healing wounds. It is a crucial component of the immune system, helping to fight infections, including the common cold.

Common uses

- Helps to prevent colds, flu and other infections.
- Helps to treat a wide range of chronic ailments, from rheumatoid arthritis and underactive thyroid to chronic fatigue and osteoporosis.
- Alleviates skin problems and digestive complaints.
- May improve fertility, build healthy hair and diminish tinnitus.

Forms

- Capsule
- Liquid
- Lozenge
- Tablet

CAUTION!

■ Do not take too much zinc. More than 30 mg daily can, in the long term, interfere with copper absorption, leading to anaemia. Daily doses of more than 100 mg of zinc can also impair immunity.

REMINDER: *If you have a medical condition, consult your doctor before taking supplements.*

What it is

Zinc is concentrated in the muscles, bones, skin, kidneys, liver, pancreas, eyes and, in men, the prostate. It is plentiful in high-protein foods such as meat and fish. The body does not produce or store zinc, so it depends on external sources for a continuous supply.

What it does

Zinc is critical for hundreds of processes that take place in the body, from cell growth to sexual maturation and immunity – even for taste and smell. Consequently, everyone who takes a daily multivitamin and mineral supplement should make sure that it contains zinc.

✪ **MAJOR BENEFITS:** Necessary for the proper functioning of the immune system, zinc helps to protect the body against colds, flu, conjunctivitis and other infections. In an American study of 100 people in the initial stages of a cold, those who sucked zinc lozenges every couple of hours recovered from their illness about three days earlier than those who sucked placebo lozenges. Zinc lozenges may also speed the healing of mouth ulcers and sore throats. Taken as a dietary supplement, zinc may support the body's natural defence and repair systems in treating more serious illnesses, such as rheumatoid arthritis, lupus, chronic fatigue syndrome and possibly multiple sclerosis, as well as other conditions, such as AIDS, which are associated with an impaired immune system.

✪ **ADDITIONAL BENEFITS:** Zinc exerts beneficial effects on the production of various hormones, including the sex and thyroid hormones. It could be helpful for enhancing the fertility of both men and women, and is also important for the health of the prostate gland. In addition, it may be effective for people with underactive thyroids and, because it improves insulin levels, it may help those with diabetes. The fact that zinc is involved in so many systems of the body means that it has other

When taken as dietary supplements, zinc tablets (below left) should always include copper; zinc lozenges (below right), which often contain vitamin C, ward off the symptoms of colds and flu.

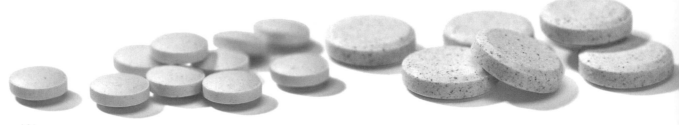

functions too. It stimulates the healing of wounds and skin irritations, which makes it a useful treatment for acne, burns, eczema, psoriasis and rosacea, and it promotes the health of the hair and scalp. Zinc has also been shown to slow vision loss in people with macular degeneration, a common cause of blindness in those aged over 50. In a recent Japanese study, tinnitus (ringing in the ears) improved with zinc supplementation. Zinc may also be useful for alleviating osteoporosis, haemorrhoids, inflammatory bowel disease and ulcers.

How much you need

The current recommended target for zinc is 7 mg for women and 9.5 mg for men daily. Higher doses are usually reserved for specific complaints.

⊟ **IF YOU GET TOO LITTLE:** Severe zinc deficiency is rare in the UK, but a mild zinc deficiency can lead to poor wound healing, more frequent colds and flu, a depressed sense of taste and smell, and skin problems such as acne, eczema and psoriasis. It can result in impaired blood sugar tolerance (and an increased diabetes risk) and a low sperm count.

⊞ **IF YOU GET TOO MUCH:** Long-term use of more than 100 mg a day has been shown to impair immunity and lower the level of HDL ('good') cholesterol. One study reported a connection between excessive zinc and Alzheimer's disease, though evidence is scant. Larger doses (more than 200 mg a day) can cause nausea, vomiting and diarrhoea.

How to take it

⊘ **DOSAGE:** The recommended target is 15 mg once a day. Taking high levels of zinc for longer than a month may interfere with copper absorption, so dietary supplements should include 2 mg of copper for every 30 mg of zinc. *For colds and flu*: Use zinc lozenges every two to four hours for a week; do not exceed 150 mg a day.

◉ **GUIDELINES FOR USE:** Take zinc an hour before or two hours after a meal; if it causes stomach upset, have it with a low-fibre food. If you are taking iron supplements for a specific condition, do not take them at the same time as zinc. Take zinc at least two hours after taking antibiotics.

Other sources

When looking for foods rich in zinc, think protein. It is abundant in beef, pork, liver, poultry (especially dark meat), eggs and seafood (especially oysters). Cheese, beans, nuts and wheat germ are other good sources, but the zinc in these foods is less easily absorbed than the zinc in meat.

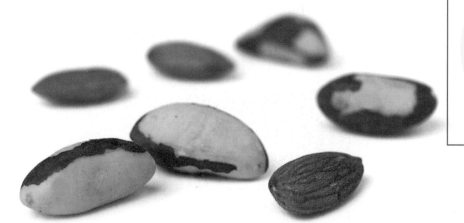

RECENT FINDINGS

A national survey in the UK found that zinc intake was below recommended targets in 43% of men and 45% of women aged 19-50.
Of children aged 4 and over, 89% had intakes below recommended levels. Among the elderly, more than 62% were not reaching their daily targets.

Adding just a little zinc to the diet greatly reduces cases of diarrhoea, pneumonia and malaria in developing countries. By boosting the immune system, zinc can prevent up to 38% of diarrhoea attacks, and cut acute respiratory infections by up to 45% and cases of malaria by 35% or more.

DID YOU KNOW?

Brazil nuts and almonds are excellent sources of zinc: for example, 100 grams of brazils yield 3-4 mg of zinc, about half the daily target for women.

Part 2

Protecting your health

This section covers more than 90 disorders, listed in alphabetical order from acne to warts and verrucas. Each entry features a chart with recommendations for vitamins, minerals, herbs and other nutritional supplements. These are the remedies that the consultants for this book have found to be most helpful and most readily available for the particular condition.

Supplements shown in blue in the charts are generally the most effective in a broad range of people, so consider starting with one or more of these. Supplements shown in black may also be beneficial or may work better for you. This section also includes special features on cancer, the growing child, later life, pregnancy, slimming, teenage health and vitality boosters.

There may be other therapies or supplements that are useful as well. It is recommended that, before taking any supplement, you turn to Part 1 of this book (pages 38–193) and read about it in detail. Take care to observe any warnings and precautions before using a supplement – and always consult your doctor if your illness has not previously been diagnosed or if your condition worsens.

ABOUT THE RECOMMENDATIONS

Specific dosage suggestions are listed in each of the profiles that follow. These are the total daily amount of a supplement that you need to treat the disorder or condition. In practical terms you may have to adjust these numbers to take account of the additional amounts of these same nutrients that you may be getting in any daily multivitamin or individual supplements that you are taking for other health reasons.

For example, we suggest taking 250 mg vitamin E daily for the promotion of a healthy prostate gland. If you are already taking a daily multivitamin tablet that supplies 250 mg vitamin E, you do not need any additional supplement of that vitamin. If you also have angina (which calls for 500 mg vitamin E),

you will have to take only 250 mg more each day to meet that requirement as well. The dosages are meant to be accurate, but each person is different. Always read the label on a supplement packet, and do not exceed recommended dosages, even though you may be treating several ailments. If you have a serious medical condition, consult your doctor about using supplements.

A final word: We have tried to include widely available dosages in the pages that follow but the strengths of individual supplement products vary greatly. If the information on a bottle or packet confuses you there are many qualified people, including health professionals and pharmacists, who can help you to choose the appropriate dose.

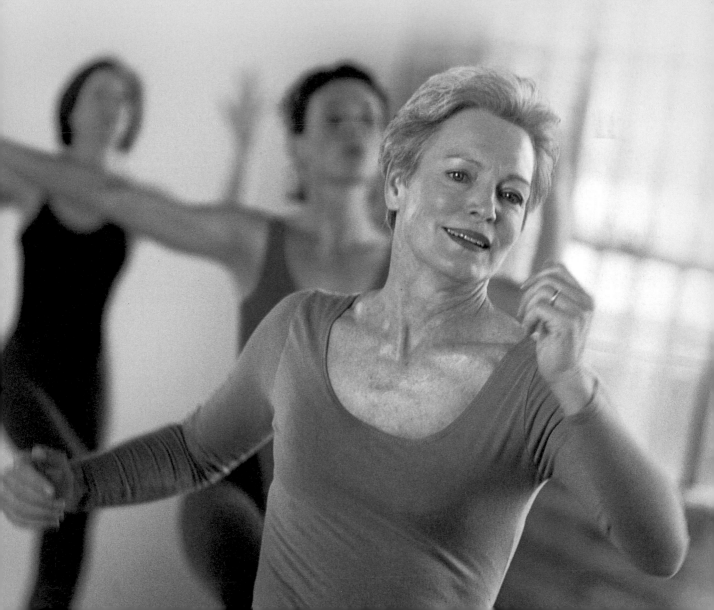

Acne

Although most people associate acne with the troublesome teenage years, it can erupt at any age. Indeed, up to 8% of those who had clear skin in their youth develop acne as adults. Fortunately, there are a variety of ways to control outbreaks – no matter how old you are when they occur.

Symptoms

- *Hard red bumps or pus-filled lesions on the skin.*
- *Red, inflamed skin with fluid-filled lumps or cysts.*

SEE YOUR DOCTOR ...

- If acne does not respond to self-care within three months.

- If severe acne develops: fluid-filled lumps, red or purple inflammation, cysts or hard nodules under the skin.

- If skin is continually red and flushed, even if no spots actually appear.

REMINDER: If you have a medical condition, consult your doctor before taking supplements.

What it is

Spots and other skin eruptions are the hallmarks of acne, a sometimes chronic condition of the face, back, chest, neck, shoulders and other areas of the body. The most common form (acne vulgaris) encompasses blackheads, whiteheads and raised red blemishes with semisolid centres. In severe cases (cystic acne), clusters of painful, fluid-filled cysts or firm, painless lumps appear beneath the skin's surface; both can lead to unsightly permanent pitting and scarring. For teenagers especially, acne can be an embarrassing and emotionally difficult condition.

What causes it

Acne occurs when the sebaceous glands at the base of the hair follicles of the skin secrete too much sebum. This thick, oily substance is normally released from the pores to keep the skin lubricated and healthy. If the sebum backs up, it can form hard plugs, or comedos, that block the pores and cause spots. Should one of these oil plugs rupture beneath the skin's surface, a localised bacterial infection can develop.

Hormonal imbalances can lead to an overproduction of sebum – a common problem during adolescence, especially in boys. In women, menstrual periods or pregnancy can also create acne-producing hormonal disturbances. Other acne triggers include emotionalstress; the friction or rubbing of clothing against the skin; andcertain medications, particularly steroids, contraceptives or drugs that affect hormone levels. Heredity may play a role as well.

Contrary to popular belief, acne is probably not caused by eating chocolate, shellfish, nuts or fatty snacks or by drinking colas. However, some doctors – and patients – contend that acne can be brought on or aggravated by certain foods or food allergies.

How supplements can help

Most people will benefit from trying all the supplements recommended in the chart; they can be safely combined. It often takes three to four weeks, or longer, to notice results. All can be used long term.

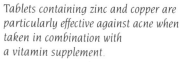

Tablets containing zinc and copper are particularly effective against acne when taken in combination with a vitamin supplement.

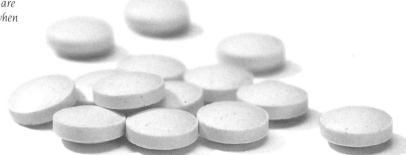

SUPPLEMENT RECOMMENDATIONS

Vitamin B$_6$	**Dosage:** 50 mg each morning. **Advice:** long-term doses of more than 200 mg a day for chronic acne can cause nerve damage.
Vitamin C	**Dosage:** 500 mg twice a day. **Advice:** reduce dose if diarrhoea develops.
Vitamin E	**Dosage:** 400 mg a day. **Caution:** consult a doctor if you take anticoagulant drugs.
Selenium	**Dosage:** 200 mcg a day. **Advice:** do not exceed a daily dose of 350 mcg.
Zinc	**Dosage:** 25 mg a day. **Advice:** supplementation with 30 mg or more of zinc should be accompanied by 2 mg copper.
Chasteberry	**Dosage:** 40 drops (½ teaspoon) of tincture a day, in a glass of water. **Advice:** often useful for premenstrual acne.
Evening primrose oil	**Dosage:** 1000 mg twice a day. **Advice:** Do not take during acute flare-ups Often useful when lesions are resolving.

Note: consider using supplements in blue first; the ones in black may also be beneficial. Some dosages may be supplied by supplements you are already taking – see page 195.

Vitamin B$_6$ may be useful for acne aggravated by menstrual cycles or the menopause. **Vitamin C**, **vitamin E** and **selenium** promote a healthy immune system, helping to keep acne-causing bacteria in check. Taken with any or all of these vitamins, **zinc** enhances immune function, reduces inflammation and promotes healthy hormone levels. Long-term use of zinc inhibits copper absorption, so it should be taken with that mineral. It may help to take zinc together with omega-3 essential fatty acids – omega-6 fatty acids, found in margarine, vegetable oil and many processed foods, tend to predominate in the modern diet, and a correct balance of omega-3 and omega-6 fatty acids helps to reduce inflammation.

Chasteberry is traditionally used to help with the treatment of menstruation-related acne. Other herbal remedies that are traditionally used for the treatment of acne include burdock, yellow dock, red clover and echinacea. **Evening primrose oil** may be used when the lesions are disappearing. It should not be used during acute flare-ups.

All of these supplements can be used long term, as well as in conjunction with conventional acne medications.

What else you can do

- ☑ Wash daily, using ordinary soap and water.
- ☑ Eat a balanced diet; avoid foods you feel may act as acne triggers.
- ☑ Choose cosmetics labelled 'noncomedogenic' or 'oil-free'.
- ☑ Avoid squeezing spots; it increases inflammation and can cause scarring.

RECENT FINDINGS

When evaluated by a group of physicians in one study, patients with acne who received 30 mg of zinc daily for two months had clearer complexions than those in a control group who had received a placebo. In another study, zinc produced results equal to those of the antibiotic tetracycline. But not many dermatologists have embraced zinc supplements because other research has failed to show that this mineral has any benefits to offer against acne.

DID YOU KNOW?

Holding the receiver of a telephone too tightly against your skin can cause acne to break out above your ear or along the side of your chin.

FACTS & TIPS

■ Fighting acne with natural supplements may be an attractive option for women of childbearing age, most of whom cannot take the powerful prescription drug isotretinoin (a derivative of vitamin A) because it may cause birth defects.

■ A 5% solution of topical tea tree oil is as effective as, but gentler than, 5% benzoyl peroxide for drying up mild acne blemishes, according to a study conducted in Australia. Higher dosages, containing up to 15% tea tree oil, may be helpful for more severe cases of acne.

Ageing

Many people live well into their 80s – and beyond. As the body ages, various systems slow down, and the risk of disease increases. You cannot halt the progress of time, but you can forestall some of the negative effects of ageing with a healthy lifestyle and well-chosen supplements.

Symptoms

- *Slowing of cognitive processes: declining memory and difficulty in remembering new people and events.*

- *Sensory decline: delay in refocusing eyes and impaired ability to hear high-pitched sounds.*

- *Weakened immune system: increased susceptibility to colds, flu and other illnesses.*

- *Decline in muscle and bone mass.*

- *Increased risk of developing heart disease and cancer.*

SEE YOUR DOCTOR ...

- **If you are 50 or over, you need a health check every year, but see your doctor straight-away if you are worried about the risk of age-related diseases.**

REMINDER: If you have a medical condition, consult your doctor before taking supplements.

People over the age of 50 may need to take extra folic acid and vitamin B$_{12}$.

What it is

Put simply, ageing is the process of growing old. Every part of the body is affected: among other changes, hair turns grey, skin wrinkles, joints and muscles lose flexibility, bones become weak, memory declines, eyesight diminishes, and immunity is impaired.

What causes it

The process of cell division and replacement that continues throughout life slows down with advancing age, and a progressive deterioration of all body systems begins. Though some decline is normal and inevitable, many researchers believe that unstable oxygen molecules called free radicals accelerate the process, making some people old before their time. A certain amount of damage is unavoidable because free radicals are produced during the normal course of cell activity, but it may be possible to slow down ageing by avoiding outside factors that foster free-radical formation – cigarette smoke, pollution, excessive alcohol, and radiation from X-rays or the sun – and by enhancing the body's own antioxidant defences. Manufactured by the cells and obtained through diet, antioxidants are powerful weapons that can disarm free radicals.

How supplements can help

Some supplements should be used daily by everyone concerned about the effects of ageing. **Vitamin C** and **vitamin E** are antioxidants that fight free radicals. Vitamin C and **flavonoids** work within the cells' watery interiors. Vitamin E protects the fatty membranes that surround cells; in addition, it improves immune function in older people and reduces the risk of some age-related conditions, including heart disease, some forms of cancer and, possibly, Alzheimer's disease. **Green tea extract** – which has long been prized for its longevity-promoting properties, and grape seed extract (100 mg twice a day) are other antioxidants that may be more potent than vitamins C and E.

    Folic acid, a B vitamin, maintains red blood cells and promotes the healthy functioning of nerves. Moreover, it protects the heart by helping the body process homocysteine, an amino acid-like compound that may

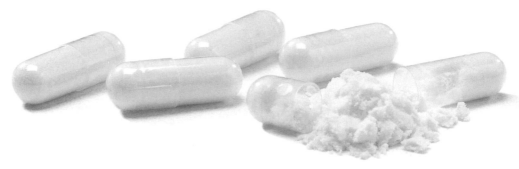

Vitamin C/ flavonoids	**Dosage:** 200 mg vitamin C and 100 mg flavonoids twice a day. **Advice:** also aim to eat five portions of fruit and vegetables a day.
Vitamin E	**Dosage:** 250 mg a day. **Caution:** consult your doctor if you take anticoagulant drugs.
Green tea extract	**Dosage:** 250 mg twice a day. **Advice:** standardised to contain at least 50% polyphenols.
Folic acid/ vitamin B_{12}	**Dosage:** 400 mcg folic acid and 1000 mcg vitamin B_{12} once a day. **Advice:** take the sublingual form for most efficient absorption.
Carnitine	**Dosage:** 500 mg L-carnitine twice a day. **Advice:** if you take a carnitine supplement for longer than one month, add mixed amino acids.
Calcium/ magnesium	**Dosage:** 500 mg calcium and 200 mg magnesium once or twice a day. **Advice:** combination supplement designed to enhance bone strength; should also include vitamin D.
Ginkgo biloba	**Dosage:** 40 mg three times a day. **Advice:** standardised to contain 24% flavone glycosides.

Some dosages may be supplied by supplements you are already taking – see page 195.

raise the risk of heart disease. Folic acid is assisted by **vitamin B$_{12}$**, which fosters healthy brain function. Vitamin B$_{12}$ supplements are useful for older people because many of them lose the ability to absorb the vitamin from food, and low B$_{12}$ levels can cause nerve damage and dementia. It is probably best to take B vitamins in the form of an 'A to Z' multivitamin and mineral formulation; these have been shown to improve the immune function and reduce infection rates in the elderly, who need more of a wide range of nutrients.

The amino acid-like substance **carnitine** contributes to a healthy heart because it helps to transport oxygen to the cells and produces energy. To protect against osteoporosis, nutritionists recommend supplementation with **calcium, magnesium** and vitamin D because adequate doses of these are not supplied by multivitamin and mineral formulations. The herb **ginkgo biloba** enhances blood flow, and may therefore improve such age-related conditions as dizziness, impotence and memory loss.

What else you can do

☑ Protect yourself from sun. Ultraviolet rays make skin age faster.
☑ If you smoke, give it up. Smoking speeds bone and lung deterioration.
☑ Build and maintain bone and muscle mass with weight-bearing exercise, such as walking and weight training.
☑ Eat a variety of fruits and vegetables – they are rich in antioxidants – and oily fish for omega-3 fatty acids.

Vitamin E may add years to your life. In a study by the US National Institute on Aging, people who took vitamin E supplements were about half as likely to die of heart disease as those not using vitamin E. In another American study, the vitamin strengthened the immune system in people aged 65 and older. Those who took 125 mg of vitamin E daily over a four-month period showed significant immune system improvement compared with people who were given other doses of the vitamin or a placebo.

A Swiss study found a link between high levels of antioxidants (such as beta-carotene and vitamin C) in the blood and better memory skills in older people.

DID YOU KNOW?
Although appetite often decreases as people grow older, the body's demand for vitamins, minerals and other nutrients actually increases.

FACTS & TIPS
■ Some practitioners advise that people over the age of 50 take a supplement of coenzyme Q$_{10}$ to minimise the effects of ageing. This substance helps to transport energy throughout the body and acts as an antioxidant, but its production by the body declines with age. If you want to add coenzyme Q$_{10}$ to your regimen, take 50 mg twice a day with food.

Alcoholism

Abstinence is the best course for those who cannot control their drinking. Although they do not offer a cure, various supplements may help heavy drinkers to overcome their craving for alcohol, support them during the taxing withdrawal process and set them on the road to recovery.

Symptoms

- *Constantly seeking opportunities to drink; being unable to cut intake; putting alcohol before family, friends and work.*

- *Needing more and more alcohol to achieve the same effect.*

- *Reacting indignantly to criticism of drinking; adamantly denying the problem.*

- *Experiencing withdrawal symptoms (tremors, hallucinations and fits) if drinking is stopped.*

SEE YOUR DOCTOR ...

- **If you drink before breakfast.**

- **If drinking binges last for 48 hours or more.**

- **If you have blackouts or falls.**

- **If you routinely turn to alcohol to relieve stress or pain.**

- **If drinking is ruining your personal relationships.**

REMINDER: If you have a medical condition, consult your doctor before taking supplements.

Extracts from the milk thistle plant can help to repair alcohol-induced liver damage.

What it is

An intense physical and psychological dependence on alcohol is the hallmark of alcoholism – which many consider a chronic disease, like diabetes or hypertension. Though alcohol appears to protect the heart when taken in moderation, excessive drinking can, over time, damage the liver, pancreas, intestine, brain and other organs. It can also cause malnutrition when 'empty' alcohol calories replace a nourishing diet.

What causes it

Drinking has a social component: it makes most people feel talkative and relaxed. Precisely why some people pursue alcohol to excess remains a mystery; psychosocial factors play a role, but there seems to be a strong genetic component as well. Indeed, children of alcoholics are at high risk of the disease, even when brought up in nondrinking households.

How supplements can help

The recommended supplements, plus an 'A to Z' multivitamin and mineral supplement – all of which can be taken together – can play several important roles in weaning problem drinkers from alcohol and helping them through the initial recovery period, which may last for weeks or even months. In addition to supplements, prescription drugs are usually needed to help alcoholics to weather withdrawal symptoms.

Most heavy drinkers are deficient in important nutrients, including B vitamins, vitamin C and minerals (especially magnesium, chromium and zinc), because they do not have healthy diets and because alcohol has toxic effects. It may be beneficial to continue therapy for several months, or even longer, to help to restore depleted nutrients. **Vitamin C**

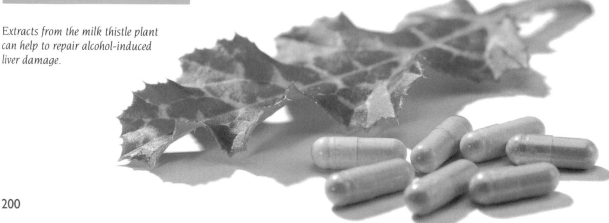

SUPPLEMENT RECOMMENDATIONS

Vitamin C/ vitamin E	**Dosage:** 500 mg vitamin C twice a day; 250 mg vitamin E daily. **Advice:** vitamin C helps to boost the effects of vitamin E.
Vitamin B complex	**Dosage:** one tablet or capsule each morning with food. **Advice:** look for a B-50 complex with 50 mcg vitamin B_{12} and biotin, 400 mcg folic acid, and 50 mg all other B vitamins.
Kudzu	**Dosage:** 150 mg extract three times a day. **Advice:** standardised to contain at least 0.95% daidzen.
Milk thistle	**Dosage:** 250 mg three times a day between meals. **Advice:** standardised to contain at least 70% silymarin.
Magnesium	**Dosage:** 200 mg twice a day. **Caution:** do not take if you have kidney disease.
Evening primrose oil	**Dosage:** 1000 mg three times a day. **Advice:** you can substitute 1000 mg borage oil once a day.

Note: consider using supplements in blue first; the one in black may also be beneficial. Some dosages may be supplied by supplements you are already taking – see page 195.

can help to strengthen the body during this difficult period, clearing alcohol from the tissues and reducing mild withdrawal symptoms; it is most useful when taken with **vitamin E**. The **B complex vitamins**, the amino acid glutamine and extracts from the **kudzu** vine appear to reduce the craving. The herb **milk thistle** and phosphatidylcholine (500 mg three times a day) strengthen the liver, helping it to rid the body of toxins.

Adequate amounts of the minerals chromium and zinc are contained in a multivitamin and mineral supplement. Chromium helps to prevent fatigue caused by low blood sugar (hypoglycaemia), a common problem in alcoholics. Zinc is a key component of many enzymes necessary for the body's metabolism. **Magnesium** is also essential for many metabolic functions, but the amounts provided by multivitamin and mineral supplements are insufficient. **Evening primrose oil** provides the fatty acid GLA (gamma-linolenic acid); this substance stimulates production of a brain chemical called prostaglandin E, which works to prevent withdrawal symptoms such as fits and depression. It also assists in protecting the liver and nervous system.

What else you can do

- ☑ Join a support group, such as Alcoholics Anonymous (AA).
- ☑ Try acupuncture. It may reduce the craving for alcohol.

RECENT FINDINGS

There is now scientific evidence to back up claims that kudzu can block alcohol cravings. Researchers at the University of North Carolina noted that in monkeys (considered good stand-ins for humans) kudzu cut alcohol intake by about 25%. Harvard scientists found that, in a strain of golden Syrian hamsters that preferred alcohol to water, kudzu cut consumption in half.

Studies confirm the protective effects of the herb milk thistle. When people with cirrhosis (liver scarring), a dangerous late-stage complication of alcoholism, took milk thistle, 58% were alive after four years, compared with only 39% who did not use the herb.

FACTS & TIPS

■ To reduce the craving for alcohol, supplements are usually safer than prescription drugs, which may have unpleasant side effects.

Alzheimer's disease

This progressive brain disorder – marked by slowly increasing memory loss and disorientation – is a wrenching experience for patients and carers. Early treatment may help to slow or temporarily reverse the course of this devastating illness.

Symptoms

- *Memory loss, including an inability to recall recent events and difficulty finding appropriate words or solving basic problems.*

- *Disorientation, including getting lost in a familiar place – for example, at home or in the neighbourhood.*

- *Personality changes, marked by agitation, anxiety, combativeness, indifference to others, social withdrawal or poor judgment.*

- *Language impairment, such as rambling speech, long pauses and repetition.*

SEE YOUR DOCTOR ...

- **If you experience or someone close to you experiences severe disorientation or a change in behaviour – seek a full medical examination, including an assessment for dementia.**

REMINDER: If you have a medical condition, consult your doctor before taking supplements.

What it is

Alzheimer's disease, a degenerative brain disorder, impairs memory and mental functioning. The onset is typically very slow. Initially, Alzheimer's sufferers have short-term memory loss and difficulty making decisions; they may forget how to perform simple tasks. Advanced stages bring loss of memory and speech, loss of bladder and bowel control, and changes in temperament, such as excessive hostility or withdrawal. About 10% of people over the age of 80 in the UK are afflicted by Alzheimer's disease.

What causes it

Scientists are still not sure what causes Alzheimer's disease. They do know that it is marked by a major loss of nerve cells in the brain, particularly in areas controlling memory and thinking. The disease is also characterised by reduced levels of brain chemicals important for memory. A family history of the disease can increase the risk of developing Alzheimer's; other possible causes include serious head injury, cardiovascular disease and slow-acting viruses. Studies indicate that aluminium (such as from cookware) is unlikely to be the cause of Alzheimer's disease.

How supplements can help

Although there is no cure for Alzheimer's disease, researchers continue to make strides in treating the symptoms. A number of supplements may help to restore mental functioning during the earlier stages of the disease and even delay the onset of advanced symptoms. Supplements should be started as soon as possible, taken individually or together. It may be at least eight weeks before results are noticed. The supplements can also be used with prescription drugs such as aricept, but this should only be done on medical advice. One promising supplement is the herb **ginkgo biloba**. Controlled trials have shown that ginkgo, which increases

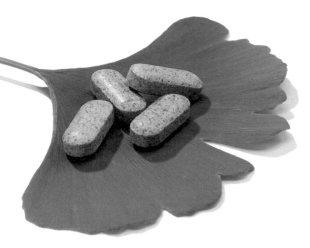

Extracts from the leaf of the ginkgo biloba tree show real promise as memory boosters.

SUPPLEMENT RECOMMENDATIONS

Ginkgo biloba	**Dosage:** 80 mg three times a day. **Advice:** standardised to contain at least 24% flavone glycosides.
Antioxidants	**Dosage:** 1000 mg vitamin C, 500 mg vitamin E and 15 mg mixed carotenoids a day. **Advice:** may be sold as a single supplement.
Vitamin B complex	**Dosage:** one tablet or capsule a day with food. **Advice:** look for a B-50 complex with 50 mcg vitamin B_{12} and biotin, 400 mcg folic acid and 50 mg all other B vitamins.
Evening primrose oil	**Dosage:** 1000 mg three times a day. **Advice:** you can substitute 1000 mg borage oil once a day.
Gotu kola	**Dosage:** 200 mg extract or 400-500 mg crude herb three times a day. **Advice:** standardised to contain 10% asiaticosides; may reduce fatigue and depression and stimulate central nervous system.
Ginseng (Siberian)	**Dosage:** 100-300 mg extract three times a day. **Advice:** standardised to contain at least 0.8% eleutherosides.
L-acetyl-carnitine(LAC)	**Dosage:** 500 mg three times a day. **Advice:** LAC is thought to be more active than other forms of carnitine.

Note: consider using supplements in blue first; those in black may also be beneficial. Some dosages may be supplied by supplements you are already taking – see page 195.

the brain's blood supply, may improve memory in some patients. It may have antioxidant properties as well, playing a key role in maintaining healthy nerve cells. Other **antioxidants** that may be beneficial include vitamin C, vitamin E and mixed carotenoids; these are often combined in convenient and economical commercial preparations.

In addition, be sure to get enough B vitamins – low levels have been linked with Alzheimer's disease; take **vitamin B complex**. Also worth trying are **evening primrose oil** and the herbs **gotu kola** and **ginseng (Siberian)**; all may benefit memory by improving the transmission of nerve impulses. Two other nutrients may help by boosting memory-enhancing brain chemicals: the amino acid-like substance **L-acetylcarnitine (LAC)**, a form of carnitine, or phosphatidylserine (100 mg three times a day). See which one works best for you.

What else you can do

☑ Exercise. Even a short daily walk may help to improve mental abilities.
☑ Keep your mind active by reading, doing puzzles or practising memory exercises.
☑ Stay relaxed to improve memory and concentration.
☑ Alzheimer's disease has a profound effect on family and friends. Support groups may be helpful.

Anaemia

Looking pale? Feeling weak and tired? A quick blood test can assess if anaemia is to blame – and, if so, whether it is caused by iron-poor blood or something else. Your doctor is the best person to ask about whether certain supplements might be right for you.

Symptoms

- Weakness, fatigue, dizziness, irritability or mental confusion.

- Paleness, especially of the gums and eyelids or under the nails.

- Palpitations; shortness of breath.

- Sores in the mouth or on the tongue; unusual bruising or bleeding.

- Numbness and tingling of the feet or legs.

- Nausea and diarrhoea.

SEE YOUR DOCTOR ...

- If you have any symptoms of anaemia – your doctor must find the underlying cause.

- If you are pregnant (or are considering pregnancy) or menstruate heavily.

- If you are following a treatment plan for anaemia – regular checkups can determine if supplements are working.

REMINDER: If you have a medical condition, consult your doctor before taking supplements.

What it is

Anaemia is a condition in which there is a shortage of red cells in the blood or a deficiency of haemoglobin (the oxygen-carrying pigment) in these cells. When anaemia occurs, the body doesn't get enough oxygen, and weakness and fatigue result. Although symptoms may not appear – or may be very mild – for a long time, the condition can be life-threatening if it is left undiagnosed and untreated. If you suspect you are anaemic, it is essential that you see your doctor promptly to ascertain the underlying cause. Treatment will vary, depending on the diagnosis.

What causes it

Iron deficiency, the most common cause of anaemia, usually results from a gradual, prolonged blood loss, which depletes the body's iron stores. Without enough iron, haemoglobin levels fall. Menstruating women, particularly those with heavy periods, are prone to iron-deficiency anaemia. However, men and women can develop iron deficiency from any condition that causes slow bleeding – including long-term haemorrhoids, rectal polyps or ulcers; stomach or colon cancer; or prolonged use of aspirin or other nonsteroidal anti-inflammatory drugs (NSAIDs), such as ibuprofen. Because so many foods are fortified with iron, iron-deficiency anaemia can rarely be attributed to a lack of this mineral in the diet.

Less common is anaemia that results from a deficiency of vitamin B_{12} (in which case it is called pernicious anaemia) or folic acid. Both nutrients are essential to red blood cell production. Alcoholics, smokers, people with certain digestive disorders, vegetarians, those over the age of 50, and pregnant or breastfeeding women are the most likely to be at risk, through either poor or inadequate nutrition or an inability to absorb these nutrients properly. Other forms of anaemia can be traced to chronic illnesses (for example, cancer, lupus or rheumatoid arthritis); hereditary disorders, such as sickle-cell anaemia, or exposure to toxic drugs, chemicals or radiation.

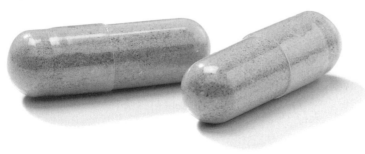

Iron supplements for so-called 'tired blood' can be dangerous if you have not got an iron deficiency.

Iron	**Dosage:** up to 17 mg a day, taken with meals. **Advice:** your doctor may prescribe a higher dose.
Vitamin C	**Dosage:** 500 mg twice a day. **Advice:** take with food.
Vitamin B_{12}/ folic acid	**Dosage:** 1000 mcg B_{12} and 400 mcg folic acid in sublingual (under the tongue) form twice a day for one month. **Advice:** always take B_{12} and folic acid together; if still anaemic after oral B_{12} supplements, you may need to try B_{12} injections.
Echinacea	**Dosage:** 200 mg extract twice a day. **Advice:** standardised to contain 3.5% echnacosides.
Nettle	**Dosage:** 250 mg nettle leaf extract twice a day. **Advice:** standardised extracts of nettle leaf are not available.

Note: consider using supplements in blue first; those in black may also be beneficial. Some dosages may be supplied by supplements you are already taking – see page 195.

How supplements can help

Before taking supplements you need to determine the underlying cause of your anaemia. It is especially important to see a doctor about iron-deficiency anaemia, which may be caused by internal bleeding. If you are advised to take supplements, have your blood tested every month to see if they are improving your condition.

If iron-deficiency anaemia is diagnosed, it may be beneficial to combine **iron** with **vitamin C**. Iron is a key component of haemoglobin, and vitamin C helps the body to absorb the mineral. Take iron only under your doctor's supervision, because too much can be dangerous.

Various herbs may also be useful. **Echinacea** has a reputation for promoting the regeneration of red blood cells, while **nettle** has been successfully used by herbalists for the treatment of anaemia. Although herbs cannot make substantial contributions to the vitamins and minerals required by the body, they provide phytonutrients to support their utilisation. Taken as a tincture, juice or tea, some herbs (dandelion, burdock, yellow dock, gentian and red clover) may enhance the body's ability to utilise iron from foods or supplements.

Vitamin C may be beneficial if anaemia is caused by a deficiency of vitamin B_{12} or folic acid as well; it aids the body in absorbing these nutrients. **Vitamin B_{12}** and **folic acid** should always be taken in tandem, and under a doctor's supervision, because a high intake of one can mask a deficiency of the other. Together they work to boost production of red blood cells. Once anaemia is corrected, and a problem with absorption has been ruled out as a cause, the amount of B_{12} and folic acid in your daily multivitamin may be sufficient to prevent recurrence.

What else you can do

☑ Eat foods rich in iron (dried beans, liver, red meat, dried fruits, nuts and shellfish); in folic acid (citrus fruits, asparagus, spinach, mushrooms, liver, soya beans and wheat germ); and in vitamin B_{12} (liver, shellfish, lamb, beef, cheese, fish and eggs).

A study involving 28 strict vegetarians found that 500 mg of vitamin C, taken after lunch and dinner for two months, raised haemoglobin levels by 8% and blood iron levels by 17%. Vitamin C increases the body's ability to absorb iron.

Studies suggest that people over the age of 50 are less able than younger people to absorb vitamin B_{12}, and are therefore more susceptible to anaemia. The US National Academy of Sciences now urges all senior citizens to take B_{12} supplements.

FACTS & TIPS

■ Most postmenopausal women, and men of all ages, get plenty of iron in their diets and should not take a multivitamin and mineral supplement that contains it. Excess iron acts as an 'oxidant', generating harmful molecules called free radicals that can raise cholesterol and block arteries. Excessive intake of iron has been linked to heart disease.

■ Some doctors believe that vitamin B_{12} is more easily absorbed by injection than in the oral forms, but studies show that oral supplements are usually just as effective.

Angina

Although conventional medications for angina may help to relieve the intense chest pain of this heart disorder, they do very little to halt the physiological mechanisms behind it. Vitamins, minerals and natural remedies may improve the condition – or at least prevent it from getting worse.

Symptoms

- *Crushing or squeezing chest pain.*
- *Weakness.*
- *Sweating.*
- *Shortness of breath.*
- *Palpitations.*
- *Nausea.*
- *Light-headedness.*

SEE YOUR DOCTOR ...

- **If you have any of the above symptoms for the first time.**
- **If there is any change in the normal pattern of your angina attacks – for example, if they increase in frequency, intensity or duration, or if they are brought on by new activities.**
- **If an angina attack lasts more than 15 minutes: this may be a heart attack – phone for an ambulance immediately.**

REMINDER: If you have a medical condition, consult your doctor before taking supplements.

What it is

When your heart is not getting enough blood and oxygen, the crushing or squeezing pain of angina is typically the result. Usually the pain begins below the breastbone and radiates to the shoulder, arm or jaw, increasing in intensity until it reaches a plateau and then diminishes. The attack can last up to 15 minutes.

What causes it

Angina is a direct result of the build-up of plaque (atherosclerosis) in the arteries that supply the heart with blood. Like the other muscles and organs in the body, the heart needs blood and oxygen to do its work – in its case, pumping blood throughout the circulatory system.

With atherosclerosis, arteries may be wide enough to provide sufficient blood flow during rest, but they cannot supply enough oxygen-rich blood when physical activity increases the demand on the heart. Any exertion – climbing stairs, running for the bus, digging the garden, even having sex – can trigger some angina attacks. Angina may also result if a coronary artery goes into spasm.

How supplements can help

The supplements listed in the chart can all be used together or alone. They can also complement your prescription angina medications, but never stop your heart medication without first consulting your doctor.

The antioxidant effect of vitamins C and E can help prevent cell damage: **vitamin C** aids in the repair of the arteries injured by plaque, and **vitamin E** blocks the oxidation of LDL ('bad') cholesterol, the initial step in the formation of plaque. In addition, some people with heart disease have low levels of vitamin E as well as of the mineral **magnesium**, which may inhibit spasms of the coronary arteries.

Amino acids can benefit the heart in several ways. **Arginine** plays a role in forming nitric oxide, which relaxes artery walls. One study found

Hawthorn extract, derived from berries or other parts of the plant, is a good heart-protective herbal treatment.

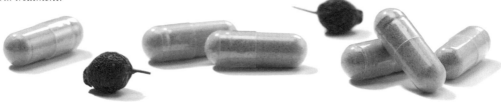

SUPPLEMENT RECOMMENDATIONS

Vitamin C	**Dosage:** 500 mg twice a day. **Advice:** reduce dose if diarrhoea develops.
Vitamin E	**Dosage:** 250 twice a day. **Caution:** consult your doctor if you take anticoagulant drugs.
Magnesium	**Dosage:** 200 mg twice a day. **Caution:** do not take if you have kidney disease.
Arginine	**Dosage:** 500 mg L-arginine three times a day, between meals. **Advice:** if you take an arginine supplement for more than a month, add mixed amino acids.
Carnitine	**Dosage:** 500 mg L-carnitine three times a day between meals. **Advice:** if you take a carnitine supplement for more than a month, add mixed amino acids.
Coenzyme Q$_{10}$	**Dosage:** 100 mg twice a day. **Advice:** for best absorption, take with food.
Hawthorn	**Dosage:** 100-150 mg extract three times a day. **Advice:** standardised to contain at least 1.8% vitexin.
Essential fatty acids	**Dosage:** one tablespoon flaxseed oil a day; 2000 mg fish oils three times a day. **Caution:** diabetics should never exceed the stated dose. **Advice:** take only if you do not eat fish at least twice a week.

Some dosages may be supplied by supplements you are already taking – see page 195.

that taking this amino acid three times a day increased the amount of time for which individuals with angina could exercise at moderate intensity without having to stop because of chest pain. **Carnitine**, an amino acid-like substance, allows heart muscle cells to use energy more efficiently.

Like carnitine, the nutritional supplement **coenzyme Q$_{10}$** enhances the heart muscle, reducing its workload, and the herb **hawthorn** improves blood flow to the heart. **Essential fatty acids** may be effective in lowering triglyceride levels and keeping arteries flexible.

What else you can do

☑ Eat a low-fat, fibre-rich diet; use a polyunsaturate spread or olive oil instead of butter.

☑ Do not smoke, and avoid smoky places.

☑ Learn to relax. Meditation, t'ai chi and yoga may reduce angina attacks.

☑ Join a support group. Determine what brought you to this point in your life and what you can do to begin reversing the disease.

CASE HISTORY
A heartfelt tale

Michael M., a surgeon, first felt twinges in his chest as he was running in a 5 kilometre race. 'It must be the heat or indigestion,' he remembers thinking. But later, when the pain literally stopped him in his tracks as he was running up some stairs, he knew something was wrong.

A year later, after many painful episodes of angina, a heart attack and a coronary bypass, he began to feel similar chest twinges again. He realised this new angina was a clear warning that the whole process could easily repeat itself unless he made some drastic changes.

Michael embraced his new lifestyle as seriously as he had ever done anything in his life. He walked every day and reduced the fat in his diet; he practised meditation and the Chinese martial art t'ai chi. In addition, he replaced his annual holiday with a number of three-day weekends rather than one long (and often stressful) trip. Finally, he learned about the potential benefits of vitamins, herbs, minerals and antioxidants.

Now, virtually symptom-free and 9 kilograms lighter, Michael looks a decade younger than his 64 years. 'I had been giving health advice for years,' he comments. 'The time finally came when I had to say, "Physician, heal thyself."'

Anxiety and panic

Everyone feels anxious from time to time, but some people are uneasy so often – or have frightening episodes called panic attacks – that anxiety interferes with their normal life. Taking B vitamins, certain minerals and calming herbs may help.

Symptoms

Acute anxiety

- Extreme fear.
- Rapid heartbeat and breathing.
- Excessive perspiration, chills or hot flushes.
- Dry mouth.
- Dizziness.

Chronic anxiety

- Muscle tension, headaches and back pain.
- Insomnia.
- Depression.
- Low sex drive.
- Inability to relax.

SEE YOUR DOCTOR ...

- **Before replacing prescription antianxiety medications, such as alprazolam, lorazepam or diazepam, with herbs or supplements – cutting back suddenly can be dangerous.**

- **To rule out the possibility of other causes: anxiety symptoms can mimic those of a serious illness, or be caused by certain medical conditions or drugs.**

REMINDER: *If you have a medical or psychiatric condition, consult your doctor before taking supplements.*

What it is

When you are faced with a potentially dangerous situation – a large barking dog, for example – anxiety is a healthy response. Sensing the danger, your brain signals for the release of hormones to prepare your body to defend itself. Muscles grow tense, heartbeat and breathing rate increase, and the blood even becomes more likely to clot (in case you are injured). In many individuals this response is set in motion even when there is no obvious threat. Such a reaction can be bad for your health, causing exhaustion, poor concentration, a sense of detachment from yourself or your surroundings, headaches, stomach problems and an increase in blood pressure.

Anxiety disorders come in two basic forms. Generalised anxiety disorder (GAD) is a chronic condition that involves a recurring sense of foreboding and worry accompanied by mild physical symptoms. A panic attack, on the other hand, comes on suddenly and unexpectedly, with symptoms so violent that the episodes are often mistaken for a heart attack or another life-threatening condition.

What causes it

Some scientists think that the central nervous systems of people with anxiety disorders overreact to stress and take a longer time than most to return to a calmer state. Anxiety may begin with an upsetting event – an accident or a divorce – or have no identifiable root. It may also have a biochemical basis. People prone to panic attacks have higher blood levels of lactic acid, a chemical produced when muscles metabolise sugar without enough oxygen. Other research suggests that anxiety may be the result of an overproduction of stress hormones by the brain and adrenal glands.

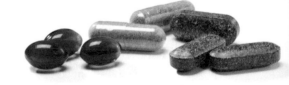

The herb valerian (below) can be used during the day as well as at night for its calming effect and in combination with St John's wort (right).

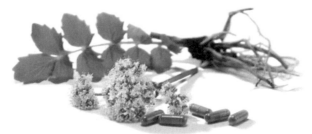

SUPPLEMENT RECOMMENDATIONS	
Calcium/ magnesium	**Dosage:** 500 mg calcium and 200 mg magnesium twice a day. **Advice:** take with food; sometimes sold as a single supplement.
Vitamin B complex	**Dosage:** one tablet or capsule each morning with food. **Advice:** look for a B-50 complex with 50 mcg vitamin B_{12} and biotin, 400 mcg folic acid and 50 mg all other B vitamins.
Valerian	**Dosage:** 250 mg extract twice a day. **Caution:** may cause drowsiness if you are short of sleep. **Advice:** standardised to contain 0.8% valerenic acid.
St John's wort	**Dosage:** 300 mg extract three times a day. **Advice:** standardised to contain 0.3% hypericin.

Note: consider using supplements in blue first; those in black may also be beneficial. Some dosages may be supplied by supplements you are already taking – see page 195.

How supplements can help

In many cases, herbal and nutritional remedies for anxiety can be used in place of prescription drugs, which may be addictive and have other unpleasant side effects. People with anxiety should try **calcium**, **magnesium** and a **vitamin B complex** supplement. These nutrients are important for the healthy functioning of the nervous system, especially for the production in the brain of the key chemical messengers called neurotransmitters.

The herb **valerian**, known as a sleep aid, can be used at low doses throughout the day for a calming effect. You can also have a night-time dose (250 to 500 mg) of valerian extract as well if you have trouble falling asleep. **St John's wort** can be added to valerian, whether you are depressed or not. It may take about a month before the full effect of St John's wort are felt; the other supplements begin working immediately.

What else you can do

☑ Cut out caffeine, alcohol and excess sugar, which may trigger anxiety.
☑ Do aerobic exercises regularly. They burn lactic acid, produce natural feel-good chemicals (endorphins) and enhance your use of oxygen.
☑ See a therapist to develop more positive ways of coping.

DID YOU KNOW?

Anxiety and panic attacks are surprisingly common: in the UK, more than one in ten people are likely to have a disabling anxiety disorder at some point in their lifetime.

FACTS & TIPS

■ Chamomile makes a pleasant floral tea that will relax you without making you sleepy. It contains apigenin, which animal tests show affects the same brain receptors as anti-anxiety drugs, yet it is nonaddictive. Chamomile can be used with other herbs.

■ Breathing techniques can often help you to manage a panic attack. Inhale slowly, to a count of four; wait, to a count of four; exhale slowly, to a count of four; and wait, to a count of four. Repeat until the attack subsides.

■ Several studies indicate that individuals with anxiety symptoms may be uniquely sensitive to caffeine. Try reducing your caffeine intake – do it slowly to minimise withdrawal symptoms such as headaches – and see if this eases your anxiety.

Arrhythmia

The heart, workhorse of the body, beats more than 100,000 times a day, pumping life-giving blood through thousands of miles of arteries, capillaries and veins. Irregular heart rhythms – or arrhythmia – can disrupt this process and require careful medical evaluation.

Symptoms

- *Heart palpitations or pounding heartbeats.*

- *Fluttering in the chest or neck.*

- *Fatigue, light-headedness.*

- *Shortness of breath, chest pain, fainting spells.*

- *Often there are no symptoms; your doctor may find an arrhythmia during a routine examination.*

SEE YOUR DOCTOR ...

- **If you are aware of frequent irregularities in your heartbeat or suddenly become light-headed, dizzy or weak.**

- **If someone suddenly loses consciousness, or has severe chest pain or shortness of breath – phone for an ambulance straightaway.**

REMINDER: If you have a medical condition, consult your doctor before taking supplements.

What it is

Arrhythmia is characterised by abnormal rhythms of the heart. The condition may be as fleeting as a single missed beat, or it may be more serious, causing the heart to beat irregularly or unusually quickly or slowly for extended periods.

What causes it

For many people with arrhythmia, the cause is unclear. However, some cases can be traced to a heart condition, such as coronary artery disease. Thyroid or kidney disease, certain drugs, and imbalances of magnesium or potassium in the body can contribute to arrhythmia. Abnormal rhythms may also be induced by a high intake of caffeine or alcohol, heavy smoking and stress.

How supplements can help

It is important to remember that some forms of arrhythmia can be serious. The supplements listed in the chart are meant to complement – not to replace – standard pharmaceutical treatments. Never discontinue a heart drug without consulting your doctor first. All the supplements can be used together, but your doctor should determine which ones you should take and in what order. They may work within a week, but often need to be used long term.

   Magnesium supplements often benefit people with heart rhythm disorders, many of whom are deficient in this mineral. Magnesium is vital for coordinating the activities of nerves (including those that initiate heartbeats) and muscles (including the heart). **Hawthorn**, a herb that has been used as a heart tonic for centuries, is also valuable: it increases blood flow to the heart, making it beat more strongly and restoring rhythm. **Coenzyme Q$_{10}$** also helps to steady heart rhythm,

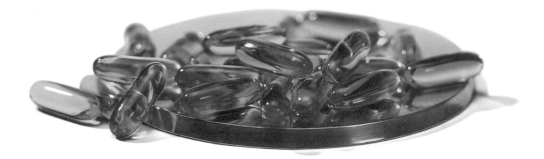

A supplement of fish oils may be helpful for people with heart rhythm disorders.

Magnesium	**Dosage:** 200 mg twice a day.
	Caution: do not take if you have kidney disease.
Hawthorn	**Dosage:** 100-150 mg extract three times a day.
	Advice: standardised to contain at least 1.8% vitexin.
Coenzyme Q₁₀	**Dosage:** 50 mg twice a day.
	Advice: for best absorption, take with food.
Fish oils	**Dosage:** 1000 mg three times a day.
	Caution: diabetics should never exceed the stated dose.
	Advice: take only if you do not eat fish at least twice a week.
Amino acids	**Dosage:** 1500 mg L-taurine twice a day; 500 mg L-carnitine three times a day.
	Caution: avoid in pregnancy and when breastfeeding.
	Advice: for long-term use, try a mixed amino acid complex.
Astragalus	**Dosage:** 400 mg twice a day, or three cups of tea a day.
	Advice: supplying 0.5% glucosides and 70% polysaccharides.

Note: consider using supplements in blue first; those in black may also be beneficial. Some dosages may be supplied by supplements you are already taking – see page 195.

and may be particularly useful for people who have previously suffered a heart attack or have another form of heart disease. In addition, **fish oils** are being extensively studied for treating heart ailments; early results strongly suggest that they are effective at relieving arrhythmia.

Other supplements may stabilise heart rhythm as well. The **amino acids** taurine and carnitine increase the oxygen supply to the heart. Taken as a tea, tablet, capsule or tincture (30 drops three times a day), the herb **astragalus** has been found to contain various substances that stabilise heart rhythm. Doctors also occasionally prescribe potassium supplements to prevent arrhythmia, although, for most people, eating fresh fruit and vegetables is a better way to obtain adequate supplies of this mineral.

What else you can do

☑ Reduce or eliminate caffeine and alcohol.
☑ If you smoke, give it up. No supplement can compensate for the long-term cardiac damage caused by smoking.
☑ Exercise regularly. Aerobic exercise strengthens the heart.
☑ Reduce stress. Relaxation techniques such as biofeedback may help.

In a recent study in Denmark, 55 heart attack survivors were given capsules of either fish oils or olive oil (placebo). After three months those receiving the fish oils did significantly better on heart tests, indicating that they were less likely to suffer from serious arrhythmia.

According to a study in the *Journal of the American College of Cardiology*, 232 people who had frequent arrhythmia significantly reduced their likelihood of abnormal heart rhythms after just three weeks by increasing their intake of magnesium and potassium.

FACTS & TIPS

■ Sipping astragalus tea may help to stabilise heart rhythm, but don't drink it all day long. Herbal teas can be potent medicine, so limit your intake to three cups a day.

■ If you dislike the taste of astragalus, try other herbal teas or tinctures. The herb barberry and its cousin Oregon grape both contain compounds known as berberines, which have been shown to reduce arrhythmia; angelica contains a mixture of substances that combat arrhythmia; and ginkgo biloba, like hawthorn, improves blood flow to the heart.

■ Many doctors recommend eating salmon, mackerel, herring or sardines at least twice a week to help to reduce the risk of fatal arrhythmia. It is a good idea: cold-water 'oily' fish may be an even better source of healing omega-3 fatty acids than fish oil capsules.

Arthritis

Osteoarthritis is usually age-related and commonly affects people over 50, while the joint inflammation and pain caused by rheumatoid arthritis often occur much earlier in life. Both conditions can be greatly relieved by the use of dietary supplements and ointment applied to the skin.

Symptoms

Osteoarthritis

- *Onset often gradual, marked by mild joint stiffness and pain – especially in the morning and following rest.*

Rheumatoid arthritis

- *Fatigue, weight loss, low fever and joint stiffness, followed several weeks later by red and painful swollen joints (wrists, fingers, knees, ankles and feet) that may feel warm.*

SEE YOUR DOCTOR ...

- If joint pain is accompanied by fever. This may signal infectious arthritis and require immediate medical attention.

- If pain and stiffness develop quickly, which may be a sign of rheumatoid arthritis.

- If you self-diagnose mild osteoarthritis, which should be confirmed by your doctor.

REMINDER: If you have a medical condition, consult your doctor before taking supplements.

What it is

In people suffering from osteoarthritis, joints gradually lose their cartilage – the smooth, gel-like shock-absorbing material that prevents adjacent bones from touching. Most commonly affected are the fingers, knees, hips, neck and spine. Rheumatoid arthritis is a chronic disorder in which the cartilage and other tissues in and around the bones become inflamed and damaged.

What causes it

Osteoarthritis may be the result of decades of joint wear and tear, though genetic factors, excess weight and impairments in the body's ability to repair cartilage may also play a role. In rheumatoid arthritis, the immune system attacks the body's own joints and associated tissues – the so-called autoimmune reaction. In some people this inflammatory condition, which often appears between the ages of 20 and 40, may be the result of a genetic predisposition.

How supplements can help

Although osteoarthritis and rheumatoid arthritis have different causes, there are many similarities in the treatments used by complementary practitioners. Antioxidants such as **vitamins C** and **E** and **zinc** are used for both conditions to protect cells, including those of the joints, from damage. **Glucosamine**, a cartilage-building sugar compound, is one of the most helpful remedies for relieving arthritis pain. It appears to slow down joint damage over time, though whether it can actually reverse the disease is unknown. To enhance the effectiveness of glucosamine, take it in combination with chondroitin. In addition, try one of the other supplements listed in the chart. Allow at least a month to assess the

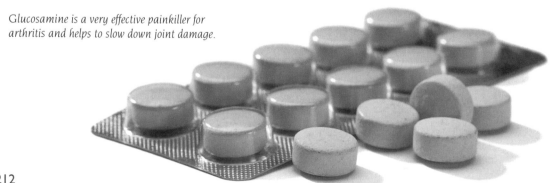

Glucosamine is a very effective painkiller for arthritis and helps to slow down joint damage.

SUPPLEMENT RECOMMENDATIONS

Vitamin C	**Dosage:** 500 mg twice a day. **Advice:** reduce dose if diarrhoea develops.
Vitamin E	**Dosage:** 250 mg twice a day. **Caution:** consult your doctor if you take anticoagulant drugs.
Zinc	**Dosage:** 15 mg a day. **Advice:** if you take a zinc supplement for more than a month, use one that includes 2 mg copper.
Glucosamine	**Dosage:** 500 mg glucosamine sulphate three times a day. **Advice:** take with food to minimise digestive upset.
Chondroitin	**Dosage:** up to 400 mg three times a day. **Advice:** take in combination with glucosamine.
Fish oils	**Dosage:** 2 teaspoons to supply 2 grams of omega-3 fatty acids a day. **Caution:** consult your doctor if you take anticoagulant drugs.
Chilli ointment	**Dosage:** apply to joints several times a day. **Advice:** standardised to contain 0.025%-0.075% capsaicin.
Niacin (nicotinamide)	**Dosage:** 1000 mg three times a day. **Caution:** high doses can cause liver damage and other serious side effects; medical monitoring is necessary during treatment.
Boswellia	**Dosage:** one tablet or capsule three times a day. **Advice:** standardised to have 150 mg boswellic acid.

Note: consider using supplements in blue first; those in black may also be beneficial. Some dosages may be supplied by supplements you are already taking – see page 195.

results; then, if necessary, substitute another supplement to use with glucosamine to see if it works better for you. These supplements can be used long term for both types of arthritis, as well as with conventional pain relievers such as aspirin and paracetamol and ibuprofen.

Supplements to try with glucosamine include **niacin** (nicotinamide), which may be especially effective in relieving knee pain; **boswellia**, a tree resin that may inhibit inflammation and build cartilage; and devil's claw, a herb from Namibia (300 mg extract three times a day). Rare side effects of taking boswellia include skin rashes, nausea and diarrhoea.

A supplement of **fish oils** may reduce inflammation, particularly in rheumatoid arthritis. For osteoarthritis, one form of the amino acid methionine called SAM (S-adenosylmethionine) has anti-inflammatory effects similar to ibuprofen and rebuilds cartilage; take 400 mg twice a day for two weeks, then 200 mg twice a day. (People with manic depressive illnesses should not take SAM.) Any of these therapies can be used with topically applied **chilli ointment** for pain relief.

What else you can do

☑ Engage in moderate low-impact exercise such as walking or swimming to strengthen muscles and improve overall joint condition.
☑ Apply heat or ice to joints for 20 minutes three times a day to help to reduce pain.

Asthma

Some 3½ million people in the UK have asthma – often a lifetime condition – and these numbers increase each year. This lung disease always requires medical management, but there are several steps you can take on your own to minimise the frequency and severity of asthma attacks.

Symptoms

- *Tightness, not pain, in the chest.*
- *Wheezing or whistling when breathing.*
- *Shortness of breath or difficulty breathing, which may improve when sitting up.*
- *Coughing (often with phlegm).*
- *Restlessness or insomnia.*

SEE YOUR DOCTOR ...

- **If you develop the symptoms of asthma for the first time.**

- **If self-care measures or prescription asthma drugs do not alleviate an attack.**

- **If you are gasping for breath or have a rapid pulse and a bluish tinge to fingers or lips – these require immediate emergency medical attention.**

REMINDER: If you have a medical condition, consult your doctor before taking supplements.

Regular supplements of vitamin B₆ are effective in relieving the symptoms of asthma, especially wheezing.

What it is

Asthma is a disease in which the airways of the lungs swell and tighten, restricting airflow and making it hard to breathe. During an asthma attack the smallest airways (the bronchioles) constrict. This causes the release of chemicals such as histamine that increase inflammation and swelling and produce excess mucus. Though many asthma attacks are mild and easily controlled at home, severe ones can cause sufferers to begin to suffocate. In the UK an estimated 1620 people die each year as a result of the disease.

What causes it

External or internal factors can provoke asthma attacks, and some people are sensitive to both. Outside triggers usually involve an allergen, such as pet hair, a food, dust and dust mites, insects, pollen, tobacco smoke and many other environmental pollutants. Internal triggers, which are usually less obvious and can be harder to avoid, include stress, anxiety, temperature changes, exercise and respiratory infections such as bronchitis.

How supplements can help

The supplements in the chart are meant to complement conventional asthma therapy. Never stop taking medication prescribed for asthma without medical advice. People with asthma may be deficient in key nutrients, especially **vitamin C**, **magnesium** and **vitamin B₆**. Vitamin C, the major anti-oxidant present in the lining of the respiratory

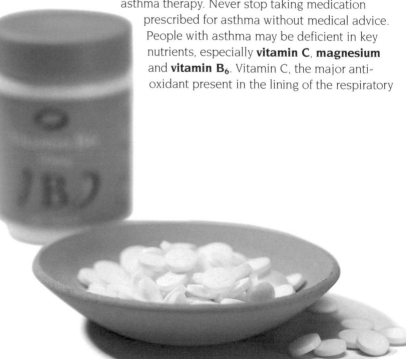

Vitamin C	**Dosage:** 500 mg twice a day. **Advice:** reduce dose if diarrhoea develops.
Magnesium	**Dosage:** 200 mg twice a day. **Advice:** take for six weeks to achieve adequate levels.
Vitamin B$_6$	**Dosage:** 50 mg twice a day. **Advice:** especially important if you take the prescription asthma drug theophylline.
Quercetin	**Dosage:** 500 mg three times a day. **Advice:** take 20 minutes before food; often sold with vitamin C.
Fish oils	**Dosage:** 2 teaspoons to supply 2 grams omega-3 fatty acids a day. **Caution:** consult your doctor if you take anticoagulant drugs.
Liquorice	**Dosage:** 200 mg standardised extract three times a day. **Caution:** consult your doctor before taking a liquorice supplement; it can raise blood pressure.

Some dosages may be supplied by supplements you are already taking – see page 195.

tract, appears to act immediately to combat inhaled oxidants. In addition, it may halt an allergic reaction by preventing the cells from releasing histamine. Furthermore, vitamin C is very effective for exercise-induced asthma; according to various studies, taking a dose before a workout may even thwart an asthma attack. As for the mineral magnesium, it can prevent attacks by inhibiting the contraction of the bronchial muscles. Other studies have shown that vitamin B$_6$ supplements reduce wheezing and other asthma symptoms.

The flavonoid **quercetin** has two main effects: it inhibits the release of histamine and, as an antioxidant, it neutralises unstable oxygen molecules which can cause bronchial inflammation. Fatty fish such as salmon, mackerel and cod, as well as **fish oils**, may help to protect against asthma as they are a rich source of the omega-3 fatty acids, which are thought to have an anti-inflammatory effect. Expectorants such as **liquorice** may benefit people with asthma, as may other herbs such as thyme, plantain, hyssop and garlic.

What else you can do

☑ Keep your home clear of dust and pollen. Avoid tobacco smoke.
☑ Stay away from cats; their hair is highly allergenic.
☑ Remain calm. Managing stress helps to fight asthma.
☑ Treat colds and flu promptly to reduce the chances of an attack.
☑ In winter, wear a scarf over your mouth and nose to warm the cold air.
☑ Keep an asthma diary to help you to determine your asthma triggers.
☑ Drink at least eight glasses of water a day to keep mucus loose.

FACTS & TIPS

■ Substances in green tea can reduce the inflammation of the airways that comes with an asthma attack. Sipping a cup of tea can be soothing and calming as well. You can safely drink several cups a day in combination with other nutritional and herbal remedies.

■ Yoga is an excellent activity for people with asthma. Not only does it enhance breathing, it is also relaxing.

■ An inexpensive device called a peak-flow meter measures how fast and how hard you can exhale air from your lungs. Its results, when compared with levels set by your doctor or with previous readings, can often predict an asthma attack, even a day or two in advance.

Athlete's foot

The most common fungal infection of the skin, athlete's foot usually begins between the toes, causing itching, scaling and sometimes painful breaks in the skin. This generally harmless but unusually troublesome condition may be relieved with various natural remedies.

Symptoms

- *Scaling and peeling between the toes. In severe cases there may be cracks between the toes.*

- *Redness, itching, scaling and tiny blisters along the sides and soles of the feet.*

- *Soft and painful skin.*

- *Infected toenails that can become thickened, discoloured or crumbly.*

SEE YOUR DOCTOR ...

- If there is no improvement a week to ten days after starting treatment with supplements.

- If home treatment does not provide a complete cure within four weeks.

- If any area becomes red and swollen, a sign of a more serious bacterial infection.

REMINDER: If you have a medical condition, consult your doctor before taking supplements.

What it is

'Athlete's foot' is the common term for a fungal infection called tinea pedis. The fungi that cause it are composed of tiny, plant-like cells found on the skin of all humans. They can sometimes multiply out of control. The fungi thrive in cramped, damp places, such as inside shoes and socks. In some people athlete's foot occurs entirely between the toes, where the skin cracks, peels and becomes scaly; in others the infection appears on the soles and sides of the feet or affects the toenails.

What causes it

The most common fungi causing athlete's foot belong to the group *Trichophyton*. Though poorly ventilated shoes and sweaty socks provide breeding grounds for the fungi, athlete's foot is not highly contagious, so walking barefoot in a changing room does not increase your risk.

How supplements can help

Many doctors prescribe conventional antifungal medications for persistent cases of athlete's foot. These drugs can be very effective – and very costly. For milder cases, supplements can be an inexpensive way to combat this infection; symptoms should begin to clear up within a week.

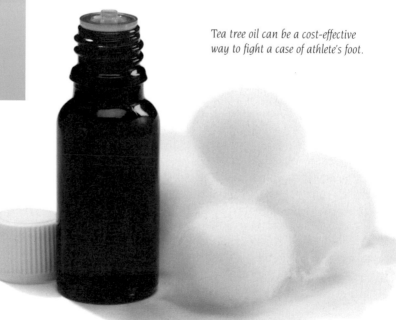

Tea tree oil can be a cost-effective way to fight a case of athlete's foot.

SUPPLEMENT RECOMMENDATIONS

Vitamin C	**Dosage:** 500 mg twice a day. **Advice:** long-term use may prevent recurrences; reduce dose if diarrhoea develops.
Tea tree oil	**Dosage:** apply to affected areas of skin twice a day. **Caution:** never ingest tea tree oil.
Garlic oil	**Dosage:** apply garlic oil, diluted 1:4 with vegetable oil, to affected areas of skin twice a day. **Advice:** can be used in place of tea tree oil.
Calendula	**Dosage:** apply cream or lotion to affected areas twice a day. **Advice:** should contain at least 2% calendula; use with caution if you are allergic to daisy-like flowers.

Note: consider using supplements in blue first; those in black may also be beneficial. Some dosages may be supplied by supplements you are already taking – see page 195.

Vitamin C, an antioxidant, promotes immune function and aids the body in fighting fungal infections. It can be taken while any of the topical supplements listed in the chart are being used.

Tea tree oil, a powerful natural antifungal agent, alters the chemical environment of the skin, making it inhospitable to fungal growth. Effective topical preparations include creams or lotions containing tea tree oil; look for products that contain it as one of the first ingredients, or make your own by adding two parts tea tree oil to three parts of a neutral oil, such as almond oil. For an antifungal foot bath, add 20 drops of tea tree oil to a bowl of warm water; soak your feet for 15 minutes two or three times a day. Dry the feet well and dab a few drops of undiluted tea tree oil on the affected areas. If pure tea tree oil irritates your skin, use one of the topical preparations described.

Rub **garlic oil**, diluted to a ratio of 1:4 with vegetable oil, directly onto the affected areas. Garlic contains a natural fungus-fighting substance called allicin that can help to clear up athlete's foot. You can also try dusting your feet with garlic powder. **Calendula**, derived from marigold, an orange daisy-like flower, is another useful option. Widely available in health-food shops, this herb relieves inflammation and soothes the skin, which promotes healing. If all else fails, try applying undiluted myrrh tincture directly to the affected area.

What else you can do

☑ Keep your feet clean and dry. Dry your feet with a hair dryer, set on low. If you prefer to use a towel, wash it after each use.

☑ Wear clean, dry socks. Air your shoes after each use, and do not wear the same pair every day.

☑ Go barefoot when you can, or opt for sandals or other well-ventilated shoes that allow your feet to breathe.

☑ Try over-the-counter antifungal lotions and powders, but avoid those that contain cornflour, which can encourage fungal growth.

☑ Cut your toenails straight across to help to prevent fungal infection.

Back pain

Humans defy gravity by standing upright, so the spine is often put under stress. This condition frequently leads to back pain, one of the most common ailments affecting people in the UK today. The secret for relieving it is to strengthen both the vertebrae and the surrounding tissues.

Symptoms

- *Aching or stiffness along the spine, especially during movement.*

- *Sharp pain in the upper or lower back or down the leg.*

- *Debilitating pain after exercise, strenuous activity or exertion.*

- *Aching and discomfort after long periods of sitting or standing.*

SEE YOUR DOCTOR ...

- If pain is disabling or accompanied by fever or vomiting.

- If tingling or numbness appears in the arms or legs, or intense pain extends down the back of the leg (sciatica).

- If pain and stiffness affect one area of the spine upon waking.

- If pain follows a fall or an accident.

REMINDER: *If you have a medical condition, consult your doctor before taking supplements.*

What it is

Though they are frequently quite uncomfortable, most backaches are not serious. Typically, the lower back, which supports almost all of the body's weight, is the area most affected. But inflammation of, or even a minor injury to, any of the bones in the spine (vertebrae) or the muscles, cartilage, nerves or other tissues connected to the spine can cause pain.

What causes it

Most back pain is the result of muscle strain. Poor posture, weakened bones or cartilage, a slipped disc, a pinched nerve or stress and emotional upset can also cause the discomfort. A disease such as arthritis or osteoporosis can predispose a person to chronic back pain.

How supplements can help

Before you begin taking a therapeutic supplement, check with your doctor to see whether medical or surgical treatment is warranted. Supplements are aimed at building stronger bones and muscles, reducing inflammation and treating pain. Effects may be felt within a week.

People prone to back problems should start with vitamins and minerals that strengthen bones and cartilage, such as **calcium**, **magnesium** and **vitamins C** and **D**. In addition, various other supplements are worth trying, either singly or in combination. Some hospitals have had success using **bromelain**, an enzyme found in pineapple, to reduce inflammation and pain from surgery, trauma, sports injuries and arthritis. The nutritional supplement **glucosamine** builds cartilage, including the tissue supporting the spinal discs, and the herb **white willow bark** has pain-relieving characteristics similar

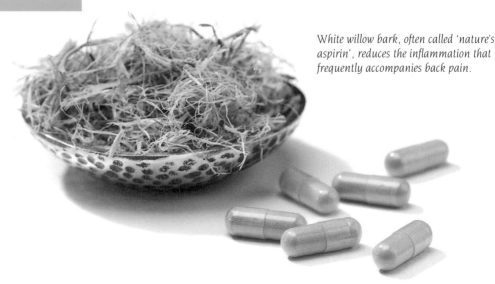

White willow bark, often called 'nature's aspirin', reduces the inflammation that frequently accompanies back pain.

Calcium/ magnesium	**Dosage:** 600 mg calcium and 250 mg magnesium a day. **Advice:** can be bought as part of a bone-building formula.
Vitamin C	**Dosage:** 500 mg twice a day. **Advice:** reduce dose if diarrhoea develops.
Vitamin D	**Dosage:** 10 mcg a day. **Caution:** avoid doses above 25 mcg a day, which may be toxic.
Bromelain	**Dosage:** 500 mg three times a day on an empty stomach. **Advice:** should provide 6000 GDU or 9000 MCU daily.
Glucosamine	**Dosage:** 500 mg glucosamine sulphate three times a day. **Advice:** take with food to minimise digestive upset.
White willow bark	**Dosage:** one or two tablets or capsules times a day (follow instructions on the packet). **Advice:** should be standardised to contain 15% salicin; do not take with conventional pain relievers.
Fish oils	**Dosage:** 2 teaspoons to supply 2 grams of omega-3 fatty acids a day. **Advice:** consult your doctor if you take anticoagulant drugs; vegetarians can use 1 tablespoon flaxseed oil instead.

Note: consider using supplements in blue first; those in black may also be beneficial. Some dosages may be supplied by supplements you are already taking – see page 195.

to those of aspirin, but with fewer side effects. **Fish oils,** rich in omega-3 fatty acids, may also have healing, analgesic and anti-inflammatory properties. All of these supplements may reduce the need for conventional pain relievers and, except for white willow bark, can be taken with them.

Other beneficial supplements include S-adenosylmethionine, or SAM, a form of the muscle-strengthening, collagen-building amino acid methionine (200 mg three times a day); boswellia, a herbal remedy from India which has anti-inflammatory properties (150 mg boswellic acid three times a day); and niacin (nicotinamide), a form of niacin that may be effective against arthritic back pain (500 mg three times a day). The herb devil's claw (400 mg three times a day) may be particularly useful for inflammatory pain from arthritis or degenerative spine disease (spondylosis). For sciatica, St John's wort (300 mg extract three times a day) may be helpful.

What else you can do

☑ To improve posture, wear comfortable footwear; consider orthotics.
☑ Try therapeutic massage, chiropractic, acupuncture, osteopathy or TENS (transcutaneous electrical nerve stimulation) for pain relief.
☑ When lifting, do not bend from the waist without bending your knees.
☑ Sit in a chair with lower-back support; take frequent breaks to stretch.

Bad breath

This troublesome complaint affects millions of people and has fuelled a thriving industry. Strict oral hygiene and natural remedies usually provide relief; if bad breath persists, careful dental or medical detective work can often uncover a correctable underlying cause.

Symptoms

- *Regular experience of a disagreeable taste is a sign that the breath leaving your mouth probably has an unpleasant odour.*

- *Many people with bad breath do not taste or smell it themselves, so look for possible clues from others: they step back when you speak, for instance. If you suspect a problem, ask someone you trust for an honest opinion.*

- *Bleeding gums signal gingivitis, an inflammation of the gums that can sometimes cause bad breath.*

SEE YOUR DOCTOR ...

- **If bad breath persists despite self-care measures. Your dentist or doctor can check for an underlying medical cause, such as gum disease or a chronic sinus infection.**

REMINDER: If you have a medical condition, consult your doctor before taking supplements.

Drinking peppermint tea can help to keep the mouth moist and fresh.

What it is

Bad breath, or halitosis, can often be traced back to smoking, drinking alcohol or eating foods notorious for their lingering odours, including garlic, onions and anchovies. Sometimes the condition may become chronic and be caused by an underlying medical condition.

What causes it

Bad breath usually results from the multiplication of odour-causing bacteria in the mouth. The drier your mouth, the more bacteria thrive there. Any condition that reduces saliva production can contribute to bad breath – including advancing age, breathing through the mouth, crash diets (the less food you chew, the less saliva is produced), certain drugs and even the time of day ('morning breath' occurs because salivation is much reduced during sleep). Bacteria may also collect on the tongue and in food debris that accumulates on dentures and teeth – especially when plaque or cavities are present. Persistent bad breath is frequently caused by gum disease or a chronic sinus infection. Many complementary practitioners believe that bad breath reflects an imbalance of micro-organisms in the bowel caused by a preponderance of 'unfriendly' bacteria whose volatile toxic products are carried on the breath.

How supplements can help

Natural strategies for bad breath work best in combination with regular and thorough oral hygiene, including flossing and cleaning the teeth and also brushing the tongue (especially the back part), where odour-causing bacteria are likely to flourish.

Place a drop or two of **peppermint** oil on the tongue a couple of times a day – larger amounts of the pure oil may cause digestive upset.

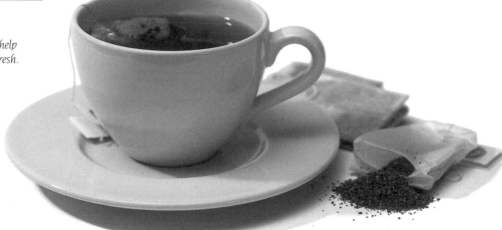

Peppermint	**Dosage:** 1 or 2 drops essential oil of peppermint, placed on the tongue. **Advice:** larger amounts of peppermint oil can cause digestive upsets; drinking peppermint tea may also be helpful.
Fennel	**Dosage:** chew a pinch of fennel seeds after meals or as needed. **Advice:** chew thoroughly for best effect; anise seeds or cloves can also be used.
Parsley	**Dosage:** chew a fresh parsley sprig after meals or as needed. **Advice:** some natural breath fresheners contain parsley oil as a key ingredient.
Spirulina	**Dosage:** rinse the mouth with a commercial chlorophyll-rich green drink (follow instructions on the packet). **Advice:** alternatively, tablets can be chewed.
Acidophilus	**Dosage:** one capsule twice a day. **Advice:** bioyoghurts may be taken instead.

Some dosages may be supplied by supplements you are already taking – see page 195.

Apart from its pleasant taste and aroma, peppermint oil is effective in killing bacteria. Drinking peppermint or spearmint teas as well as plenty of plain water may also help to fight bad breath by keeping the mouth moist. Another approach is to chew several **fennel** seeds, anise seeds or cloves to freshen the breath; they can be carried conveniently in a small sealed container. Fresh **parsley** has a similar effect; it is also high in chlorophyll (the chemical that gives plants their green colour), which has long been recognised as a powerful breath freshener.

Chlorophyll is also found in commercially available 'green' drinks containing **spirulina**, wheat grass, chlorella or other herbs. These chlorophyll-rich liquids are best when swished around the mouth before being swallowed. Alternatively, try spirulina tablets, which should be chewed thoroughly. As well as having an effect in the mouth, both the herbs and these chlorophyll-rich products may encourage the growth of 'friendly' bacteria in the large intestine. Probiotics, which are cultures of 'friendly' bacteria such as **acidophilus** and bifidus, also help to normalise the balance of the intestinal micro-organisms. They are available in capsule form and in certain yoghurts, normally labelled 'bioyoghurts'. The bacteria in normal yoghurts do not influence the balance of gut flora in the way that acidophilus and bifidus do.

What else you can do

☑ Clean your teeth after each meal and floss at least once a day. When you cannot use a toothbrush, rinse your mouth out with some water.
☑ Use a moist toothbrush, a tongue scraper (available at some chemists and health-food shops) or a metal spoon held upside down to scrape off any coating on the back of the tongue and cleanse that area.
☑ Avoid strong-smelling foods and alcohol; do not smoke.
☑ Eat an orange every day; phytochemicals in citrus fruit help to normalise the bowel flora.

FACTS & TIPS

■ Liquorice-flavoured anise seeds can easily be made into a breath-freshening mouthwash or drink. Boil several teaspoons of seeds in 250 ml of water for a few minutes, then strain and cool.

■ You can ensure that your toothbrush remains free of bacteria by storing it in grapefruit seed extract or hydrogen peroxide; rinse it well before using it.

■ Commercially available mouthwashes may reduce bacteria in the mouth, but their effect is only temporary and they do not provide a satisfactory substitute for regular flossing and brushing.

■ Some practitioners advise adding extra fibre, such as psyllium, and fluid to the diet to avoid constipation. Colon-cleansing herbal formulas, available at health-food shops, may also be recommended.

Breast problems

Painful and lumpy breasts, which increase in discomfort before a menstrual period (fibrocystic breasts) are extremely common in women under the age of 50. Selected supplements and a change of diet may help to diminish the symptoms of this disorder.

Symptoms

- *Breast lumps or nodules that may be tender or not painful at all.*

- *An increase in the size of lumps or in breast discomfort a week or so before a menstrual period.*

SEE YOUR DOCTOR ...

- **If a new lump develops, especially if you have not always had lumpy breasts.**

- **If a lump hardens, grows larger or does not diminish after your menstrual period ends.**

- **If you have any discharge from either nipple.**

- **If your breast pain is severe.**

REMINDER: If you have a medical condition, consult your doctor before taking supplements.

What it is

Normal breasts vary in density and texture. Before the menopause, women tend to have more tissue (which can make the breasts feel firm or lumpy) and less fat in their breasts than they do in their later years. Occasionally women develop fluid-filled cysts or fibrous areas, which can be tender just before menstruation. Though most women experience some mild breast discomfort in their life, some have monthly pain so severe that it interferes with daily activities.

Such premenstrual changes are labelled 'fibrocystic breast disease'. Although this condition does not increase your risk of breast cancer, having lumpy breasts may make identifying a cancerous growth more difficult if one develops. Normal lumps can usually be distinguished from cancerous ones because they move freely in the breast, changing with the menstrual cycle.

What causes it

Fibrocystic changes in the breast are associated with the rise and fall of hormones that occur during the menstrual cycle. Women who produce a particularly high level of oestrogen in conjunction with a low level of progesterone after ovulation may suffer more. This combination is linked with too much prolactin, a hormone that triggers milk production in new mothers but increases breast tenderness in women who are not breastfeeding. Many researchers think

The essential fatty acids in evening primrose oil often reduce breast inflammation.

Vitamin E	**Dosage:** 500 mg a day. **Caution:** consult a doctor if you take anticoagulant drugs.
Chasteberry	**Dosage:** 225 mg standardised extract each morning. **Advice:** also called vitex; should contain 0.5% agnuside.
Essential fatty acids	**Dosage:** 1000 mg evening primrose oil three times a day, and 1 tablespoon flaxseed oil a day. **Advice:** alternatively, replace evening primrose oil with 1000 mg borage oil once a day.
Magnesium	**Dosage:** 400 mg a day. **Advice:** take with food; reduce dose if diarrhoea develops.
Vitamin B$_6$	**Dosage:** 50 mg a day for one week. **Advice:** if taken long term, high daily doses (greater than 200 mg) can cause nerve damage.

Note: consider using supplements in blue first; the one in black may also be beneficial. Some dosages may be supplied by supplements you are already taking – see page 195.

that caffeine stimulates the growth of lumps or fluid-filled breast cysts (and some women show improvement when they eliminate caffeine), but others maintain that there is no firm evidence of any connection between caffeine and breast tenderness.

How supplements can help

All the supplements listed can be used together and as needed; you should see improvement in a month or two. Many women report relief from breast pain after taking **vitamin E**. Just how it works is unknown, but some practitioners believe that this vitamin blocks the changes in breast tissue which are possibly caused by caffeine.

The herb **chasteberry** works to reduce prolactin levels and to restore the hormonal balance between oestrogen and progesterone, so it may be useful in reducing menstrual-related breast changes. **Essential fatty acids** often act as anti-inflammatory compounds; they may also help the body to absorb iodine (low iodine levels have been linked to fibrocystic breasts). **Magnesium** may also reduce inflammation and pain. **Vitamin B$_6$** may be beneficial for women who experience post-menstrual syndrome symptoms with breast pain; it may also help the liver to process excess oestrogen.

What else you can do

☑ Eat a healthy diet high in whole grain cereals, fruits and vegetables.
☑ Eliminate caffeine and see if that helps. As well as coffee and tea, caffeine is found in chocolate, colas and some over-the-counter medications. Be patient: six months may pass before you notice any significant improvement.
☑ Wear a bra with good support when your breasts are tender.

Bronchitis

This generally temporary illness often develops after a cold or flu. However, for some people (particularly smokers), bronchitis is a serious, recurring disease. Acute and chronic symptoms are similar and may be effectively relieved with the use of certain supplements.

Symptoms

Acute bronchitis
- *Cough that produces white, yellow or green phlegm.*
- *Low fever (37.8°C or less).*
- *Coarse breathing sounds (called rhonchi) that change or disappear when coughing.*
- *Chest muscle pain from coughing.*

Chronic bronchitis
- *Persistent cough producing yellow, white or green phlegm for at least three months of the year for two consecutive years.*
- *Wheezing, breathlessness.*
- *Coughing during exertion, no matter how slight.*

SEE YOUR DOCTOR ...

- If a persistent cough interferes with your sleep or your normal daily activities.
- If mucus becomes darker or thicker or increases significantly in volume.
- If your fever is above 37.8°C.
- If your breathing becomes increasingly difficult, or if you cough up blood.
- If your symptoms last longer than 48 hours.

REMINDER: *If you have a medical condition, consult your doctor before taking supplements.*

What it is

Bronchitis is an inflammation of the windpipe and bronchial tubes, the large airways that lead to the lungs. These airways swell and thicken, paralysing the cilia, the tiny hairs that line the respiratory tract and sweep away dust and germs. Mucus builds up, resulting in a cough. There are two types of bronchitis: acute and chronic. Acute is marked by a slight fever that lasts for a few days and a cough that goes away after several weeks. In chronic bronchitis, a hacking cough along with discoloured phlegm persists for several months and may disappear and recur.

What causes it

Acute bronchitis often follows a cold or flu. It is seldom caused by a bacterial infection, so it may not be helped by antibiotics; indeed, these can lower the body's level of 'friendly' bacteria, making individual bacterial strains more resistant to the antibiotics. Chronic bronchitis occurs when the lungs have been irritated for a long time. The primary cause of chronic bronchitis is smoking. People with long-term exposure to tobacco smoke, workers routinely exposed to chemical fumes, and individuals with chronic allergies are also susceptible.

How supplements can help

A daily multivitamin and mineral supplement may help to ward off colds and related infections which can initiate bronchitis. In addition, other

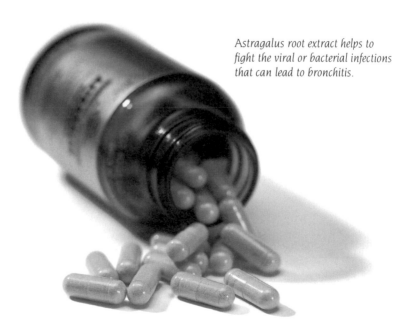

Astragalus root extract helps to fight the viral or bacterial infections that can lead to bronchitis.

supplements can help to strengthen your body's immune response, and also stimulate its normal process of loosening and bringing up phlegm. The supplements for acute bronchitis should be taken only while you are ill. Those for chronic bronchitis require long-term use.

Vitamin C is particularly helpful in fighting off viruses that attack the respiratory system and assists in the healing of damaged lung tissue. Take it coupled with powerful antioxidants called **flavonoids** (or bioflavonoids), which are natural antivirals and anti-inflammatories.

For an acute attack, drink **thyme** tea to thin mucus secretions. Other herbs that can be combined with thyme, or used as alternatives, are elecampane, hyssop, plantain and angelica. Take singly or as mixtures, and use them as described for thyme in the chart. The amino acid-like substance **NAC** (N-acetylcysteine) also thins mucus and has been reported to reduce the recurrence rate of bronchitis.

The herbs **echinacea** and **astragalus** have antibacterial, antiviral and immune-strengthening properties, and they can be used to ward off acute bronchitis. For chronic or seasonal bronchitis, try taking the following herbs in rotation: echinacea (200 mg extract twice a day), astragalus (200 mg extract twice a day), pau d'arco (250 mg extract twice a day), and 1500 mg of reishi or 600 mg of maitake mushrooms a day. Use one herb for one week, then switch to another; continue this cycle for as long as you need it.

What else you can do

☑ Stop smoking – and avoid situations where others smoke.
☑ Drink plenty of fluids, such as diluted fruit juices and herbal teas. Dehydration can cause mucus to thicken and be difficult to cough up.
☑ Eliminate the use of aerosol products (hair sprays, deodorants and insecticides), which can irritate airway passages.
☑ If you have chronic bronchitis, stay indoors when the air quality is poor.

FACTS & TIPS
■ People with bronchitis often find it hard to breathe at the same time as they are eating. For this reason sufferers should try to avoid foods that are difficult to chew, such as meats and raw vegetables.

■ Lung symptoms will not be alleviated by antihistamines or decongestants. Indeed, these drugs may actually make your condition worse because they tend to dry up and thicken mucus, making it more difficult to cough up.

Burns

Most burns are not serious and can be managed with simple care at home. Soothing herbal ointments such as aloe vera or calendula can be applied to mild ones. In addition, a number of vitamins, minerals and other supplements can be taken orally to promote healing and prevent infection.

Symptoms

Mild burns
- *Tenderness, redness.*
- *Possible swelling.*

Moderate burns
- *Pain, redness, blisters.*
- *Mild to moderate swelling.*

Severe burns
- *No immediate pain or bleeding because nerves are damaged.*
- *Skin that is charred or black, white or red.*
- *No blisters, but serious swelling.*

SEE YOUR DOCTOR ...

- **If you suffer a severe burn, including a chemical or an electrical one – go at once to an accident and emergency unit.**
- **If a mild burn covers a large area or is very painful.**
- **If a moderate burn occurs on your face or hands, or covers 5 cm or more of skin.**
- **If you have a fever, vomiting, chills or swollen glands; if pus forms in blisters; or if an unpleasant odour emanates from the burn: these may be signs of infection.**
- **If you are in doubt about the severity of a burn.**

REMINDER: If you have a medical condition, consult your doctor before taking supplements.

What they are

A burn is damage to the skin caused by wet or dry heat, chemicals or electricity. Most burns occur at home, and occasionally they require emergency hospital treatment. A burn can be mild, moderate or severe. Those resulting from overexposure to sunlight are generally considered mild because they involve only the outer layer of skin, whereas moderate burns injure part of the underlying skin layer. Severe burns affect all the skin layers, causing harm to the muscles, bones, nerves and blood vessels below. They always represent a medical emergency and require sophisticated treatment, such as skin grafting, to aid recovery and minimise scarring.

What causes them

Burns are commonly caused by scalding water, hot oil or grease, hot foods or overexposure to sun. More serious injuries may result from fire, steam or chemicals. Electrical burns, usually occurring from contact with faulty or uninsulated wiring, can be deceptive: skin damage may be minimal, but internal injuries can be extensive.

How supplements can help

Self-care is appropriate for mild and some moderate burns covering a small area (more serious burns demand medical attention). To treat, immerse the burnt area in cold water for about 15 minutes (be careful not

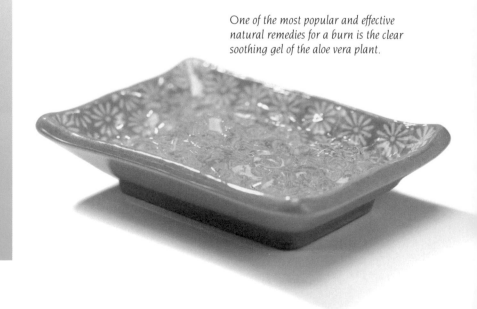

One of the most popular and effective natural remedies for a burn is the clear soothing gel of the aloe vera plant.

Aloe vera gel	**Dosage:** apply gel to affected areas of skin as needed. **Advice:** use fresh aloe leaf or commercial gel.
Calendula cream	**Dosage:** apply cream to burns. **Advice:** also known as marigold cream.
Gotu kola	**Dosage:** 200 mg extract or 400-500 mg crude herb twice a day. **Advice:** use extract standardised to contain 10% asiaticosides.
Vitamin C	**Dosage:** 500 mg twice a day until burn has healed. **Advice:** reduce dose if diarrhoea develops.
Vitamin E	**Dosage:** 250 mg a day until burn has healed. **Advice:** creams containing vitamin E are available and may prevent scarring when applied topically.
Zinc	**Dosage:** 25 mg a day. **Advice:** if you use a zinc supplement for more than a month, choose one that includes 2 mg copper.
Chamomile	**Dosage:** use a strong tea: 2 or 3 teaspoons dried herb for each 250 ml of hot water; cool quickly in freezer or with ice cubes. **Advice:** apply a clean tea-soaked cloth to the area of the burn for about 15 minutes.

Note: consider using supplements in blue first; the one in black may also be beneficial. Some dosages may be supplied by supplements you are already taking – see page 195.

Aloe vera gel greatly speeds up healing, according to a study of 27 people with moderate burns. Those patients treated with aloe vera healed in 12 days on average, compared with 18 for those who used a standard gauze dressing.

DID YOU KNOW?
Butter is an old folk remedy for burns – but don't use it. Like other oils or greasy ointments, butter traps moisture, slows healing and increases the risk of later infection.

FACTS & TIPS

■ If you don't have any aloe vera or chamomile easily available to treat a burn, try a potato instead. Put several slices of raw potato on the affected skin; replace them several times – every two or three minutes – before applying a dressing. The starch in the potato forms a protective layer that may help to soothe the burn.

■ Milk can also be a fairly effective first-aid remedy for minor burns. Soak a terry-cloth towel or piece of cotton flannel in milk and use it as a compress for 15 minutes or so. Repeat this procedure every two to six hours. Be sure to rinse the skin between applications to avoid the smell of sour milk.

to break any blisters) or apply cold compresses. Once the burn has cooled, apply **aloe vera gel**, a dressing soaked in **chamomile** tea or lavender oil directly to the injured area to relieve pain and inflammation and soothe the skin. Then use infection-fighting **calendula cream** or goldenseal cream on any raw areas and cover with a light dressing.

During the healing process the body needs extra nutrients which should be taken for a week or two, until the burn heals. Taken in combination, the herb **gotu kola** (which stimulates the growth of connective tissue in the skin), **vitamins C** and **E** and the mineral **zinc** all work together to boost the immune response, repair skin and tissues and prevent scarring.

What else you can do

☑ Gently cleanse burns daily, using mild soap and taking care not to break any blisters; rinse well. Use sterile gauze dressings to keep burns dry and protected from dirt and bacteria.

☑ Drink plenty of fluids while your skin is healing.

☑ Avoid exposing your burnt skin to hot showers or the sun.

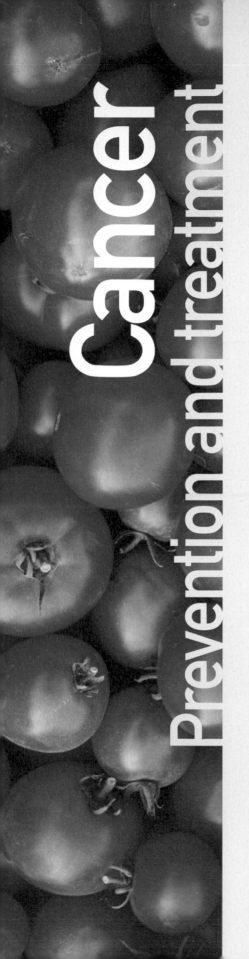

Cancer
Prevention and treatment

A healthy diet is the best protection against cancer, but, if a diet falls short of ideal, some supplements can have protective effects. Others may enhance conventional cancer treatments and help to alleviate the side effects.

One in three people in the UK is likely to develop cancer at some time in his or her life, but it is estimated that up to 70% of these cancers could be prevented by making lifestyle changes (see pages 15-22).

A PROLIFERATION OF ABNORMAL CELLS

If the body's processes of cell multiplication, or replication, are disrupted, cells proliferate at random, invading and damaging healthy tissue. The immune system normally identifies these changes and destroys the abnormal cells, but an abnormal cell that escapes this surveillance may develop into a tumour.

Tumours can break up and spread through the blood or the lymphatic system to other parts of the body, and trigger further growths. If untreated, cancer cells can overpower normal cells and sap the body's vital nutrients, resulting in serious, life-threatening illness.

THE ROLE OF FREE RADICALS

It is not fully understood why healthy cells turn cancerous, but it is known that molecules known as free radicals can damage the genetic material in cells and trigger cancer by disrupting cell replication. Levels of free radicals produced by normal metabolism are well controlled, but their production is increased by factors such as poor diet, smoking, heavy alcohol consumption and over-exposure to the sun.

Cell replication can also be disrupted by certain viruses, stress, and hereditary factors.

REDUCING THE RISK:
DO

■ *Maintain a healthy body weight* (see pages 358-61). Fats should make up only one third of your daily calories.

■ *Eat at least five portions of fruit and vegetables a day* for the antioxidants they provide. Include cooked tomatoes.

■ *Eat more fibre;* it removes carcinogens from the body.

DON'T

■ *Smoke.* Smoking is the main cause of lung cancer and raises

---

BODY MASS INDEX
To check if you are over-weight, divide your weight in kilograms by your height in metres squared to calculate your body mass index, or BMI: it should be 20-25 throughout adult life.

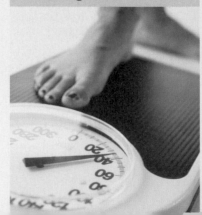

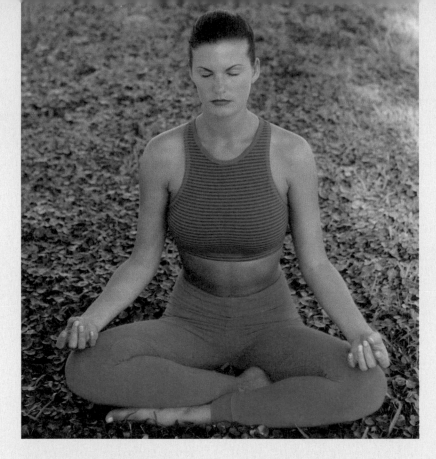

your risk of developing cancers of the oesophagus, larynx, pharynx, bladder, stomach, pancreas and cervix.

■ *Sunbathe without protection.* Excessive exposure to the sun can lead to skin cancer.

■ *Eat more than 80 grams a day of red meat;* it increases the risk of bowel cancer.

■ *Eat too much salt-cured or barbecued food.* High salt intakes have been linked to stomach cancer, and charred foods are known to contain carcinogens.

■ *Drink too much alcohol.* Keep consumption within the recommended safe limits (*see page 22*).

USING SUPPLEMENTS FOR PREVENTION

■ Vitamin C and flavonoids offer protection against cancers of the cervix, lung, mouth, oesophagus, pancreas and stomach.

■ Vitamin E and compounds contained in flaxseed oil called lignans help to ward off breast, colon and prostate cancer.

■ Selenium and green tea extract have a generally protective effect.

■ Coenzyme Q_{10} and mixed natural carotenoids complement the action of other dietary antioxidants.

GAINING MAXIMUM BENEFIT FROM CANCER TREATMENT

Surgery, radiotherapy and chemotherapy can be highly effective in combating cancer. Natural therapies for treating cancer are unproven, and should be used only to boost conventional treatment and relieve side effects.

Appetite loss is common, so a well-formulated multivitamin and mineral formula will ensure a good intake of micronutrients.

Radiotherapy and chemotherapy damage healthy cells while attacking cancer cells. Vitamin A and the antioxidants vitamin C, vitamin E, mixed carotenoids (especially beta-carotene and lycopene), selenium and coenzyme Q_{10} can help to protect cells from uncontrolled free radicals, and may inhibit the further growth of cancerous cells.

Phytochemicals with cancer-fighting properties, found in plants such as echinacea and maitake mushrooms, can be taken in parallel with radiotherapy or chemotherapy to help to maintain blood levels of leucocytes (infection-fighting white blood cells).

THE WARNING SIGNS

Early detection is vital. If you experience any of the symptoms listed below for more than two weeks, see your doctor at once.

■ A lump beneath the skin – most are harmless, but breast lumps in particular must be examined.

■ A change in the size or shape of a mole.

■ A sore, scab or ulcer that will not heal.

■ Abnormal bleeding.

■ Sudden or unexplained weight loss or fatigue.

■ A persistent cough or hoarseness.

■ A change in bowel or bladder habits.

Carpal tunnel syndrome

If wrist pain wakes you at night, or you feel pins and needles in your hands while driving, you may be suffering from carpal tunnel syndrome. The syndrome, often regarded as a condition of modern times, has been recognised since the 1880s.

Symptoms

■ *Numbness or tingling in the thumb and the first three fingers.*

■ *Shooting pains in the wrist and forearm, which may radiate into the shoulder and neck.*

■ *Weakness in the hand; difficulty in picking up and holding objects.*

■ *A feeling that the fingers are swollen when no swelling is visible.*

SEE YOUR DOCTOR ...

■ **If your fingers feel stiff and painful – you may be suffering from arthritis.**

■ **If wrist pain interferes with daily activities.**

■ **If numbness and pain continue despite rest and treatment with supplements – you may need a local steroid injection or a minor operation to relieve the pressure on the median nerve.**

REMINDER: *If you have a medical condition, consult your doctor before taking supplements.*

What it is

The bones and ligaments in the wrist (medically known as the carpus, from the Greek *karpos*) form a pathway called the carpal tunnel. The tunnel channels the median nerve, which controls movement and feeling in most of the hand, and the tendons that connect the arm and hand muscles, from the forearm into the hand. It can be narrowed by bone spurs or dislocation, fluid retention or the swelling of ligaments or tendons. If the narrowing compresses the median nerve, pain, numbness and weakness develop in the thumb and fingers.

Symptoms may become apparent gradually or suddenly, and are usually most painful at night – 95% of patients with this condition report being woken up by the pain. The symptoms may last for a few days and disappear without treatment, or persist for months and require medical intervention.

What causes it

Carpal tunnel syndrome is usually a stress injury induced by prolonged repetitive movements of the hands or fingers. Overuse of the hands while typing, working on an assembly line or playing a musical instrument, for example, can inflame the tendons or ligaments inside the wrist, causing them to swell and compress the median nerve.

The changes in hormone levels associated with birth control pills, pregnancy or the menopause can cause fluid retention, which often provokes or worsens symptoms – the syndrome occurs three times more often in women than it does in men, and is particularly common in overweight women between the ages of 30 and 60 who have been pregnant. Trauma to the wrist, or underlying conditions such as diabetes, hypothyroidism, Raynaud's disease or rheumatoid arthritis, may also cause symptoms.

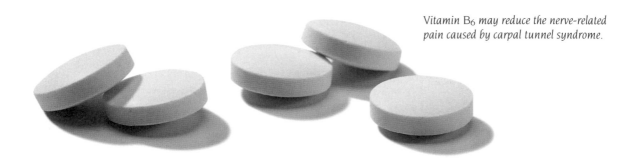

Vitamin B$_6$ may reduce the nerve-related pain caused by carpal tunnel syndrome.

Vitamin B$_6$	**Dosage:** 50 mg three times a day until symptoms subside. **Advice:** taking 200 mg daily over a long period can cause nerve damage; do not exceed the recommended dose.
Bromelain	**Dosage:** 1000 mg twice a day during acute phase; reduce to 500 mg twice a day when symptoms subside. **Caution:** consult your doctor if you take anticoagulant drugs. **Advice:** take between meals; provides 8000 GDU or 12,000 MCU in acute phase.
Turmeric	**Dosage:** 400 mg three times a day. **Advice:** standardised to contain 95% curcumin; should be used in combination with bromelain.

Some dosages may be supplied by supplements you are already taking – see page 195.

How supplements can help

Several studies have suggested that a **vitamin B$_6$** deficiency can make you susceptible to the numbness and pain of carpal tunnel syndrome. This vitamin is important in maintaining healthy nerve tissue, relieving inflammation and improving circulation. It is also thought to increase the brain's production of the nerve chemical GABA (gamma-aminobutyric acid), which helps to control pain sensations.

If you do not notice any improvement after taking vitamin B$_6$ for three weeks, try taking the same dosage of pyridoxal-5-phosphate (P-5-P) instead. This is a substance that the body eventually produces as it breaks down vitamin B$_6$. Some people find that this form is more effective in relieving their symptoms.

In addition to B$_6$, **bromelain**, a powerful enzyme found in pineapple, is very effective in counteracting inflammation and any resulting pain. A combination of bromelain and vitamin B$_6$ works better than either supplement alone. **Turmeric**, a member of the ginger family, also eases swelling – the herb contains a yellow pigment, curcumin, with anti-inflammatory properties. When turmeric is taken with bromelain, each substance enhances the actions of the other. Turmeric is expensive, but is safe for long-term use. The dose should be halved when the symptoms begin to subside.

What else you can do

☑ Take frequent breaks when performing any repetitive activity with your hands, such as knitting or typing. Stop at least once an hour to flex your fingers and shake your hands.

☑ Apply ice to your wrists when pain strikes. Use a flexible ice pack – or even a bag of frozen peas – for 10 minutes every hour to ease the pain and reduce the inflammation.

☑ Elevate your wrists with a pillow when you lie down.

Cataracts

Fifty per cent of people over 50 and three-quarters of the over-75s develop cataracts, but the visual impairment they cause does not have to be an inevitable part of the ageing process. Recent studies show that lifestyle changes can lessen your chance of developing this disorder.

Symptoms

- *Gradual and painless blurring or dimming of vision.*
- *Increased sensitivity to sun glare or car headlights at night.*
- *Seeing halos around lights.*
- *Changes in colour perception.*

SEE YOUR DOCTOR ...

- **If you begin to develop cataract symptoms.**

REMINDER: If you have a medical condition, consult your doctor before taking supplements.

What it is

The lens of the eye is a transparent disc which refracts light and focuses it on the retina, allowing a clear image to form. Cataracts are opaque spots on the lens created when proteins inside it break down and clump together. These spots reduce the amount of light transmitted to the retina, causing cloudy or blurred vision. The degree of visual impairment depends on the size and density of the spot and its location on the lens.

What causes it

Cataracts may develop as a result of an injury to the eye or through age-related body changes. A congenital cause is rare, affecting about one in 10,000 children. Some scientists believe that the majority of cases can be attributed to a lifetime's exposure to ultraviolet (UV) light from the sun, or to smoking. A low level of antioxidants such as vitamins C and E, beta-carotene and selenium in the diet may be a contributing factor. Antioxidants neutralise free radicals (unstable oxygen molecules) that can damage the lens. The risk of cataracts is increased in those who are diabetic or overweight – both conditions involve high blood-sugar levels, which may contribute to the destruction of lens proteins.

How supplements can help

Taking supplements before a cataract develops may postpone its formation or prevent it altogether; in the early stages of a cataract, supplements may slow its growth. Once a cataract has appeared it can only be removed by surgery.

The antioxidants **vitamin C** and **vitamin E** may protect against lens damage caused by UV light and cigarette smoke. **Selenium** also helps to neutralise free radicals. The herb **bilberry** is rich in antioxidants in the form of flavonoids – natural compounds which help to eliminate toxins from the lens and retina. In one study, bilberry combined with vitamin E stopped the progression of cataracts in 48 out of 50

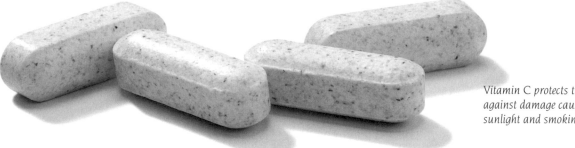

Vitamin C protects the lens against damage caused by sunlight and smoking.

SUPPLEMENT RECOMMENDATIONS

Vitamin C	**Dosage:** 500 mg twice a day. **Advice:** reduce dose if diarrhoea develops.
Vitamin E	**Dosage:** 250 mg a day. **Caution:** consult your doctor if you take anticoagulant drugs.
Selenium	**Dosage:** 200 mcg a day. **Advice:** do not exceed the recommended dose; higher doses may be toxic.
Bilberry	**Dosage:** 80 mg extract three times a day. **Advice:** standardised to contain 25% anthocyanosides; may be included in nutritional supplement eye formulas.
Ginkgo biloba	**Dosage:** 40 mg three times a day. **Advice:** standardised to contain at least 24% flavone glycosides.
Alpha-lipoic acid	**Dosage:** 150 mg a day. **Advice:** take in the morning, with or without food.
Grape seed extract	**Dosage:** 100 mg twice a day. **Advice:** standardised to contain 92-95% proanthocyanidins.
Fish oils	**Dosage:** 2 teaspoons to supply 2 grams of omega-3 fatty acids a day. **Caution:** consult your doctor if you take anticoagulant drugs.
Flaxseed oil	**Dosage:** 1 tablespoon a day. **Advice:** can be mixed with food; take in the morning.

Note: consider using supplements in blue first; those in black may also be beneficial. Some dosages may be supplied by supplements you are already taking – see page 195.

see page 195

participants. **Ginkgo biloba**, which improves the circulation and has strong antioxidant properties, can be substituted for bilberry. This may be a good choice for people who are already taking ginkgo for memory problems. **Alpha-lipoic acid** shows promise as a cataract preventive and also boosts the effectiveness of vitamins C and E. Because **grape seed extract** can have a therapeutic effect on even the tiniest blood vessels, it benefits circulation in the eye.

Consider adding omega-3 fatty acids, in the form of **fish oils** or **flaxseed oil**, to this regimen, as they nourish the eye. Riboflavin (vitamin B$_2$) is also important, as it helps antioxidants to function; take 25 mg a day if you do not take a multivitamin or a B-complex supplement that provides at least this amount.

What else you can do

☑ Stop smoking.
☑ Protect your eyes from UV rays by wearing sunglasses and a wide-brimmed hat when you are outdoors.
☑ Eat plenty of fresh fruit and vegetables – they are good sources of antioxidants.

RECENT FINDINGS

In a study of people aged 55 and older, those who took vitamin E supplements were only half as likely to develop cataracts as those who didn't. The participants took at least 250 mg of vitamin E daily.

The risk of developing cataracts can be reduced by eating fruits and vegetables that are rich in antioxidants. In a study of almost 500 women, those with the highest intakes of vitamins C and E, lutein, zeaxanthin and beta-carotene had a lower risk of cataracts than those with the lowest intakes. Those who took vitamin C supplements for 10 or more years had a 64% reduction in lens cloudiness.

FACTS & TIPS

■ The only way to remove a cataract is surgically to replace the cloudy lens with an artificial lens, but surgery is not necessary unless your vision is so impaired that you cannot work, drive, read or participate in leisure activities that you usually enjoy.

Chronic fatigue syndrome

About a million people in Britain are suffering from CFS at any one time. Controversy over its cause has led to many names for the disorder, from 'post-viral fatigue syndrome' to 'yuppie flu'. Supplements can often ease the symptoms.

Symptoms

- *Continuing or recurring fatigue lasting at least six months and not relieved by sleep or rest.*

- *Memory loss, inability to concentrate, headaches.*

- *Low-grade fever, muscle or joint aches, sore throat or swollen lymph nodes in neck or armpits.*

- *Persistent muscular pain, in addition to the symptoms listed above, may indicate fibromyalgia.*

SEE YOUR DOCTOR ...

- If the fatigue lasts longer than two weeks or is accompanied by sudden weight loss, muscle weakness or other unusual symptoms.

- If you take other medication. Fatigue is a side effect of some drugs – your doctor can rule out other possible and often correctable causes.

- If fatigue worsens despite home treatment.

REMINDER: If you have a medical condition, consult your doctor before taking supplements.

What it is

Profound and persistent exhaustion characterises chronic fatigue syndrome (CFS), known until the mid 1990s as myalgic encephalomyelitis (ME). Sufferers often have difficulty in sleeping, concentrating and performing daily tasks; many have underlying depression. Doctors disagree about whether CFS is a specific condition or a group of largely unrelated symptoms. The syndrome is sometimes diagnosed as fibromyalgia, a similar illness but with the additional symptom of muscular pain. Both conditions affect more women than men.

What causes it

The specific cause of CFS is unknown, but an impaired immune response may play a role. People with CFS often have other immune disturbances: about 65% are allergy sufferers (compared with 20% of the general population), and some have autoimmune disorders, such as lupus, in which the immune system attacks the body's own healthy tissues.

Many patients recall a flu-like illness before their fatigue began, and symptoms do suggest a lingering viral condition. Suspected infectious agents have included Epstein-Barr (the virus which causes glandular fever) and candida (the cause of thrush). These infections can have severe effects if the body is under-nourished or stressed. CFS has also been attributed to exposure to environmental toxins, low blood pressure, brain inflammation or abnormal hormone levels.

Compounds in pau d'arco fight infection by destroying invading micro-organisms.

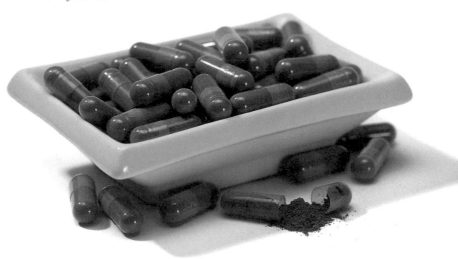

Vitamin C	**Dosage:** 500 mg twice a day. **Advice:** reduce dose if diarrhoea develops.
Carotenoids	**Dosage:** two tablets mixed carotenoids a day with food. **Advice:** each tablet should contain 15 mg mixed carotenoids.
St John's wort	**Dosage:** 300 mg extract three times a day. **Advice:** standardised to contain 0.3% hypericin.
Echinacea	**Dosage:** 200 mg extract twice a day. **Advice:** standardised to contain at least 3.5% echinacosides.
Magnesium	**Dosage:** 400 mg once a day. **Advice:** take with food; reduce dose if diarrhoea develops.
Siberian ginseng	**Dosage:** 100-300 mg twice a day. **Advice:** standardised to contain at least 0.8% eleutherosides.
Liquorice	**Dosage:** 200 mg three times a day. **Caution:** consult your doctor if you take blood pressure drugs. **Advice:** standardised to contain 22% glycyrrhizin or glycyrrhizinic acid; can raise blood pressure.
Astragalus	**Dosage:** 200 mg standardised extract twice a day. **Advice:** rotate in three-week cycles with echinacea and pau d'arco.
Pau d'arco	**Dosage:** 250 mg twice a day. **Caution:** avoid during pregnancy and breastfeeding. **Advice:** standardised to contain 3% naphthoquinones.

Note: consider using supplements in blue first; those in black may also be beneficial. Some dosages may be supplied by supplements you are already taking – see page 195.

How supplements can help

Any nutritional deficiency can exacerbate fatigue, so take a high-potency multivitamin and multimineral supplement in addition to those listed above. Supplement therapy aims to restore a healthy immune system, so begin with **vitamin C**, **carotenoids** and **St John's wort**, which has powerful antiviral properties and relieves depression. Another immunity-enhancer, **echinacea**, can be alternated with the herbs **astragalus**, which has antiviral and immunity-enhancing effects, **pau d'arco**, which fights microbes, or the tonic goldenseal. Tea or tincture of sarsaparilla root also has a tonic effect. For muscle spasm use **magnesium**. **Siberian ginseng** and **liquorice** bolster the adrenal glands, which secrete hormones such as cortisol to counteract stress and boost energy. Allow a month for the supplements to take effect.

What else you can do

☑ Eat a healthy diet, including at least five portions of fresh fruit and vegetables a day and oily fish twice a week.

☑ Try relaxation techniques such as meditation or yoga to manage stress and treat any underlying depression.

☑ Get a good night's sleep. If necessary, use supplements for insomnia, such as valerian or 5-HTP.

Mild aerobic exercise may be excellent for CFS, according to a recent study in the *British Medical Journal*. After a 12-week programme of walking, swimming or cycling for between 5 and 30 minutes a day, 55% of CFS patients felt 'much' or 'very much' better. Too much exercise may cause a setback, so proceed slowly.

———

Preliminary research is being conducted into the effects on CFS of coenzyme NADH, a substance involved in energy metabolising. In a recent study in the USA, patients who took NADH for a period of 18 months reported improvements in symptoms.

FACTS & TIPS

■ Lingering fatigue was known as neurasthenia in the 19th century, when remedies included liquorice extract. From the 1930s to the 1950s many countries reported outbreaks of prolonged fatigue. The Centers for Disease Control and Prevention in the USA set guidelines for diagnosis in 1988, opening the way for further mainstream medical research into the disorder. These guidelines are not currently in use in the UK.

■ In the 1980s CFS was incorrectly perceived as an illness cause by the 'work hard, play hard' lifestyle of young business people and nicknamed 'yuppie flu'.

Cold sores

Once the cold sore virus has infected the body, painful lip blisters can reappear whenever the immune system is depressed. The action of the virus is inhibited by antioxidants, immunity boosters and the amino acid lysine, remedies which also help to heal the skin.

Symptoms

- Initial outbreak: tender blisters on or near the mouth, sometimes accompanied by flu-like symptoms and swelling in nearby lymph nodes.

- Recurrences: an itchy or a tingling sensation on the lips, followed in a day or two by one or more fluid-filled blisters.

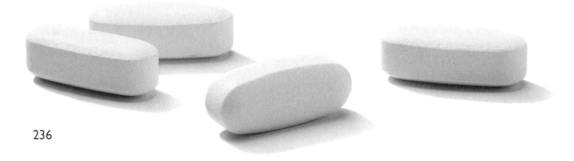

Lysine, the amino acid that helps to prevent cold sores, is available in easy-to-swallow tablets.

What they are

Cold sores are fluid-filled blisters that usually appear on the lips, though they can also develop as ulcers on the gums or inner cheeks, on the roof of the mouth, on the skin around the nostrils or in the nostril lining. The cold sore virus can spread by touch to the mucous membranes of the eyes, nose and genitals, and onto broken skin. The blisters break and form a scab before disappearing after a week to ten days.

What causes them

Cold sores are usually caused by herpes simplex type 1 virus (HSV-1). This virus is different from the one responsible for genital herpes – herpes simplex type 2 – which is generally transmitted through sexual contact. Because the cold sore virus lies dormant in nerve cells after the first outbreak, new sores are likely to recur as frequently as every few weeks or as infrequently as every few years. Sores often reappear when the immune system is depressed by a fever or a viral infection such as a cold. Recurrences can also be triggered by fatigue, menstruation or stress, or by exposure to sun, wind and salt water.

How supplements can help

A deficiency of any nutrient can impair the performance of the immune system, and anyone troubled by cold sores should regularly take a high-potency multivitamin and multimineral supplement. The supplements listed opposite help to minimise outbreaks and speed up the healing process. They should be used in combination at the first sign of a cold sore, and should take effect within two or three days.

The amino acid **lysine** suppresses the growth of HSV-1 when taken orally or applied to a sore in the form of a cream. It can be used long term and may help to prevent cold sores from forming. **Melissa cream**, made from the potent antiviral herb *Melissa officinalis* (lemon balm), should be used at the first sign of tingling. **Vitamin C** and **flavonoids** are powerful antioxidants which facilitate healing by eliminating the naturally occurring cell-damaging compounds known as free radicals;

Lysine	**Dosage:** 1000 mg three times a day for flare-ups.
	Caution: avoid during pregnancy and breastfeeding.
	Advice: take on an empty stomach; not suitable for children.
Melissa cream	**Dosage:** apply cream to sores two to four times a day.
	Advice: melissa is also called lemon balm.
Vitamin C/ flavonoids	**Dosage:** 500 mg vitamin C and 200 mg flavonoids twice a day.
	Advice: use for flare-ups; reduce dose if diarrhoea develops.
St John's wort	**Dosage:** 300 mg extract three times a day.
	Advice: standardised to contain 0.3% hypericin.
Echinacea/ goldenseal	**Dosage:** 200 mg echinacea and 125 mg goldenseal four times a day.
	Advice: sold singly or as combination supplement.
Zinc	**Dosage:** 15 mg a day.
	Advice: if you take a zinc supplement for more than one month, choose one that includes 2 mg copper.

Note: consider using supplements in blue first; the one in black may also be beneficial. Some dosages may be supplied by supplements you are already taking – see page 195.

both boost virus-fighting immune system cells. **St John's wort** may also improve immune performance, and has strong antiviral properties. Clinical studies have shown that **zinc** helps the healing process, probably because it also enhances immunity. Flare-ups can be treated with the immunity-enhancing herbs **echinacea** and **goldenseal**, which are natural antivirals and antibiotics. It's often beneficial to alternate herbs. Try 200 mg of echinacea a day for a week, followed by 200 mg a day of astragalus the following week, and an immunity-enhancing mixture of reishi (1500 mg a day), shiitake (1200 mg a day) and maitake mushrooms (600 mg a day) for the third week.

Topical application of vitamin E oil sometimes helps; other useful preparations are creams containing liquorice extract and oil extract of St John's wort (often called hypericum oil). Apply twice a day for as long as the symptoms persist.

What else you can do

☑ Apply sunscreen (SPF 15 or higher) to the lips to prevent recurrences. In a study involving people with recurrent cold sores, those who did not use sunscreen developed a cold sore after 80 minutes in the sun.

☑ Do not touch the blisters. This can spread the virus, as can sharing personal items such as towels, razors, drinking glasses or toothbrushes.

☑ Try meditation, yoga or other forms of relaxation to reduce stress, which is thought to precipitate cold sores.

☑ Avoid chocolate, gelatine, nuts and whole grain cereals. They contain a large amount of the amino acid arginine, which some doctors believe may trigger cold sores. Lysine is thought to counteract its effect.

Vitamin C may be effective when applied topically, according to a recent study in Finland. Researchers soaked cotton-wool pads in a solution of vitamin C and applied them to cold sores. In those who were treated with vitamin C, blisters cleared up faster (3.4 days) than in those who received a placebo (5.9 days).

―᠊᠊᠊᠊᠊―

The juice of the frangipani plant (*Plumeria rubra*) is a traditional African remedy for herpes infections. It is reputed to destroy the virus completely when applied to lesions, without leaving a scar; benefits are said to be felt within 20 minutes.

DID YOU KNOW?
Holding an ice cube to the affected area for a few minutes several times a day can help to reduce pain and dry out the cold sore.

FACTS & TIPS

■ As an alternative to commercial melissa cream, try lemon balm tea, applied externally, to hasten the healing of cold sores. First, prepare a strong tea: steep 2 or 3 teaspoons of the herb in a cup of very hot water for 15 minutes, then cool. Dab it on the sores with a cotton-wool pad three times a day.

■ Supplements can be safely used with over-the-counter or prescription antiviral creams, such as acyclovir or penciclovir, which also promote healing.

Colds and flu

Sooner or later just about everyone comes down with a miserable cold or a bout of flu – and some unfortunate people seem to get infected again and again. Vitamin C is probably the most familiar natural remedy for these viruses, but it is not the only one.

Symptoms

- *Congestion in the head and chest.*
- *Sneezing and coughing.*
- *Sore throat.*
- *Watery nasal discharge.*
- *Muscle aches.*
- *Fever and chills.*
- *Headache.*
- *Fatigue.*

SEE YOUR DOCTOR ...

- If your temperature is above 38°C for three days or ever goes to 39°C or higher.

- If you have a sore throat combined with a fever that stays above 38°C for 24 hours – it may indicate strep throat, a severe infection which needs treatment with antibiotics.

- If mucus is green, dark yellow or brown – this may be a sign of a bacterial infection in the sinuses or lungs.

- If you have chest pain and shortness of breath – you may have pneumonia, especially if you also have a high fever.

REMINDER: If you have a medical condition, consult your doctor before taking supplements.

What they are

As the common cold and flu are both respiratory infections, determining which one you have may be hard. Generally, a cold takes hold gradually but flu strikes suddenly – you can feel healthy in the morning but very unwell by the afternoon. The classic cold symptoms – congestion, sore throat and sneezing – are usually less severe than those of flu, which include fever, extreme fatigue, muscle aches and headaches.

Recovery times for the two infections are different. In general, a cold lasts for about a week, but symptoms may trouble you for only three or four days if your immune system is working efficiently; flu can last for up to ten days, and the accompanying fatigue may persist for a further two to three weeks. A cold rarely produces any serious complications, but flu can lead to bronchitis or pneumonia.

What causes them

Both colds and flu are caused by viruses that attach themselves to the lining of the nose or throat and spread throughout the upper respiratory system, occasionally to the lungs. In response, the immune system floods these areas with infection-fighting white blood cells. The symptoms of a cold or flu are not produced by the viruses but are actually the result of the body trying to stave off the infection. Colds and flu are more common in winter, when indoor heating reduces the humidity in the air; this may be because the lack of moist air dries out the nasal passages and creates the perfect breeding ground for the viruses.

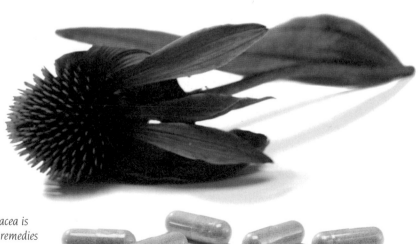

The herb echinacea is one of the best remedies for microbial infections.

Vitamin C	**Dosage:** 1000 mg three times a day until symptoms improve; if you need to take vitamin C for longer than three days, reduce dose to 500 mg twice a day. **Advice:** reduce dose if diarrhoea develops.
Echinacea	**Dosage:** 200 mg extract five times a day. **Advice:** for prevention, take 200 mg a day in three-week rotations with 400 mg a day of the herb astragalus.
Zinc lozenges	**Dosage:** one lozenge three times a day, or as instructed on the packet. **Advice:** do not continue taking for more than five days.
Garlic	**Dosage:** 400-600 mg concentrate four times a day with food. **Advice:** each tablet should provide 4000 mcg of allicin potential.
St John's wort	**Dosage:** 300 mg extract three times a day. **Advice:** standardised to contain 0.3% hypericin.

Some dosages may be supplied by supplements you are already taking – see page 195.

How supplements can help

A multivitamin and multimineral supplement taken throughout winter will support the immune system and help to fend off infection. The supplements listed above help your body to fight cold and flu viruses; they do not suppress symptoms. For this reason you may not feel better immediately after taking them, but you will probably recover faster. In some cases prompt treatment may prevent a cold or flu from fully developing. Start the supplements when symptoms first appear, and, unless otherwise stated, continue until the illness has passed.

Contrary to popular belief, **vitamin C** will not prevent a cold, but it may shorten its duration or minimise the symptoms. The herb **echinacea** stimulates the immune system to mount an attack against the virus. **Zinc lozenges** may also help to halt a cold, possibly by destroying the virus itself. A few drops of eucalyptus oil in hot water make a useful decongestant. An infusion of elderflower is also anti-catarrhal, and it strengthens the respiratory system. Limeflower and yarrow teas aid the elimination of toxins.

If you frequently develop a bacterial infection such as sinusitis or bronchitis from a cold or from flu, add **garlic** when you first notice symptoms – it contains compounds that may prevent bacteria from invading tissues. To give the immune system an extra boost, combine **St John's wort** with echinacea for the treatment (but not prevention) of colds and flu.

What else you can do

☑ Wash your hands often to reduce your chances of catching infections.

☑ Use a humidifier in winter to keep indoor air moist.

☑ Consider having a flu vaccination. It takes six to eight weeks to build up a viral immunity, so arrange your vaccination for autumn, before the flu season begins. Different flu strains emerge each year, so you will need to have an annual injection.

When it comes to cold prevention, it apparently helps to have plenty of friends. In a study of 276 men and women, those with wide social networks developed fewer cold symptoms – even after researchers deposited a cold virus directly into the nose.

———

Smokers are twice as likely to catch colds as non-smokers, according to a study by the Common Cold Unit of the Medical Research Council in Salisbury, Wiltshire.

———

In one study, faster recovery from flu was seen in men and women who took elderberry. Symptoms improved within two days in 93% of those using the herb; in the group given a placebo, six days passed before any improvement occurred.

FACTS & TIPS

■ When buying zinc lozenges read the ingredients list with care. Only zinc ascorbate, gluconate and glycinate seem to work against colds. Don't waste your money on products that contain sorbitol, mannitol or citric acid. When combined with saliva these chemicals make zinc ineffective.

■ Yarrow, peppermint and elderflower teas can help to alleviate flu symptoms. Mix equal amounts of the herbs, then add 200 ml of boiling water to 10 grams of the herb mixture, infuse for 10 minutes and strain. Drink three times a day. A ginger infusion using 10 grams of ginger root to 100 ml of boiling water is also effective.

Constipation

Regular exercise and a diet including plenty of fibre and fluids are vital for a healthy digestive system, and should keep bowel movements regular. For the occasional times when the body may need some assistance, natural supplements can be gentle and effective remedies.

Symptoms

- *Infrequent bowel movements.*
- *Hard, dry stools.*
- *Difficulty or pain when defecating.*
- *Swelling of the abdomen.*

What it is

Bowel habits can vary widely from person to person, but most doctors agree that anyone who passes hard stools and does so less than three times a week is constipated. If you frequently have to strain to defecate, you may also benefit from the therapies aimed at relieving constipation.

What causes it

In the majority of cases constipation occurs because of a lack of fibre and fluids in the diet. Inadequate liver function is another important cause – bile salts produced in the liver are natural laxatives, and are essential for the proper functioning of the digestive system. Other factors include insufficient exercise or prolonged inactivity, severe depression, and medical disorders such as high blood calcium levels, colon cancer, diabetes, irritable bowel syndrome, muscular spasm or an underactive thyroid. Overuse of laxatives or some antacids can impair bowel activity, and certain medications (including drugs for high blood pressure, anti-depressants and narcotic pain relievers) can also cause constipation.

How supplements can help

Any abrupt change in the usual pattern of bowel movements may be a sign of a more serious underlying disorder, such as cancer or a bowel obstruction, and requires medical evaluation. For occasional irregularity, various natural supplements may help. Benefits should be experienced within a day or two. With the exception of cascara sagrada, the following supplements can be taken on a long-term basis if required. **Psyllium,**

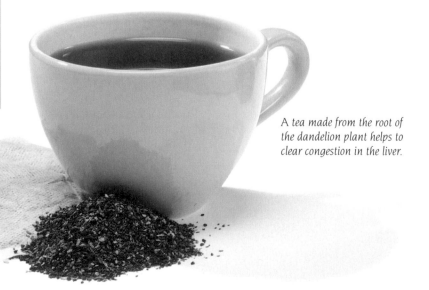

A tea made from the root of the dandelion plant helps to clear congestion in the liver.

Psyllium	**Dosage:** 1-3 tablespoons of powder a day, dissolved in water or juice. **Advice:** alternatively, take 1-3 tablespoons of ground flaxseeds or 2 teaspoons of ground fenugreek seeds; whichever herb you choose, drink eight glasses of water a day.
Prunes	**Dosage:** drink ½ cup of prune juice or eat three or four prunes each morning. **Advice:** can be taken on a daily basis.
Dandelion root	**Dosage:** one cup of tea three times a day. **Advice:** use 1 teaspoon of dried powdered root per cup.
Cascara sagrada	**Dosage:** 100 mg extract at bedtime. **Caution:** avoid during pregnancy and breastfeeding. **Advice:** standardised to contain 25% hydroxyanthracene derivatives.

Note: consider using supplement in blue first; those in black may also be beneficial. Some dosages may be supplied by supplements you are already taking – see page 195.

ground flaxseed or ground fenugreek seeds provide fibre and make the stools larger, softer and easier to pass; they can be used on a daily basis. Be sure to take plenty of water with them to facilitate the passage of extra bulk through the digestive tract. You can also try **prune** juice or dried prunes for extra fibre; these are gentle enough to use with other supplements. **Dandelion root** tea has a stimulating effect on the liver, giving it mild laxative properties, and yellow dock tea, which acts gently on the bowel itself, is a useful alternative.

If a combination of these remedies does not bring relief within a day or two, consider the herb **cascara sagrada** as a last resort. This herb is a powerful laxative which stimulates the bowel muscles to contract, and should be used for no longer than one or two weeks at a time.

As a preventative strategy, remember that wheat bran is an excellent source of insoluble fibre which readily binds water to provide bulk. Bran is difficult to eat by itself, so try to eat bran-rich cereals every day, and choose wholewheat bread rather than white or granary, neither of which contains as much fibre.

What else you can do

☑ Eat foods high in fibre, including raw fruits and vegetables, pulses and whole grains. Oranges (at least one a day) are particularly helpful as the citric acid they contain is a natural laxative.

☑ Drink at least eight glasses of water or juice a day.

☑ Exercise regularly and, whenever possible, go to the lavatory as soon as the urge strikes.

RECENT FINDINGS

Taking psyllium significantly increased the frequency of bowel movements in patients with constipation, according to a recent study from the University of Nebraska. Those consuming psyllium also reported that their stools were softer and easier to pass.

A recent study from Seattle found that men and women with frequent constipation were much more likely to develop colon cancer. The researchers concluded that the stools of those with constipation remain in the intestine for a relatively long period, thus exposing the bowel to potentially cancer-causing chemicals for a longer period of time. The results offer another example of the potential benefits to constipation sufferers of a daily intake of psyllium or other natural supplements.

FACTS & TIPS

■ If you are constipated, it is very important to drink plenty of fluids – but not all drinks are equally beneficial. Alcohol and caffeinated beverages actually cause fluid loss, making constipation worse. On the other hand, water, vegetable and fruit juices and clear soups are excellent fluid replenishers. A hot drink in the morning may help to trigger the reflex that gets the bowels moving.

Coughs

Each year millions of people seek their doctors' help to rid themselves of coughs. Home treatment with a natural remedy is often all that is necessary to relax the muscles of the respiratory system and help the body to expel an irritant, or to soothe the lining of a sore or inflamed throat.

Symptoms

- A *cough is in itself a symptom – it usually indicates the presence of a respiratory infection or an irritation of the throat, lungs or air passages.*

- A *cough can be dry (nonproductive) or wet (productive).*

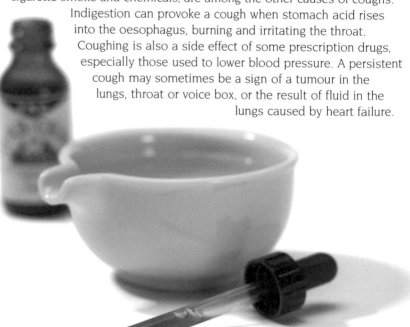

Tincture of liquorice root is an expectorant, which means that it makes a cough more productive.

What they are

Despite its seemingly unhealthy sound, a cough is actually a vital bodily function. Although you may not realise it, you probably cough once or twice every hour to clear your throat and air passages of debris. Coughing causes trouble only when a substance found in the environment or an illness makes it uncontrollable.

Coughs can be dry and nonproductive, meaning that they do not bring up fluids or sputum, or they can be wet and productive, expelling mucus and the germs or irritants it contains.

What causes them

When an irritant enters your respiratory system, tiny cough receptors in the throat, lungs and air passages begin producing extra mucus. This action stimulates nerve endings and sets in motion a sequence that culminates in a forceful expulsion of air and foreign material through the mouth: a cough. A variety of factors can trigger this reaction. Bacteria or viruses – such as those that cause flu or the common cold – lead to an overproduction of mucus, which initiates a cough reflex (particularly at night, when the sinuses drain and set off tickly coughs).

Asthma, bronchitis, hay fever and environmental pollutants, such as cigarette smoke and chemicals, are among the other causes of coughs. Indigestion can provoke a cough when stomach acid rises into the oesophagus, burning and irritating the throat. Coughing is also a side effect of some prescription drugs, especially those used to lower blood pressure. A persistent cough may sometimes be a sign of a tumour in the lungs, throat or voice box, or the result of fluid in the lungs caused by heart failure.

SUPPLEMENT RECOMMENDATIONS

Angelica/ coltsfoot/ horehound/ thyme	**Dosage:** as a tea, I cup up to three times a day, as needed. **Advice:** use I or 2 teaspoons of dried herb per cup of hot water; each herb can be taken alone or mixed with one or more of the other three herbs.
Liquorice	**Dosage:** 45 drops of tincture or I cup of tea three times a day. **Caution:** may raise blood pressure – consult your doctor if you suffer from hypertension. **Advice:** add tincture to water, or steep I teaspoon of dried herb in hot water with slippery elm or marshmallow.
Slippery elm	**Dosage:** as a tea, I cup up to three times a day as needed. **Advice:** use I teaspoon of dried herb per cup of hot water.
Marshmallow leaf	**Dosage:** as a tea, I cup up to three times a day, as needed. **Advice:** use 2 teaspoons of dried herb per cup of hot water; can be blended with slippery elm.

Some dosages may be supplied by supplements you are already taking – see page 195.

How supplements can help

There are two distinct goals when treating a cough, depending on whether it is productive or nonproductive. Productive coughs must not be repressed – expectorants should be used to thin the mucus, making it easier to bring up. This allows the body to flush out the irritant, helping the mucous membrane to heal. Nonproductive coughs may need to be subdued, especially when the cough causes pain or lack of sleep.

Angelica, **coltsfoot**, **horehound** and **thyme** all act as expectorants, and can be used to make teas. **Liquorice** tincture can be added to these teas to relax the bronchi further and loosen phlegm. Different combinations of these herbs are available in commercially prepared tea bags. They can also be taken as tinctures: follow the instructions on the packet, or add your chosen tincture to a small glass of warm water, and drink three times a day.

Tea made from **slippery elm** will soothe the throat and suppress dry coughs. **Marshmallow leaf** can be added: when steeped in water it releases mucilage – a gel-like plant substance – that coats the throat and calms the cough receptors. If you prefer, substitute mullein flowers, which also contain mucilage. Tinctures of aniseed, wild lettuce and wild cherry can also be taken in water for suppressing irritating dry coughs.

The inhaling of steam from hot water suffused with a few drops of eucalyptus or chamomile oil can open clogged sinuses, clear respiratory passages and minimise bronchial spasms. Cough drops or hard sweets containing eucalyptus, peppermint, anise or fennel increase saliva: this causes you to swallow more, which also suppresses the cough reflex.

What else you can do

☑ Drink lots of water, warm soup, tea and room-temperature fruit or vegetable juice to thin the mucus.
☑ Use a humidifier to moisten the air.
☑ Don't smoke, and avoid contact with irritating fumes or vapours.

Cuts and grazes

Minor everyday injuries can become more serious if they are neglected. Basic hygiene, prompt first aid and the application of natural antiseptics and anti-inflammatories can help to prevent infection and accelerate the skin's ability to repair itself.

Symptoms

- *Narrow slices through the skin that usually bleed.*
- *Superficial skin abrasions that show redness or some bleeding.*
- *Punctures or holes that may penetrate deep into the skin.*

SEE YOUR DOCTOR ...

- If a cut or graze is dirty and cannot be cleaned at home.
- If the cut will not close.
- If you are not sure of the severity of the wound.
- If blood spurts out or the bleeding cannot be stopped.
- If signs of infection appear (pus in a cut or graze, red streaks spreading from the injury, an unusual discharge or fever).
- If you get a dirty cut or graze or any puncture wound, and have not had (or cannot remember having had) a tetanus vaccination in the past ten years.

REMINDER: *If you have a medical condition, consult your doctor before taking supplements.*

What they are

Cuts and grazes are injuries that break the outer protective layer of skin. A cut describes skin that has been pierced or sliced; a graze skin that is visibly abraded or roughened.

What causes them

Sharp implements such as a knives and razor blades, the edge of a piece of paper or jagged pieces of glass or metal can easily cut the top layer of the skin. A puncture wound is a small circular penetration by an instrument with a sharp point such as a pin, nail or pencil point. A graze occurs when the skin is literally rubbed away by a rough surface such as gravel or a concrete pavement.

How supplements can help

Many topical supplements can ease or relieve pain, promote healing, prevent infection and reduce the risk of scarring, but they should be used for minor cuts and grazes only; gaping wounds that will not close and injuries that become infected require medical attention. After stopping any bleeding and thoroughly cleaning the wound, apply **lavender oil** to the fresh cut or graze to kill germs and help it to heal. **Tea tree oil** diluted with a little water will help to halt infection and minimise scarring. Diluted **echinacea**, marigold or myrrh tincture also fight infection, and comfrey ointment can quicken the healing process. Once you have completed these first-aid measures, bandage the wound. Change the bandage three or four times a day, and spread

Diluted with a little water, echinacea tincture is a potent infection-fighter when applied directly to skin wounds.

Lavender oil	**Dosage:** apply 1 or 2 drops of oil to wound after cleansing. **Advice:** dab directly onto any superficial wound.
Aloe vera gel	**Dosage:** apply gel liberally to wound three or four times a day. **Advice:** use fresh aloe leaf or shop-bought gel.
Vitamin C	**Dosage:** 500 mg twice a day for five days. **Advice:** reduce dose if diarrhoea develops.
Tea tree oil	**Dosage:** apply 1 or 2 drops of diluted oil after cleaning wound. **Advice:** can be used in place of lavender oil.
Echinacea	**Dosage:** add 3 drops tincture to 1 teaspoon of water; apply to wound. **Advice:** a substitute for tea tree oil; can also be taken orally: drink 1 cup of echinacea or goldenseal tea three times a day until wound has healed.
Calendula cream	**Dosage:** apply cream to wound three times a day. **Advice:** goldenseal cream or a combination of calendula and goldenseal is also effective.
Bromelain	**Dosage:** 500 mg three times a day on an empty stomach, over a period of five days. **Caution:** consult your doctor if you take anticoagulant drugs. **Advice:** should provide 6000 GDU or 9000 MCU daily.

Note: consider using supplements in blue first; those in black may also be beneficial. Some dosages may be supplied by supplements you are already taking – see page 195.

see page 195

either soothing **aloe vera gel** or **calendula cream** on the wound each time to alleviate or limit inflammation, stop infection and speed up the process of healing.

Take the oral supplements together for five days after the injury. **Vitamin C** inhibits inflammation and accelerates healing, and **bromelain**, an enzyme found in fresh pineapple, has similar beneficial effects. Teas made with the herbs **echinacea** and goldenseal boost immunity and decrease the risk of infection.

What else you can do

☑ Stop any bleeding by applying steady pressure to the wound for a few minutes with a clean tissue or cloth. If the injury is a puncture wound, let it bleed for several minutes first to make sure that it has flushed out any embedded germs.

☑ Thoroughly clean the skin around the cut or graze. Bandage the wound, especially if it is in an area likely to get dirty, such as a finger or a knee. Antibiotics are not necessary unless signs of infection appear.

RECENT FINDINGS

In a study of people with scars, those who wore silicon bandages containing vitamin E during the night showed greater improvement than patients not using vitamin E. Additional studies are needed to assess the role of this vitamin in halting or reversing the scarring process.

A small study of people who underwent surgery to remove tattoos found that those who took 3000 mg of vitamin C and 900 mg of pantothenic acid (vitamin B5) daily healed faster than those who consumed only 1000 mg of vitamin C and 200 mg of pantothenic acid a day.

DID YOU KNOW?
In Australian munitions factories during the Second World War, tea tree oil was added to machine oils to minimise infections when workers received cuts from metal filings.

FACTS & TIPS
■ An aloe vera plant is easily grown on a windowsill and makes an invaluable first-aid treatment for minor skin injuries. Break off one of the plumper leaves, slice it open lengthways, and scrape or squeeze out the clear gel.

Depression

Each year in the UK about 15 people in every thousand visit their GPs complaining of depression – one in a thousand is hospitalised with the condition. Recent research has uncovered a role for supplements, alongside new prescription medications, in managing the symptoms.

Symptoms

- *Persistent sad or 'empty' mood.*

- *Loss of pleasure in ordinary activities, including sex.*

- *Sleep disturbances, decreased energy, fatigue.*

- *Poor or increased appetite; weight loss or weight gain.*

- *Feelings of guilt, worthlessness and helplessness.*

- *Difficulty concentrating; irritability; excessive crying.*

- *Chronic aches and pains.*

- *Thoughts of death or suicide.*

SEE YOUR DOCTOR ...

- **If you or someone you know exhibits clear symptoms for at least two weeks.**

- **If you or someone you know has suicidal thoughts – get emergency help immediately.**

REMINDER: If you have a medical or psychiatric condition, consult your doctor before taking supplements.

What it is

Depression is more than just feeling blue – it is a devastating illness that affects a person's life on a physical, mental and emotional level. It not only influences self-esteem and the sufferer's perceptions of other people but also makes ordinary, daily activities difficult to perform. There are various forms of depression, ranging from mild, long-term melancholy (known as dysthymia) to alternating moods of elation and despair (bipolar, or manic, depression) and the most serious form, despondency. Despondency leads to a total inability to function and to thoughts of suicide.

What causes it

Depression does not have a single underlying cause, although scientists believe that the illness is caused by an imbalance in the brain's levels of neurotransmitters – chemical messengers that send signals from one nerve cell to another. A depressive episode can be triggered by the death of a loved one, a divorce, a life-threatening illness, the loss of a job or another serious difficulty. Food allergies and nutritional deficiencies, reaction to medication (such as beta-blockers), stress, overconsumption of alcohol or smoking can all contribute to depression. Dysfunctional ways of coping with anger, guilt and other emotions may also be implicated. Depression is a characteristic of Seasonal Affective Disorder (SAD), a condition which affects thousands of people as daylight hours shorten towards the end of the year. The lack of daylight causes sadness, fatigue and lethargy, and sufferers become socially withdrawn until the number of daylight hours increases again.

St John's wort may be as effective an antidepressant as prescription drugs.

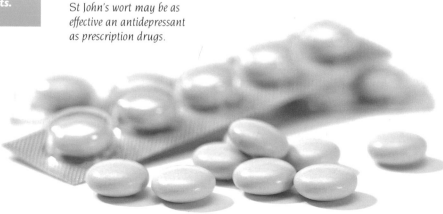

Vitamin B complex	**Dosage:** one tablet each morning with food. **Advice:** look for a B-50 complex with 50 mcg vitamin B_{12} and biotin, 400 mcg folic acid and 50 mg all other B vitamins.
Vitamin C	**Dosage:** 500 mg twice a day. **Advice:** reduce dose if diarrhoea develops.
Calcium/ magnesium	**Dosage:** 500 mg calcium and 200 mg magnesium once or twice a day. **Advice:** extra dose can be taken before bedtime to aid sleep.
St John's wort	**Dosage:** 300 mg extract three times a day. **Advice:** standardised to contain 0.3% hypericin.
5-HTP	**Dosage:** 100 mg three times a day **Caution:** do not take for longer than three months without consulting your doctor.
Ginkgo biloba	**Dosage:** 80 mg extract three times a day. **Advice:** standardised to contain at least 24% flavone glycosides.
Fish oils	**Dosage:** 2 teaspoons to supply 2 g of omega-3 fatty acids a day. **Caution:** consult your doctor if you take anti-coagulant drugs.

Note: consider using supplements in blue first; those in black may also be beneficial. Some dosages may be supplied by supplements you are already taking – see page 195.

How supplements can help

Vitamins and minerals can often help those taking antidepressants. Herbs or 5-HTP (5-hydroxytryptophan) – but not both – can be added, but should not be combined with drugs without your doctor's agreement. Do not stop taking prescription drugs without consulting your doctor.

Low levels of the **B vitamins** and **vitamin C** have been associated with depression. These play a part in the brain's production of neurotransmitters and may enhance the effectiveness of antidepressant medications. **Calcium** and **magnesium** soothe the nerves and can be particularly helpful when depression interferes with sleep. Teas or tinctures of melissa or rosemary also relieve tension; oat extract is a particularly useful nerve tonic in cases of exhaustion.

St John's wort may be a safe alternative to prescription drugs, which often have side effects. For people over the age of 50, **ginkgo biloba** combats depression more effectively than some orthodox drugs. **5-HTP** is a form of the amino acid tryptophan, which boosts serotonin levels in the brain and improves mood. **Fish oils** may also be beneficial in treating depression.

What else you can do

☑ Exercise regularly. This may be the best natural antidepressant.
☑ Avoid tobacco, excessive caffeine and alcohol.
☑ Seek counselling. Many current therapeutic techniques can help to break the cycle of depressive behaviour.

FACTS & TIPS

■ Eating turkey, salmon and milk products may help to ease depression because they contain the amino acid tryptophan. Low tryptophan levels reduce the brain's production of the neurotransmitter serotonin, which helps to regulate mood. Women may be particularly susceptible to low levels of tryptophan.

■ Women with depression may have porous bones, because imbalances in brain chemicals may be associated with a reduction in bone density. This increased risk of osteoporosis may be offset by taking 10 mcg a day of vitamin D with extra calcium and magnesium.

Diabetes

Diabetes is a condition that should always be managed by a doctor, though many herbs and supplements complement conventional medical treatment. Natural remedies can help to prevent some of the longer-term complications of this chronic but manageable disease.

Symptoms

- *Excessive thirst.*
- *Frequent and excessive urination.*
- *Extreme fatigue and weakness.*
- *Unintentional weight loss.*
- *Slow healing of cuts and wounds.*
- *Recurring infections, such as urinary tract infections or thrush.*
- *Blurred vision.*
- *Numbness or tingling in the hands and feet.*

SEE YOUR DOCTOR ...

- **If you experience any of the symptoms listed above.**

REMINDER: If you have a medical condition, consult your doctor before taking supplements.

What it is

In diabetics the hormone insulin, which regulates blood sugar, is not produced in sufficient quantities or is not used effectively by the body – a situation which creates high blood sugar levels. Over time this imbalance can lead to heart or kidney disease, nerve damage, vision loss and other complications. There are two types of diabetes: the less common is insulin-dependent diabetes (type I), which usually develops before the age of 30. Non-insulin-dependent diabetes (type II), which usually appears after the age of 40, accounts for 90% of cases.

What causes it

Type I diabetes occurs when the pancreas stops producing insulin. No one knows exactly why this happens, but some researchers believe that a virus or an autoimmune response, in which the body attacks its own pancreatic cells, is responsible. People with type I diabetes must take insulin for life. Type II diabetes develops from insulin resistance – the pancreas may secrete insulin, but the body's cells don't always respond to it. The most common cause of type II diabetes is obesity. Genetic factors can contribute to the onset of both types.

How supplements can help

Diabetes must always be tightly controlled under the management of a doctor. The supplements listed can be used alongside prescription drugs and by people with both types of diabetes. Some supplement dosages may require altered dosages of insulin or hypoglycaemic drugs (drugs which lower blood sugar levels) used for type II diabetes, and dosage changes must be supervised by your doctor.

The **B vitamins** help to produce enzymes that convert glucose into energy and may help to prevent nerve damage. The mineral **chromium** lowers blood glucose and reduces cholesterol levels in diabetics. **Gymnema sylvestre**, a herb from India, improves blood sugar control, sometimes reducing the need for insulin or hypoglycaemic medication.

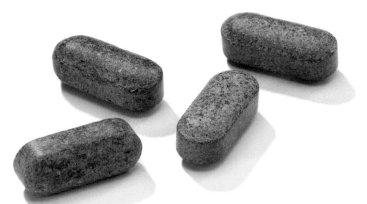

Bilberry can help to protect the eyes against complications of diabetes such as cataracts.

SUPPLEMENT RECOMMENDATIONS

Vitamin B complex	**Dosage:** one tablet each morning with food. **Advice:** look for a B-50 complex with 50 mcg vitamin B_{12} and biotin, 400 mcg folic acid and 50 mg all other B vitamins.
Chromium	**Dosage:** 200 mcg once a day with food. **Caution:** may alter insulin requirements: consult your doctor.
Magnesium	**Dosage:** 200 mg twice a day. **Caution:** do not take if you have kidney disease.
Zinc	**Dosage:** 25 mg a day. **Advice:** buy a supplement that includes 2 mg copper.
Gymnema sylvestre	**Dosage:** 200 mg extract twice a day. **Caution:** may alter insulin requirements: consult your doctor.
Fish oils	**Dosage:** 2 teaspoons to supply 2 grams of omega-3 fatty acids a day. **Caution:** consult your doctor if you take anticoagulant drugs.
Antioxidants	**Dosage:** 1000 mg vitamin C, 400 IU vitamin E and 150 mg alpha-lipoic acid each morning. **Caution:** consult your doctor before you take alpha-lipoic acid, as it may affect blood sugar.
Bilberry	**Dosage:** 160 mg extract twice a day. **Advice:** standardised to contain 25% anthocyanosides.
Taurine	**Dosage:** 500 mg L-taurine twice a day on an empty stomach. **Advice:** if using for longer than a month, add mixed amino acids.

Note: consider using supplements in blue first; the one in black may also be beneficial. Some dosages may be supplied by supplements you are already taking – see page 195.

Essential fatty acids protect against nerve damage and keep arteries supple. **Fish oils** in particular may raise levels of HDL (high density lipoproteins – 'good' cholesterol) in the blood, thereby reducing the risk of heart disease. **Antioxidants** prevent damage to the nerves, eyes and heart: vitamin E may block the build-up of plaque, and alpha-lipoic acid improves the metabolising of glucose.

Many diabetics have low levels of **magnesium** and **zinc**, which help the body to use insulin and heal wounds (a function impaired by high glucose levels). Long-term zinc use may mean that you also require extra copper. **Bilberry** helps to prevent diabetes-induced eye damage, and the amino acid **taurine** aids insulin release and can prevent abnormal blood clotting, a factor in heart disease.

What else you can do

☑ Exercise regularly. Those who burn more than 3500 calories a week through exercise are half as likely to develop type II diabetes as those burning less than 500. People with type I can benefit from exercise too.
☑ Lose weight to prevent the onset of type II diabetes.
☑ Eat whole grains, fruits and vegetables to keep blood sugar in check.

RECENT FINDINGS

Nutritional researchers in California have recently recommended that people with type II diabetes should take a daily supplement of 500 mg of vitamin E. The supplement is thought not only to combat the raised levels of free radicals associated with diabetes but also to improve blood sugar control by enhancing the action of insulin.

FACTS & TIPS

■ People suffering from diabetes may find it beneficial to add soya foods to their diet. These products – which include soya flour, soya milk and tofu – may improve glucose control, protect against heart disease and lessen stress on the kidneys.

■ The herb ginkgo biloba is useful for two common side effects of diabetes: nerve damage and poor circulation in the extremities. If you have signs of either complication, or if you have trouble controlling your blood sugar levels, try taking ginkgo biloba extract at a dose of 40 mg three times a day.

Diarrhoea

Unpleasant as it may be, diarrhoea provides your body with a way to flush out harmful toxins. This common ailment usually subsides on its own in a day or so, but it can be uncomfortable and inconvenient. Treatment should prevent dehydration and restore bulk to the stools.

Symptoms

- *Frequent loose watery stools.*
- *Abdominal cramps.*
- *Nausea, fever or thirst.*

SEE YOUR DOCTOR ...

- If diarrhoea persists for more than **48 hours.**
- If fever is higher than **38°C** and is accompanied by severe abdominal cramps, dizziness and light-headedness, or no urination.
- If there is blood in the stool or the stool is black.
- If there are signs of dehydration, such as persistent thirst, dry lips or sunken eyes.
- If diarrhoea recurs often – this could be a sign of a serious condition, such as colon disease.

REMINDER: If you have a medical condition, consult your doctor before taking supplements.

What it is

An increase in the frequency of stools or the passage of loose watery stools is called diarrhoea. It is not a disease itself but a symptom of a variety of disorders – most benign, some serious. Diarrhoea is a sign of disruption in the normal passage of food and waste through the large intestine. Ordinarily, water is absorbed through the intestinal walls as food passes through the large intestine, and faecal matter leaves the body as a solid mass. If something speeds up or otherwise interferes with this process, the fluid will be expelled from the body with faecal matter.

What causes it

Diarrhoea is caused by the inflammation or irritation of the intestine, and is usually the result of a bacterial or viral infection from contaminated food or drinking water. Most people travelling to less developed areas of the world are aware of the risk of food or water contamination and take steps to avoid diarrhoea, but they may not be so careful at home. Often the diarrhoea blamed on a 24-hour flu bug is more likely to be a consequence of food poisoning.

There are several other causes. Eating more fruit or vegetables than your digestive tract is accustomed to can sometimes lead to diarrhoea: citrus fruits and beans are typically the culprits. When consumed in large amounts the low-calorie sweetener sorbitol may also cause diarrhoea. The condition is sometimes a side effect of taking therapeutic doses of vitamin C or magnesium (if this occurs, reduce the dose). People with lactose intolerance – an

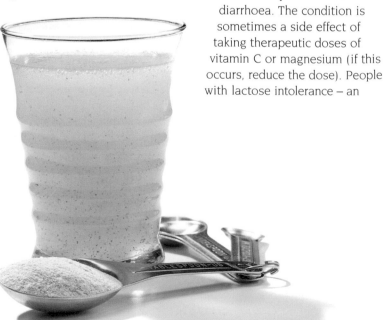

Psyllium is a soluble fibre, and is easy to take dissolved in a glass of water or juice.

SUPPLEMENT RECOMMENDATIONS	
Agrimony	**Dosage:** as a tea, I cup up to six times a day. **Advice:** use I tablespoon of leaves per cup; let it steep for 15 minutes and strain; drink throughout the day as required.
Blackberry/ raspberry leaf	**Dosage:** as a tea, I cup up to six times a day. **Advice:** use I tablespoon of leaves per cup; let it steep for 15 minutes and strain; drink throughout the day as required.
Psyllium	**Dosage:** 1-3 tablespoons of powder a day, dissolved in water or juice. **Advice:** drink extra water throughout the day.
Probiotics	**Dosage:** two tablets three times a day on an empty stomach; or try eating two or three pots of bioyoghurt throughout the day. **Advice:** choose acidophilus or bifidus cultures, or a mixture of the two.

Some dosages may be supplied by supplements you are already taking – see page 195.

inability to digest lactose, the sugar in dairy products – usually suffer from wind, bloating and diarrhoea after eating any food in which it can be found. Antibiotics can cause diarrhoea because they destroy the intestine's 'friendly' bacteria. In some people, stress is a trigger.

Diarrhoea can also be a symptom of a gastrointestinal disorder such as colitis, colon cancer, Crohn's disease, irritable bowel syndrome or pancreatic disease.

How supplements can help

Try drinking **agrimony**, **blackberry leaf** or **raspberry leaf** tea. These contain tannins, chemicals that have a sealing effect on the mucous membranes in the intestine and help the body to retain fluids. The teas also replenish lost fluids, which is important in preventing the dehydration that may result from a prolonged bout of diarrhoea.

If none of the teas provides relief, consider **psyllium**. Though this soluble fibre is more familiar as a treatment for constipation, it absorbs excess fluid in the intestine and adds bulk to the stool. **Probiotics** help to restore adequate levels of healthy bacteria to the intestine and are especially important if the diarrhoea is related to antibiotic use. All of these remedies can be substituted for over-the-counter preparations (except acidophilus, which can be used with them but should not be taken at the same time of day).

If food poisoning is to blame, wait a few hours before trying to treat the problem so that your body has enough time to get rid of the offending organism. Otherwise, start using the remedies immediately.

What else you can do

☑ Drink plenty of water and clear liquids to prevent dehydration.
☑ Avoid citrus fruits, milk and high-fibre foods for a day or two after having diarrhoea; eat bland foods, such as bananas and white rice.
☑ When travelling to areas where diarrhoea is likely to occur, eat cooked foods only. Avoid ice cubes and use bottled water, even to clean teeth.

RECENT FINDINGS

Wine has long been touted as a healing remedy for infection and disease. Now, some research indicates that drinking wine can also help to combat diarrhoea. In a recent study, both white wine and red wine were shown to be more effective in getting rid of harmful intestinal bacteria such as *Salmonella* and some strains of *E. coli* than a variety of over-the-counter antidiarrhoea products.

FACTS & TIPS

■ Blackberry leaf tea is often considered the strongest herbal remedy for diarrhoea. But read the labels on the packaging carefully – many products contain blackberry-flavoured black tea, not blackberry leaf tea.

■ Most people experience occasional diarrhoea caused by bacteria, viruses or other organisms in food. You can eliminate most risks by taking sensible precautions. Wash your hands with warm water and soap before preparing foods and after handling raw meats. Defrost foods only in the refrigerator or microwave; marinate meats only in the refrigerator. Wash plates and utensils used with raw poultry or meat before using them for cooked meats or other foods. Refrigerate all leftovers promptly.

Diverticular disorders

Many people over the age of 40 and up to 50% of those over 70 have a diverticular disorder. Diverticulosis is a disease of lifestyle, resulting particularly from a lack of fibre in the diet and inadequate exercise. A few simple measures can help.

Symptoms

Diverticulosis

- *Often there are no symptoms.*

- *In some cases, bloating, wind, nausea and constipation alternate with diarrhoea.*

Diverticulitis

- *Abdominal pain, usually on the lower left side (unlike appendicitis, which affects the right side).*

- *Fever, nausea, constipation or diarrhoea.*

- *Blood or mucus in the stool.*

SEE YOUR DOCTOR ...

- If you have fever, chills and abdominal swelling, or are vomiting – these may be signs of a ruptured diverticulum.

- If you have blood or mucus in the stool or any other symptoms of diverticulitis.

- If diverticular pain does not subside despite self-care.

REMINDER: If you have a medical condition, consult your doctor before taking supplements.

Acidophilus boosts levels of 'friendly' bacteria in the gut, improving general bowel health in those with diverticular disease.

What they are

There are two main types of diverticular disorder: diverticulosis and the more serious diverticulitis. In diverticulosis the inner lining of the large bowel pushes through the muscular layer that usually confines it, forming pouches (diverticula) ranging from pea-size to more than an inch in diameter. Though diverticulosis often has no symptoms, food can get trapped in these pouches, which then become inflamed and infected. The result is diverticulitis, the symptoms of which are impossible to ignore.

What causes them

Most cases of diverticulosis probably stem from a low-fibre diet. A lack of fibre means that the colon must work harder to pass the stool, and straining during bowel movements can aggravate the condition. A diet low in fibre also increases the likelihood of diverticulitis because waste moves slowly, allowing more time for food particles to become trapped and cause inflammation or infection. Lack of exercise also makes the colon sluggish. A tendency towards these disorders may run in families.

How supplements can help

Although supplements cannot reverse diverticulosis once a pouch has developed, they (and changes in your diet) can help to prevent or ease flare-ups of infection. Providing fibre that forms bulk, **psyllium** acts to relieve or prevent constipation. Ground **flaxseeds** are also rich in fibre and ward off infection by keeping intestinal pouches clear. These two can be taken together first thing in the morning to assist with the initial bowel movement, along with **probiotics** such as acidophilus. The fibre helps to protect the acidophilus from stomach acids and carries it into the intestine, where it alters the balance of bacteria in the digestive tract, enabling

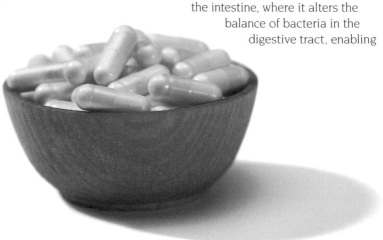

Psyllium	**Dosage:** I tablespoon of powder dissolved in water or juice twice a day. **Advice:** drink extra water throughout the day.
Flaxseeds	**Dosage:** 2 tablespoons of ground flaxseeds in water twice a day. **Advice:** drink extra water throughout the day.
Probiotics	**Dosage:** two tablets three times a day on an empty stomach; or try eating two or three pots of bioyoghurt throughout the day. **Advice:** Choose acidophilus or bifidus cultures, or a mixture of the two.
Aloe vera juice	**Dosage:** ½ cup of juice twice a day. **Advice:** the juice should contain 98% aloe vera and no aloin or aloe-emodin.
Glutamine	**Dosage:** 500 mg L-glutamine twice a day on an empty stomach. **Advice:** if you take it for more than a month, add a mixed amino acid complex (follow instructions on the packet).
Slippery elm	**Dosage:** 2 heaped teaspoons of bark powder, prepared with hot water and eaten like hot cereal each morning. **Advice:** or use tea (I teaspoon per cup) three times a day.
Chamomile	**Dosage:** as a tea, one cup three times a day. **Advice:** use 2 teaspoons of dried herb per cup; steep for 10 minutes, then strain; or try lemon balm or meadowsweet tea.
Wild yam/ peppermint/ valerian	**Dosage:** one cup of tea three or four times a day. **Advice:** use two parts wild yam, one part peppermint and one part valerian per cup of hot water; steep for 10 minutes, then strain; sweeten to taste.

Note: consider using supplements in blue first; those in black may also be beneficial. Some dosages may be supplied by supplements you are already taking – see page 195.

the body to fight off intestinal infections. Acidophilus is especially important if you are taking antibiotics during a flare-up.

Additional supplements, which may be particularly useful for treating flare-ups, are best taken at least 2 hours after taking psyllium, as it can interfere with their absorption. **Aloe vera juice** promotes the healing of inflamed areas, as does the amino acid **glutamine**, which is essential for regenerating the cells that line the intestine. These two can be combined with one or more relieving herbs. **Slippery elm** is a mild laxative that soothes infected diverticula. **Chamomile** and **wild yam** are anti-inflammatories. **Peppermint** relaxes digestive spasms, and **valerian**, lemon balm and meadowsweet soothe the digestive tract.

What else you can do

☑ Eat plenty of fruit, vegetables and whole grains to boost your fibre intake to between 20 and 30 grams a day.

☑ Drink at least eight glasses of water or other fluids every day.

Harvard University researchers monitored more than 43,000 men between the ages of 40 and 75. Those who later developed diverticular disease ate significantly less fibre than those who did not get the disease.

DID YOU KNOW?

Diverticulosis is almost unknown in rural areas of Africa and in non-industrialised nations, where a high-fibre diet and regular exercise are part of normal life.

FACTS & TIPS

■ Although fibre can make you feel bloated and full of wind, especially if you are not used to it, it is a good remedy for the bloating and wind of diverticular disease because its bulk keeps waste moving quickly through the bowel. Many studies show that a high-fibre diet prevents symptoms from returning for five years or longer.

■ People who are prone to suffering from diverticulitis are often warned not to eat seeds, including the tiny ones found in fruits such as strawberries, because it is thought that seeds can get caught in diverticula and cause inflammation. Studies have shown this fear to be groundless.

■ Regular exercise helps to prevent constipation. If you become constipated take advantage of natural laxatives, such as prunes.

Earache

Whether it is a middle ear infection, located deep in the ear, or 'swimmer's ear', affecting the outer ear canal, earache hurts. It is most often a problem in children, but adults get earache too. Although some conditions disappear of their own accord, supplements can hasten the healing process.

Symptoms

- *Throbbing or steady pain in the ear; pain when pulling on the lobe.*
- *Pressure or itching in the ear.*
- *A bloody, green, yellow or clear discharge from the ear.*
- *Muffled hearing; popping in the ear.*
- *Fever.*
- *Dizziness.*

SEE YOUR DOCTOR ...

■ If earache is accompanied by fever above 38°C, stiff neck, severe headache or seepage of pus or other fluids; or if the ear or the area behind it appears red or swollen – it is probably an infection requiring antibiotics.

■ If pain or hearing loss is severe or worsens despite self-care.

■ If an object is lodged in the ear or you have symptoms of a ruptured eardrum, such as sudden pain, partial hearing loss, bleeding or ringing in the ears.

REMINDER: If you have a medical condition, consult your doctor before taking supplements.

What it is

Earache results from inflammation, infection or swelling in either the outer canal of the ear or in the space adjoining the eardrum, which is the thin membrane separating the outer and the middle ear. The eustachian tube, which extends from the middle ear to the throat, normally drains fluids from the ear, keeping it clear; but inflammation or infection can irritate the ear canal or block the eustachian tube, leading to the build-up of pus or other fluids and causing pain and other unpleasant symptoms.

What causes it

Earache is caused by harmful bacteria, viruses or fungi, usually preceded by an upper respiratory infection or seasonal allergies, or by moisture trapped in the ear. Other causes include excessive ear wax, sudden changes in air pressure, a perforated eardrum or exposure to irritating chemicals, such as hair dyes and the chlorine in swimming-pool water.

How supplements can help

The recommended supplements can aid in the healing of earache. They can be used in conjunction with antibiotics, pain relievers and other conventional remedies for short-term treatment of mild to moderate ear discomfort. All severe, lingering or recurrent ear pain, however, requires medical evaluation. Start with natural eardrops made from **garlic oil** or **mullein flower oil**. Eardrops should not be used, however, if ear pain is severe or if it is accompanied by partial hearing loss or pus-like drainage from the ears; consult your doctor because the eardrum may

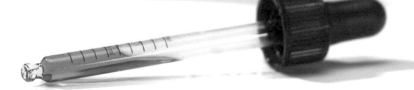

Echinacea can help to relieve earache caused by infections such as colds and flu.

Garlic oil	**Dosage:** 1 or 2 drops on a cotton wool ear-plug. **Advice:** a little may be mixed with mullein flower oil and applied directly.
Mullein flower oil	**Dosage:** a few drops in the ear twice a day. **Advice:** may be used alone or mixed with a little garlic oil.
Lavender oil	**Dosage:** apply a few drops to the outer ear and rub in gently. **Advice:** can be used as needed throughout the day.
Eucalyptus oil	**Dosage:** add several drops essential eucalyptus oil to pan of water. **Advice:** bring oil and water to boil and remove from heat; place towel over head and pan and inhale steam through the nose.
Vitamin C/ flavonoids	**Dosage:** 500 mg vitamin C and 250 mg flavonoids twice a day until infection clears. **Advice:** reduce vitamin C dose if diarrhoea develops.
Echinacea	**Dosage:** 200 mg three times a day until infection clears. **Advice:** standardised to contain at least 3.5% echinacosides.

Some dosages may be supplied by supplements you are already taking – see page 195.

be ruptured. Garlic and mullein flower oils help to fight disease-causing microbes and reduce inflammation, and may relieve pain and itching. If the outer ear appears irritated, **lavender oil**, rubbed in gently, can be very soothing. In addition to applying topical herbal oils, prepare a **eucalyptus oil** steam bath, which will aid in opening the eustachian tube; this will ease pressure and facilitate the drainage of infectious fluids from the ear. Repeat several times a day until the pain subsides.

Supplements should also be taken internally. Immunity-boosters such as **vitamin C** play an important role in fighting infections and preventing recurrences. Take vitamin C with the plant-based anti-inflammatories called **flavonoids**, which enhance its effectiveness. The immunity-enhancing herb **echinacea** can be valuable as well, especially when earache is the result of an upper respiratory infection.

Herbalists use elderflowers, mullein leaves, marshmallow leaves and chamomile flowers, either singly or combined, for treating earache. To make a tea, add 200 ml boiling water to about 10 g of the dried herb or a mixture of the herbs, and infuse for 10 minutes before straining. Sip this tea twice a day.

What else you can do

☑ Place a warm compress on the outside of your ear; use a heating pad or warm face flannel. Heat can bring quick pain relief and it also facilitates healing.

☑ Never insert a cotton bud into your ear. It can perforate the eardrum. Avoid using hydrogen peroxide as a cleaner; it can irritate the ear canal.

RECENT FINDINGS

A study looking at the link between tobacco smoke and ear infections reported that exposure to smoke can affect the ears. Children who lived in households with at least two smokers were 85% more likely to suffer from middle ear infections than those who lived in nonsmoking homes. Although some studies have shown no link, it is always a good idea not to smoke, and to avoid smoke-filled rooms, especially if you are prone to earache.

In a recent Finnish study, children who chewed gum sweetened with xylitol, a type of natural sugar (sometimes called birch sugar) found in a number of commercial chewing gums, had almost half as many ear infections as those who chewed other types of gum. The researchers speculate that xylitol may help to prevent harmful microorganisms at the back of the mouth from reaching the ear, where they can cause infections.

FACTS & TIPS

■ Herbal eardrops often bring rapid pain relief – within 10 minutes of administration. To make the application of drops more comfortable, warm the bottle under hot, running tap water before placing the liquid in the ear.

Eczema

Applied to the skin, soothing creams can help to relieve the red and often intensely itchy rashes of eczema. Various nutrients taken internally may also hasten healing. They may even be effective in preventing recurrences of this all-too-common – and bothersome – skin complaint.

Symptoms

- *Areas of itchy skin that are red, dry, scaly, rough or cracked.*
- *Tiny pimple-like blisters.*
- *Thickened, dry patches of skin in persistent cases of eczema.*

SEE YOUR DOCTOR ...

- **If eczema is especially widespread or recurrent.**
- **If oozing or crusting sores appear – they may indicate a bacterial infection.**
- **If eczema does not respond to self-care measures within three or four days.**

REMINDER: If you have a medical condition, consult your doctor before taking supplements.

What it is

Known medically as dermatitis, eczema produces inflamed patches of red, scaly skin on the face, scalp, hands and wrists; in front of the elbows and behind the knees; and in other areas of the body. Although eczema frequently itches a great deal, scratching can aggravate it.

What causes it

Eczema is often triggered by an allergy to foods, pollen, animal fur or other substances, and is likely to run in allergy-prone families. In fact, many people with eczema have (or later develop) hay fever. Those with eczema have in their bodies higher than normal amounts of histamine, a chemical that produces an allergic reaction when released in the skin. Some cases occur after contact with allergens, such as poisonous plants, jewellery made of nickel or chrome, dyes, cosmetics, topical medications and cleaning agents. People who have poor circulation in their legs may suffer from a type of eczema called stasis dermatitis, which causes scaly patches around the ankles. Eczema can also be triggered or aggravated by dry air, too much sun and stress.

How supplements can help

Used individually, in combination with other supplements or in conjunction with conventional drugs, various supplements can offer relief from flare-ups of eczema. Benefits should begin to appear within three or four days. The recommended supplements can also be taken long term to prevent recurrences.

A number of supplements taken internally are useful in countering inflammation and tempering the allergic response. Try a few and see which ones work for you. The various sources of omega-3 fats, such as **fish oils**, **evening primrose oil** and flaxseed oil, contain different types of skin-revitalising essential fatty acids that can relieve itching and inflammation, and **vitamin E** can mitigate skin dryness and itchiness.

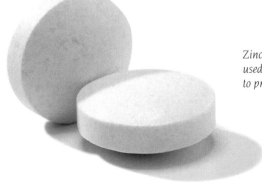

Zinc – which should be taken with copper if used over a long period – helps to relieve and to prevent red and itchy flare-ups of eczema.

SUPPLEMENT RECOMMENDATIONS

Fish oils	**Dosage:** 2 teaspoons to supply 2 grams omega-3 fatty acids a day. **Caution:** consult your doctor if you take anticoagulant drugs. **Advice:** vegetarians can substitute 1 tablespoon of flaxseed oil.
Evening primrose oil	**Dosage:** 1000 mg three times a day. **Advice:** you can substitute 1000 mg borage oil once a day.
Zinc	**Dosage:** 15 mg daily. **Advice:** if you take a zinc supplement for more than a month, choose one that includes 2 mg copper.
Vitamin E	**Dosage:** 250 mg a day. **Caution:** consult your doctor if you take anticoagulant drugs.
Grape seed extract	**Dosage:** 100 mg twice a day. **Advice:** standardised to contain 92%-95% proanthocyanidins.
Chamomile	**Dosage:** apply cream or lotion to affected areas three or four times a day. **Advice:** available ready-made in health-food shops.
Liquorice	**Dosage:** apply cream to affected areas three or four times daily. **Advice:** also called glycyrrhetinic acid cream.

Note: consider using supplements in blue first; those in black may also be beneficial. Some dosages may be supplied by supplements you are already taking – see page 195.

The mineral **zinc** aids the healing process and boosts the functioning of the immune system; it is also necessary for the processing of essential fatty acids. When used long term or at high doses, zinc should be taken with copper because it depletes the body's copper reserve. In addition, **grape seed extract** is rich in antioxidant substances called flavonoids, which inhibit the body's allergic responses.

It is frequently beneficial to apply a topical cream containing **chamomile** or **liquorice**. These herbs reduce skin inflammation and can be surprisingly soothing when applied directly to lesions. Herbs that may be helpful when taken as teas include nettle leaf, red clover, sarsaparilla and burdock root, used singly or in combination. Add 200 ml boiling water to about 15 grams of the dried herb (or a mixture) and infuse for 10 minutes before straining. Drink at once or in split doses during the day.

What else you can do

☑ Eliminate from your diet any foods that may cause an allergic reaction. These often include milk, eggs, shellfish, wheat, chocolate, nuts and strawberries.

☑ Wear loose-fitting clothing made of cotton, which is less likely than other fabrics to irritate the skin.

☑ Bath or shower less frequently to prevent the skin from drying out. Use lukewarm water and avoid deodorant soaps, bubble baths and perfumed products. Pat your skin dry instead of rubbing it.

RECENT FINDINGS

Many conventional doctors question the effectiveness of evening primrose oil as a treatment for eczema, and studies conflict. One recent study, however, found that adults and children with eczema who took evening primrose oil for six months experienced less itching and decreased inflammation.

FACTS & TIPS

■ As topical treatments for eczema, herbal liquids or lotions work best on oozing lesions. Ointments and creams are most effective on dry patches of eczema.

■ Liquorice cream is very effective for people who also use prescription or over-the-counter cortisone creams to treat eczema. Liquorice contains glycyrrhetinic acid, which both increases the effectiveness of cortisone and also reduces possible side effects, such as burning, itching and irritation.

■ Another product worth considering is witch hazel cream, which has been shown to be as beneficial as 1% hydrocortisone cream for the treatment of eczema.

■ Traditional Chinese herbalists prescribe a tea for eczema containing liquorice and, depending on symptoms, some nine other herbs. The treatment can be very effective, but analysis of preparations sold in the UK found that many of them contained extremely high doses of the potent steroid dexamethasone.

Endometriosis

In the past, many women suffering from the pain and heavy bleeding of endometriosis were told their complaints were 'just cramps' or 'all in the head'. The condition is now taken more seriously, but conventional medicine does not always alleviate all the symptoms.

Symptoms

- *Intense menstrual cramps that begin before the period starts and reach their peak after it ends.*

- *Abnormally heavy menstrual bleeding, often with large clots.*

- *Nausea and vomiting just before a menstrual period.*

- *Sharp pain during sexual inter-course at any time of the month.*

- *Diarrhoea, constipation or pain during bowel movements.*

- *Blood in the stool or urine during menstrual period.*

- *Infertility.*

SEE YOUR DOCTOR ...

- **If you have any of the above symptoms.**

REMINDER: If you have a medical condition, consult your doctor before taking supplements.

What it is

In endometriosis, bits of the uterine lining (endometrium) migrate out of the uterus and embed themselves in other abdominal tissues, often the ovaries, uterine ligaments or intestines. Each month, as oestrogen and other hormones cause the lining of the uterus to thicken with blood, the wayward cells also expand. The uterine tissues then slough off normally. But the stray cells have nowhere to release the blood they have amassed, which leads to cysts, scarring or adhesions (fibrous tissue that binds parts of the body that are normally not attached to each other). Although not all women with endometriosis have symptoms, the condition can cause severe pain. Endometriosis is a leading cause of female infertility.

What causes it

No one knows why endometriosis develops, but speculation abounds. According to the 'reflux menstruation' theory, menstrual blood travels backwards through the fallopian tubes, funnelling endometrial cells into other abdominal areas where they seed and grow. Another hypothesis suggests that endometriosis is congenital – meaning that some endometrial cells have been outside the uterus since birth. Still another idea is that endometriosis is caused by a faulty immune system, which neglects to destroy the out-of-place cells.

How supplements can help

All the recommended supplements can be used together and with any medications prescribed by your doctor. Start by taking the traditional combination of **chasteberry** and **black cohosh**. These herbs aid in correcting the hormonal imbalances that can intensify the pain of

Black cohosh contains substances that mimic the effects of natural hormones and can rectify hormonal imbalances in the human body.

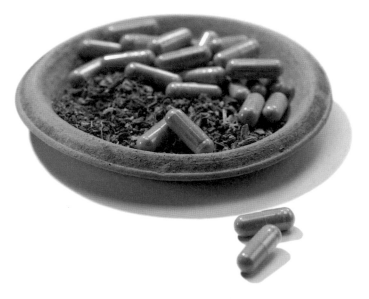

SUPPLEMENT RECOMMENDATIONS

Chasteberry	**Dosage:** 225 mg standardised extract three times a day. **Advice:** also called vitex; should contain 0.5% agnuside.
Black cohosh	**Dosage:** 250 mg extract, or 30 drops tincture, three times daily. **Advice:** standardised to contain 5% deoxyactein.
Wild yam	**Dosage:** 500 mg twice a day. **Advice:** take with food to minimise risk of stomach upset.
Lipotropic combination	**Dosage:** one or two tablets three times a day. **Advice:** should contain milk thistle, choline, inositol, methionine, dandelion and other ingredients.
Calcium/ magnesium	**Dosage:** 500 mg calcium and 200 mg magnesium once or twice a day. **Advice:** take throughout the menstrual cycle.
Vitamin C	**Dosage:** 500 mg twice a day. **Advice:** reduce dose if diarrhoea develops.
Vitamin E	**Dosage:** 250 mg twice a day. **Caution:** consult your doctor if you take anticoagulant drugs.
Fish oils	**Dosage:** 2 teaspoons to provide 2 g of omega-3 fatty acids a day. **Caution:** consult your doctor if you take anticoagulant drugs. **Advice:** vegetarians can substitute 1 tablespoon flaxseed oil.
Evening primrose oil	**Dosage:** 1000 mg three times a day. **Advice:** you can substitute 1000 mg borage oil once a day.

Note: consider using supplements in blue first; those in black may also be beneficial. Some dosages may be supplied by supplements you are already taking – see page 195.

RECENT FINDINGS

Women who do not get enough omega-3 fatty acids – found in fish oils and flaxseed oil – often have increased menstrual discomfort. In a Danish study that included 181 women, those who ate a lot of fish had milder menstrual cramps than the women who ate very little fish.

endometriosis, and also relax the uterus, as does **wild yam**. In addition, take a **lipotropic combination**, which stimulates the liver to eliminate excess oestrogen from the body.

For best results these supplements should be taken throughout the menstrual cycle. If menstrual cramps are painful, take the high doses of **calcium** and **magnesium** listed. These minerals help to lower the body's production of prostaglandins, substances made by endometrial cells that cause menstrual cramps. If a few months of taking these supplements does not help, try adding **vitamin C** to promote healing of the tissues damaged by cysts and scarring; **vitamin E** to balance hormone production further; and **fish oils**, **evening primrose oil** or flaxseed oil to help to control inflammation.

What else you can do

☑ Eat soya products, which contain phytoestrogens (plant oestrogens) that may offset the effect of oestrogen on symptoms of endometriosis.
☑ Take regular exercise. It has been shown in several studies to suppress symptoms, and may actually prevent endometriosis.

Epilepsy

Throughout history, people prone to seizures have been thought to be possessed by demons, to have special powers or to be mentally ill. Today we know that all these ideas were wrong: epilepsy is a condition that does not diminish intellectual capacity, creativity or productivity.

Symptoms

Many and various, including:

- Short periods of blackout, confusion or altered memory.

- Repetitive blinking, chewing or lip smacking, with or without a lack of awareness.

- Lack of attention: a blank stare, no response when spoken to.

- Loss of consciousness, sometimes with a loud cry, jerking muscles, or loss of bladder or bowel control; often followed by extreme fatigue.

SEE YOUR DOCTOR ...

- If you experience any of the above symptoms.

- If you have a seizure for the first time. However, for later seizures, only a fall causing an injury or one episode followed closely by another need a doctor's immediate attention.

REMINDER: If you have a medical condition, consult your doctor before taking supplements.

What it is

Epilepsy is a disorder that results from excessive electrical activity in the brain and nervous system. Normally, brain cells transmit electrical impulses in a highly regulated manner. People with epilepsy, however, experience periods when many brain cells all fire at once. This uncontrolled discharge produces symptoms that can range from a blank stare to a loss of consciousness with convulsions. These episodes are called seizures (epilepsy is also known as seizure disorder). Having a single seizure is not necessarily a sign of epilepsy, which is actually defined as having recurrent seizures. In fact, only about a quarter of those people who have a seizure will have another within three years.

What causes it

In more than half of epilepsy cases the cause of the disorder is unknown. In the remaining cases, seizures can sometimes be traced to a previous head injury, stroke, brain tumour or brain infection. Neurologists think that anyone may be susceptible to seizures but, for some reason, certain individuals are particularly vulnerable. Heredity seems to play some role.

In people with epilepsy, low blood sugar levels (hypoglycaemia) and low levels of certain nutrients (such as magnesium or B vitamins) can induce seizures. In addition, lack of sleep, drinking too much alcohol, stress or an illness may trigger a seizure even in people who do not have epilepsy.

How supplements can help

Under no circumstances should individuals using anticonvulsant drugs for epilepsy stop taking them or reduce the dosage on their own. The supplements in the chart are not a substitute for prescription drugs. Instead, they may help to correct nutritional deficiencies that can contribute to seizures, or aid in controlling seizures in people who

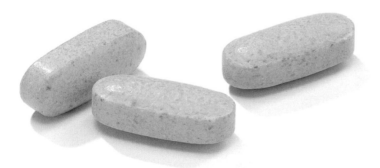

People with epilepsy may benefit from a balanced B-complex vitamin, which helps to keep the brain and nerve tissues healthy.

Vitamin B complex	**Dosage:** one tablet or capsule each morning with food. **Advice:** look for a B-50 complex with 50 mcg vitamin B_{12} and biotin, 400 mcg folic acid and 50 mg all other B vitamins.
Calcium/ magnesium	**Dosage:** 500 mg calcium and 200 mg magnesium twice a day with food. **Advice:** sometimes sold in a single supplement.
Valerian	**Dosage:** 300 mg extract once or twice a day. **Advice:** standardised to contain at least 0.5% valerenic acid.
Taurine	**Dosage:** 500 mg L-taurine three times a day on an empty stomach. **Advice:** if you take this for more than one month, add mixed amino acids.

Note: consider using supplements in blue first; those in black may also be beneficial. Some dosages may be supplied by supplements you are already taking – see page 195.

continue to have them despite medication. Supplements may eventually allow a physician to reduce the dosage of anticonvulsant drugs, which often have unpleasant side effects.

Adequate amounts of B vitamins, especially B_6 and folic acid, are important because they are involved in the manufacture of the brain chemicals (called neurotransmitters) that transmit messages throughout the nervous system. It's best to take a **vitamin B complex** supplement, because B vitamins work closely together. Other nutrients that promote brain and nerve health are **calcium**, **magnesium**, zinc and selenium; sufficient amounts of the trace elements should be provided by a good quality 'A to Z' multivitamin and mineral formulation.

Valerian also has a calming effect on the nervous system. Low levels of the chemical GABA (gamma-aminobutyric acid) in the brain appear to be linked to seizures; valerian, like the amino acid **taurine**, increases GABA levels.

What else you can do

☑ Get plenty of sleep. Fatigue can predispose you to seizures.
☑ Avoid alcohol. It can interfere with anticonvulsant medications and possibly contribute to seizures.

Preliminary research suggests that vitamin E can help people with epilepsy. One theory about seizures suggests that they are triggered by damage to the fatty membranes that surround nerve cells. With its antioxidant properties, vitamin E can inhibit the chemical changes in the body that lead to this damage. Although more study is needed, people with epilepsy can safely take 250 mg of vitamin E a day, either in a multivitamin or as a separate supplement.

FACTS & TIPS

■ Do not try to restrain a person having a seizure or insert a gag or anything else into the mouth to prevent the tongue from being bitten. This could cause serious injury to the person or to you if he or she bites your fingers. Instead, cushion the person's fall and clear away any sharp or hard objects. When the seizure is over, turn him or her on the side to prevent possible choking.

■ About 420,000 people in the UK suffer from various forms of epilepsy – one in 130. This makes epilepsy the second most common neurological condition in the country after migraine.

Eye infections

Automatically reaching for over-the-counter eyedrops when your eyes become watery, itchy, red or inflamed can actually make matters worse. Instead, give one of nature's gentle remedies a try – it may prove to be much more effective.

Symptoms

- *Pinkness or redness in the whites of the eyes.*
- *Thick, oozing greenish-yellow or white discharge from the eye.*
- *Excessive watering.*
- *Dried crusts on the eyelid and eyelashes that form during sleep.*
- *Sensation of sand or grit in the eye when blinking.*
- *Swollen or flaking eyelids.*
- *A small, painful red bump at the base of an eyelash (stye).*

SEE YOUR DOCTOR ...

- If the eye is red or swollen, with a thick discharge – you may need antibiotics for a bacterial infection. If you wear contact lenses, remove them.

- If the eye is painful or sensitive to sunlight, or you have blurring or loss of vision.

- If the pupils are different sizes or an object is lodged in an eye.

- If mild symptoms do not begin to wane after four days of self-care.

REMINDER: If you have a medical condition, consult your doctor before taking supplements.

What they are

Eye infections are usually related to conjunctivitis, an inflammation of the sensitive mucous membranes that line the eyelids. Other causes of redness and irritation are a persistent scaliness on the eyelid edges (called blepharitis) and inflamed, painful bumps at the base of the eye-lashes (known as styes). A doctor should evaluate eyes that are red and painful to determine the proper course of treatment and rule out more serious ailments, such as glaucoma.

What causes them

Viruses and bacteria cause eye infections. Inflammation and redness may also occur as a result of injuries to the eye, allergies or irritants (such as smoke, make-up or chlorine in a swimming pool).

How supplements can help

Any serious eye infection or injury requires immediate medical care. Mild eye infections can be treated at home with natural remedies, but see your doctor if the symptoms don't begin to clear up within three or four days.

First, use a herbal eyewash several times a day. **Eyebright** (as its name suggests) may reduce redness, swelling or irritation from conjunctivitis, blepharitis, styes or eye injuries. Eyewashes made from the herbs **chamomile** or **goldenseal** offer similar relief and are good alternatives to eyebright. Finely filter all eyewashes through a sterile gauze pad or clean piece of cheesecloth. To promote healthy eyes, try

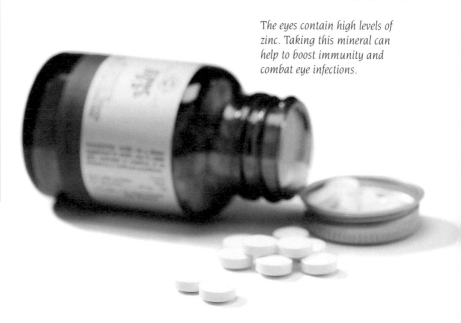

The eyes contain high levels of zinc. Taking this mineral can help to boost immunity and combat eye infections.

Eyebright	**Dosage:** 1 teaspoon dried herb per 500 ml of hot water; cool and strain. **Advice:** store in sealed container; prepare fresh daily; use an eye bath to wash affected eye three times a day.
Vitamin C	**Dosage:** 500 mg twice a day. **Advice:** reduce dose if diarrhoea develops.
Zinc	**Dosage:** 25 mg a day for one month. **Advice:** supplementation with 30 mg zinc (the maximum) should be accompanied by 2 mg copper.
Chamomile	**Dosage:** 2 or 3 teaspoons dried herb per 250 ml hot water; cool and strain. **Advice:** store in sealed container; prepare fresh daily; use an eye bath to wash affected eye three times a day.
Goldenseal	**Dosage:** 1 teaspoon dried, powdered herb per 500 ml of hot water; cool and strain. **Advice:** store in sealed container; prepare fresh daily; use an eye bath to wash affected eye three times a day.

Note: consider using supplements in blue first; those in black may also be beneficial. Some dosages may be supplied by supplements you are already taking – see page 195.

taking **vitamin C**, as well as the mineral **zinc**, for a month. Both these nutrients enhance immunity, helping to clear away an infection and prevent recurrences. Vitamin C may speed healing and protect the eye from further inflammation, and zinc, which is found in one of its highest concentrations in the eye, may boost its effectiveness.

Bloodshot eyes are often caused by leaking or dilated blood vessels in the eyeball. Bilberry extract (taken internally) may be helpful in preventing this by strengthening the capillaries of the eyes. Drinking eyebright tea will help to reduce inflammation of the eyes, as will the application of a chamomile tea bag (cooled after being infused).

What else you can do

☑ Wash your hands often with an antiseptic soap, and do not touch or rub your eyes. Change pillowcases and towels frequently; do not share them with others. Most eye infections are highly contagious.

☑ Avoid wearing eye make-up or contact lenses during an eye infection.

☑ Wipe the discharge from the infected eye with a tissue and dispose of it immediately to prevent the infection from spreading.

☑ For styes, apply a warm, moist compress for 10 minutes three or four times a day until the stye comes to a head and drains.

☑ For blepharitis, try a warm, moist compress; apply for 15 minutes to loosen the infected scaliness on the eyelids. Then scrub the eyelid gently with water and baking soda, or with diluted baby shampoo.

☑ Use a separate compress or eye bath for each eye to prevent any infection from spreading.

A French study found that when zinc was combined with antihistamines, 78% of the patients with symptoms of conjunctivitis from seasonal allergies showed considerable improvement.

———

Nonprescription eyedrops meant to relieve red, tired eyes have been shown to cause some forms of conjunctivitis, according to a recent report in the *Archives of Ophthalmology*. Overuse of eyedrops that reduce redness by narrowing blood vessels may be especially problematic for some people.

FACTS & TIPS

■ Make sure herbal teas are sterile when you use them as eyewashes or you could cause further infection. To avoid contamination, strain the cooled teas through a sterile gauze pad or cheesecloth and store them in sealed containers. Prepare a fresh batch of teas every day.

■ In addition to their use as eyewashes, herbal teas made from eyebright, chamomile or fennel are good to drink and will help to relieve your symptoms. Have two or three cups a day.

Fatigue

Hippocrates wrote about it – and so did Shakespeare. Fatigue has doggedly plagued humankind through the ages. Today TATT ('tired all the time') is one of the most common nonspecific diagnoses in general practice, and Britons consistently rank it as one of their main health concerns.

Symptoms

- *Persistent, lingering weariness, either intermittent or continuous, that lasts for more than two weeks.*

- *Personality changes, particularly a tendency to become angry, impatient or depressed because of feeling tired all the time.*

- *Diminished concentration; difficulty in accomplishing familiar tasks; less interest in activities that were once appealing.*

SEE YOUR DOCTOR ...

- **If fatigue lasts longer than two weeks or is accompanied by other symptoms, such as fever, weight loss, nausea, hoarseness or muscle aches.**

- **If fatigue causes daytime drowsiness that interferes with normal everyday activities.**

REMINDER: If you have a medical condition, consult your doctor before taking supplements.

What it is

Not a true ailment in itself, fatigue is usually a classic symptom of some other problem: poor nutrition; overwork; lack of (or too much) exercise; insomnia or poor sleeping habits; or a specific medical disorder, such as premenstrual syndrome or depression. Fatigue is a generalised feeling of exhaustion that is hard to shake off, but it is distinct from the more intractable chronic fatigue syndrome, in which fatigue persisting for at least six months is not relieved by sleep or rest and is often accompanied by symptoms such as memory loss, fever and muscular aches.

What causes it

In many sufferers, fatigue can be traced to stress, anxiety, depression or lowered immunity and chronic infections. It has been linked to diabetes, to thyroid or adrenal gland imbalance; and to heart, liver or kidney disease. Deficiency of almost any vitamin and mineral can depress the immune system, causing fatigue. Deficiency of the nutrients involved in red blood cell formation (iron, folic acid, vitamins B_{12} and B_6) can lead to fatigue because these cells transport oxygen used for energy. In women, fatigue can result from fluctuating hormone levels in pregnancy and menopause, or from anaemia caused by heavy menstrual periods. Medications, including blood pressure drugs, and sleeping disorders can also bring it on.

How supplements can help

The supplements listed here should be used only when an underlying fatigue-causing medical condition has been ruled out. A two-month course should bring relief. Start with the vitamins and one of the two ginsengs. Then add magnesium and flaxseed oil if fatigue persists. The

In Asia, ginseng has been prescribed as an energy tonic for thousands of years.

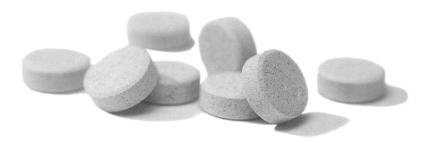

B vitamin complex	**Dosage:** one capsule twice a day with food. **Advice:** use a B-50 complex with 50 mcg vitamin B_{12} and biotin, 400 mcg folic acid and 50 mg all other B vitamins.
Vitamin C	**Dosage:** 500 mg twice a day. **Advice:** reduce dose if diarrhoea develops.
Ginseng (panax)	**Dosage:** 100–250 mg extract twice a day. **Advice:** standardised to contain at least 7% ginsenosides.
Ginseng (Siberian)	**Dosage:** 100–300 mg extract twice a day. **Advice:** standardised to contain at least 0.8% eleutherosides.
Magnesium	**Dosage:** 400 mg a day for two months. **Advice:** take with food; reduce dose if diarrhoea develops.
Fish oils	**Dosage:** 2 teaspoons to supply 2 grams omega-3 fatty acids a day. **Caution:** consult a doctor if you take anticoagulant drugs. **Advice:** vegetarians can use 1 tablespoon flaxseed oil.

Note: consider using supplements in blue first; the one in black may also be beneficial. Some dosages may be supplied by supplements you are already taking – see page 195.

B-complex vitamins support the nervous and immune systems. They enhance the effectiveness of white blood cells, which fight bacteria and viruses, and they are also needed for proper replication of red blood cells. Also important is **vitamin C**; it promotes immune function, helps to repair tissues and supports the adrenal gland, which controls production of stress hormones in the body.

One of the most popular uses of ginseng is to boost the body's own energy levels. **Panax ginseng** has long been used for this purpose in Asia. **Siberian ginseng** contains compounds that have been shown to fight fatigue. American ginseng has similar, but milder, properties and may be used as an alternative to Panax and Siberian ginseng. A mild **magnesium** deficiency may be the cause of fatigue in some people. A two-month course of the mineral should address any shortage. **Fish oils** (or flaxseed oil for vegetarians) help by supplying essential omega-3 fatty acids, which protect the integrity of cell membranes and enhance the immune system.

What else you can do

☑ Take a 20 minute nap in the afternoon or after work. But set the alarm: a longer nap can interfere with night-time sleep.

☑ Do not skip breakfast. Near bedtime, avoid large meals, fatty foods, alcohol and caffeinated beverages.

☑ Go to bed and get up at the same time every day; get at least 8 hours of sleep a night.

☑ Keep active. Moderate exercise is a prescription for feeling less tired.

☑ Do not expect an energy boost from sugary foods. Instead eat complex carbohydrates (pasta, whole grains, beans), fruit and vegetables.

☑ Have blood tests for thyroid problems or anaemia if fatigue persists.

Flatulence

Breaking wind may not be life-threatening, but it can be uncomfortable – and embarrassing – especially if it happens too often. Commonsense changes in your diet and some helpful supplements can provide welcome relief for you – and for those around you.

Symptoms

- *Frequent emission of wind through the rectum.*
- *Stomach discomfort and bloating.*

SEE YOUR DOCTOR ...

- If flatulence is accompanied by stomach pain that persists for several days.

- If you start losing weight for no apparent reason – this could be a sign of a more serious condition.

REMINDER: If you have a medical condition, consult your doctor before taking supplements.

What it is

Passing intestinal wind is normal: a typical adult does it as often as 15 times a day, generating up to 1.5 litres of gas. But normal does not necessarily mean worry-free. Even the average amount of wind can cause discomfort for some people, and in others the frequency of flatulent episodes and the amount of wind emitted are much greater than average. The only good thing about flatulence is that by itself it is not a symptom of cancer or any other serious intestinal disease.

What causes it

Flatulence results when excess gases build up in the digestive tract and are then expelled through the rectum. Chemical reactions that occur after eating certain foods are the most common cause. The most likely culprits are broccoli, Brussels sprouts, cabbage, cauliflower, onions and beans. These foods contain complex carbohydrates, which are often incompletely digested in the stomach and small intestine. After they arrive in the large intestine they are broken down by the harmless bacteria that live there, and certain gases – carbon dioxide, hydrogen and methane – are by-products of this bacterial action. In some people milk and milk products induce wind and bloating; this milk-related flatulence is often the result of lactose intolerance.

Hydrogen sulphide and other compounds containing sulphur are responsible for the unpleasant odour of some intestinal wind. Excessive flatulence can be a symptom of disorders that hinder normal digestion, such as coeliac disease. It may also be caused by stress. Stress interferes with the digestive process, with the result that incompletely digested food passes into the large intestine. Air swallowed at times of stress can also pass down the gut and cause flatulence.

How supplements can help

If flatulence is more than an occasional problem, try a combination of the first four supplements in the chart. **Ginger**, in tablet form or as freshly

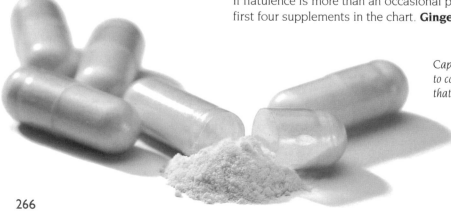

Capsules of acidophilus culture help to control intestinal tract bacteria that can produce excess gases.

Ginger	**Dosage:** 100 mg extract two or three times a day as needed. **Advice:** standardised to contain gingerols.
Peppermint	**Dosage:** one or two capsules two or three times a day; alternatively, drink peppermint tea two or three times a day. **Advice:** capsules to contain 0.2 ml oil.
Artichoke	**Dosage:** 500 mg extract three times a day. **Advice:** standardised to contain 15% cynarin.
Probiotics	**Dosage:** two capsules three times a day on an empty stomach; alternatively, eat two or three pots of bioyoghurt a day. **Advice:** choose the acidophilus or the bifidus culture, or a mixture of the two.
FOS	**Dosage:** 2000 mg twice a day. **Advice:** use in combination with probiotics.
Activated charcoal	**Dosage:** 500 mg after each meal and every 2 hours as needed. **Advice:** do not exceed 4000 mg a day.

Note: consider using supplements in blue first; the one in black may also be beneficial.
Some dosages may be supplied by supplements you are already taking – see page 195.

grated root (mixed with a little lime juice), is a good all-purpose digestive aid. It soothes the digestive tract and is useful for relieving flatulence. Many herbs, including **peppermint**, caraway seed, fennel and aniseed, have carminative properties, which means that they improve coordination of the digestive processes and so less gassy fermentation occurs in the large bowel. Similarly, herbs with bitter properties, such as wormwood and gentian, stimulate the secretion of digestive juices and can be taken as tinctures; place 20 drops on the tongue about half an hour before each meal. Taking tablets of **artichoke** extract has a similar effect.

Probiotics are cultures of the 'friendly' bacteria that inhabit the large intestine and help to keep in check the growth of gas-producing bacteria; they can be taken as capsules or in 'bioyoghurts' containing either of the beneficial bacteria acidophilus and biphidus. **FOS** (fructo-oligosaccharides), indigestible carbohydrates that are present in certain foods, promote the growth of 'friendly' bacteria. Replenishing intestinal populations of the beneficial bacteria will often relieve wind, bloating and other digestive complaints. If this course of action is unsuccessful, use **activated charcoal** to absorb gas in the intestine and help to reduce the accompanying odour. It is also available in tablet form or as a tasteless powder which can be mixed in a glass of cold water and sipped through a straw to avoid staining the teeth.

What else you can do

☑ Avoid carbonated drinks.
☑ Chew food thoroughly. Large lumps of food cause wind when they pass into the large intestine without being completely digested.
☑ Eat slowly. If you eat too quickly, you tend to swallow more air.
☑ Soak beans before cooking; this removes some indigestible sugars. Discard the soaking water and cook the beans in fresh water.

An American study of young and middle-aged men dispelled the myth that flatulence increases with age. It also confirmed that indigestible carbohydrates are at the root of the problem. While on their normal diets, both groups of men broke wind an average of ten times a day. This frequency nearly doubled when they were also given 10 grams of such carbohydrates each day.

DID YOU KNOW?

Aperitifs such as campari and martini are more than just sweet-tasting alcoholic drinks: they contain the herbs wormwood and gentian, whose bitter properties stimulate the secretion of digestive juices.

FACTS & TIPS

■ Before you consider taking supplements for flatulence, try giving up all dairy products for a few days and see if you feel better. If you do, you may be lactose intolerant. You may be able to minimise the effects of this intolerance by eating dairy products in small portions with other foods or by choosing lactose-reduced or soya products.

■ Be cautious about using the sweeteners sorbitol and xylitol, found in many commercial products. They often induce flatulence.

Gallstones

Some 10% of adults develop gallstones, crystallised pellets in the gall bladder that can suddenly cause painful spasms a few hours after eating a meal. A high-fibre diet, along with certain supplements, can help to prevent, relieve or even dissolve these troublesome stones.

Symptoms

- *Intermittent pain on the right side of the upper abdomen. The pain typically develops after a meal, lasts from 30 minutes to 4 hours, and may move to the back, chest or right shoulder.*

- *Nausea and vomiting may accompany pain. Indigestion, flatulence or bloating may also be present.*

SEE YOUR DOCTOR ...

- **If you develop severe abdominal pain, or pain with nausea, vomiting or fever. Either symptom may signal gall bladder inflammation or a blockage of the bile duct. Both are medical emergencies.**

REMINDER: If you have a medical condition, consult your doctor before taking supplements.

What they are

Gallstones are rock-like clumps of cholesterol, calcium or other substances that form in the gall bladder, the pear-shaped organ that sits in the upper right section of the abdomen, just under the liver. The gall bladder stores and concentrates bile – a thick greenish-yellow fluid that is produced by the liver – and eventually releases it through the bile duct into the small intestine to aid in the digestion of fats. Gallstones can develop if the bile contains very high levels of cholesterol, bile acids, pigments or other substances. Whether they are really tiny or as big as golf balls, gallstones often produce no symptoms and need no special care. Sometimes, though, they can block the bile duct or inflame the gall bladder, causing intense abdominal pain and requiring prompt treatment.

What causes them

Though the exact cause of gallstones is not known, several factors may contribute to their formation, including: a low-fibre, high-fat diet; intestinal surgery; inflammatory bowel disease or other disorders of the digestive tract. Gallstones tend to occur in people over the age of 40 and are three times more common in women than in men. Obesity is also strongly linked to gallstones, as is rapid weight loss. There may be a genetic component as well: among the Pima Native Americans, nearly 70% of women over the age of 30 have gallstones.

How supplements can help

The supplements recommended in the chart may all aid in preventing or dissolving gallstones. Three months of treatment may be effective in dissolving small existing stones, though the supplements in blue can also be used long term to help to prevent gallstone attacks.

Extra **vitamin C** is important because it lowers bile cholesterol levels, decreasing the chance that cholesterol-laden bile will clump to form stones. Vitamin C should be combined with various other

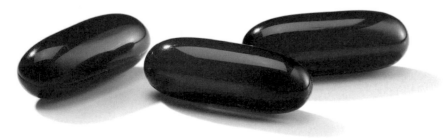

Gallstone-fighting flaxseed oil comes in capsule form for those who dislike the taste of the 'neat' oil.

Vitamin C	**Dosage:** 500 mg twice a day. **Advice:** reduce dose if diarrhoea develops.
Lipotropic combination	**Dosage:** one or two tablets or capsules twice a day. **Advice:** should contain 250 mg milk thistle extract (take extra if necessary); may also include choline, inositol, methionine and dandelion.
Lecithin	**Dosage:** two capsules (1200 mg) twice a day. **Advice:** or 2 teaspoons granular form twice a day before meals.
Flaxseed oil	**Dosage:** 1 tablespoon a day. **Advice:** can be mixed with food; take in the morning; also available as capsules.
Peppermint oil	**Dosage:** two capsules (containing 0.2 ml of oil each) twice a day. **Advice:** buy enteric-coated capsules; take between meals.
Psyllium	**Dosage:** 1 tablespoon powder, dissolved in water or juice, twice a day. **Advice:** drink extra water throughout the day.

Note: consider using supplements in blue first; those in black may also be beneficial. Some dosages may be supplied by supplements you are already taking – see page 195.

supplements. A good general choice is a **lipotropic** ('fat-metabolising') **combination**, containing milk thistle, choline, inositol and methionine, which bolsters liver function and promotes a healthy flow of fats and bile from the liver and gall bladder. The herb milk thistle, for example, alters bile composition, thus helping to dissolve gallstones and eliminate stones that may have formed. Choline and inositol (related to the B vitamins) and the amino acid methionine aid in fat and cholesterol metabolism as well. They also strengthen liver and gall bladder function. Methionine may increase levels of another amino acid, taurine, which improves bile flow and helps to dissolve existing stones. Choline and inositol are also vital to the fatty bile component **lecithin** (inadequate levels of lecithin may precipitate gallstones).

Other supplements may be worth adding to the mix, either singly or together. **Flaxseed oil** contains essential fatty acids that may be useful in preventing or even dissolving gallstones. **Peppermint oil**, taken in enteric-coated capsules, also has gallstone-dissolving effects. And daily doses of **psyllium** can promote bowel movements, which may be of value in blocking the formation of gallstones. Herbs which may be helpful include dandelion root (make a tea from 1 teaspoon of powdered root and drink three times a day) and artichoke (take 500 mg extract, standardised to contain 15% cynarin, three times a day).

What else you can do

☑ Eat a diet high in fibre and low in refined carbohydrates, sugar and fat. Fruit and vegetables, oat bran and pectin (found in apples, bananas, cabbage, carrots, oranges, peas and okra) may be especially important in preventing and dissolving gallstones.

☑ Keep your weight down and drink plenty of water daily.

An American study found that a combination of vitamin C supplements and an occasional alcoholic drink halved the incidence of gallstones in postmenopausal women. Scientists speculate that moderate alcohol intake may boost the ability of vitamin C to lower bile cholesterol levels. These lower levels, in turn, reduce the incidence of gallstones.

In a study of the effect of milk thistle on gallstones, researchers discovered that patients treated with this herb had significantly reduced levels of cholesterol in their bile – which may decrease the likelihood of gallstones.

DID YOU KNOW?
Though the typical high-fat, low-fibre modern diet appears to contribute to gallstones, they are not a new disorder. When X-rayed, the mummified corpse of an Egyptian priestess from about 1500 BC was found to have some 30 gallstones.

FACTS & TIPS

■ The first operation to remove a gall bladder was performed in 1882. Such surgery is still the medical treatment of choice for symptom-producing gallstones. Both conventional abdominal surgery and keyhole surgery (in which the gall bladder is removed through very small incisions) are performed. However, natural supplements may be an excellent alternative to such invasive procedures.

Gout

About one man in a hundred over the age of 40 suffers from gout. Women can develop it too, mainly after the menopause. Although people with gout feel fine much of the time, an attack can occur without warning, bringing on acute joint pain that demands fast-acting, effective relief.

Symptoms

- *Sudden and severe joint pain, usually involving the big toe, heel, ankle or instep first. Subsequent attacks may affect the knee, wrist, elbow, fingers or other areas.*

- *Redness and swelling in affected joint or joints.*

- *Kidney stones develop occasionally, causing fever, severe low back pain, nausea, vomiting or a swollen abdomen.*

SEE YOUR DOCTOR ...

- **If you experience symptoms of an acute gout attack – your doctor can prescribe drugs to ease the initial pain.**

- **If you suffer the severe pain of passing a kidney stone.**

REMINDER: If you have a medical condition, consult your doctor before taking supplements.

What it is

Gout is a metabolic disorder linked to high levels of uric acid in the blood. A waste product of various body processes, uric acid is also formed after eating certain foods. The body rids itself of uric acid through the urine, but some people produce too much uric acid or cannot dispose of it fast enough – and levels build up. Often the excess is converted into sharp crystals that settle in and around joints and other tissues, triggering inflammation and the excruciating pain associated with gout.

What causes it

It is not clear what precipitates a gout attack, but some factors increase risk. A quarter of those who suffer from gout have a family history of the illness, and three-quarters have high triglyceride levels. Men who gain a lot of weight between the ages of 20 and 40 are particularly vulnerable. Excessive alcohol intake (including 'binge' drinking), high blood pressure, kidney disease, exposure to lead, crash diets and certain drugs (including antibiotics, diuretics and cancer chemotherapy drugs) may also play a role. For a few people, eating foods high in chemicals called purines (such as liver or anchovies) can also cause flare-ups.

How supplements can help

Uric acid can accumulate in the body for years with no symptoms. An acute attack often happens suddenly and is best treated with conventional drugs. The main supplement that seems to help in acute attacks is **bromelain**. The others, taken together, may prevent future attacks. All can be used for long periods. Omega-3 fatty acids (from **fish oils** or flaxseed oil) reduce levels of inflammatory leukotrienes, which are

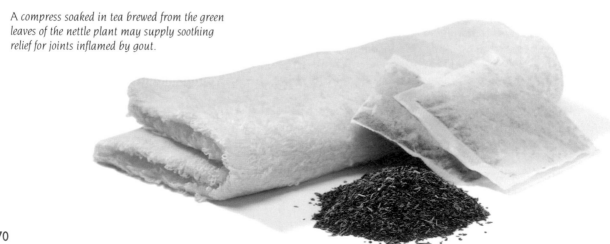

A compress soaked in tea brewed from the green leaves of the nettle plant may supply soothing relief for joints inflamed by gout.

SUPPLEMENT RECOMMENDATIONS	
Bromelain	**Dosage:** 500 mg every three hours during an attack; reduce to twice a day to help to prevent further attacks. **Advice:** each dose should provide 2000 GDU or 3000 MCU.
Fish oils	**Dosage:** 2 teaspoons daily to supply 2 g of omega-3 fatty acids. **Caution:** consult your doctor if you take anticoagulant drugs. **Advice:** vegetarians can substitute 1 tablespoon flaxseed oil.
Vitamin C	**Dosage:** 500 mg a day. **Advice:** add 100 mg every five days until you reach 500 mg twice a day; reduce dose if diarrhoea develops.
Vitamin E	**Dosage:** 250 mg twice a day. **Caution:** consult your doctor if you take anticoagulant drugs.
Quercetin	**Dosage:** 125-250 mg twice a day between meals. **Advice:** take with bromelain to help to prevent gout attacks.
Cherry fruit extract	**Dosage:** 1000 mg three times a day following an acute attack. **Advice:** reduce dosage to 1000 mg a day for maintenance.
Nettle leaf	**Dosage:** 250 mg standardised extract three times a day. **Advice:** also effective when taken as nettle tea, which can also be used as a compress applied to sore joints; use 1 or 2 teaspoons dried herb per 250 ml of hot water.

Note: consider using supplements in blue first; the one in black may also be beneficial. Some dosages may be supplied by supplements you are already taking – see page 195.

see page 195.

associated with tissue damage in gout. Antioxidants such as **vitamin C** and **vitamin E** help to reduce inflammation. When taken in incremental doses, vitamin C helps uric acid to free itself from the tissues and be excreted in the urine. (High initial doses may release so much uric acid that a kidney stone develops.)

Bromelain, an enzyme derived from pineapples, is a popular natural anti-inflammatory that may relieve gout pain. When you are not using it for acute flare-ups, decrease the dosage and add **quercetin**. This flavonoid reduces uric acid levels and is better absorbed if taken with bromelain. Cherries, an old folk remedy for gout, are rich in flavonoids and are often effective at lowering uric acid levels. **Cherry fruit extract** is available at many health-food shops; cherry or blueberry juice (125 ml a day) also works well. **Nettle leaf** can be helpful internally and externally: capsules or tea clear out excess uric acid, and topical nettle tea compresses may relieve inflamed joints. Other natural therapies to reduce uric acid levels include eating celery or bilberries (or bilberry extract) or drinking teas made from the herbs devil's claw or olive leaf.

What else you can do

☑ Drink at least eight glasses of water a day to dilute the urine and help to lower uric acid levels. Avoid alcohol, which can trigger attacks.
☑ Keep weight down. Obesity may play an important role in gout attacks.
☑ Avoid fats, refined carbohydrates, excess protein and, if you are sensitive to purines, foods containing them (including offal, anchovies, legumes, oatmeal, spinach, asparagus, cauliflower and mushrooms).

DID YOU KNOW?
Although gout is linked to high levels of uric acid in the blood, only a small percentage of people with high levels ever actually develop gout.

FACTS & TIPS
■ Eating fresh or canned cherries (250 grams a day) may help to keep gout at bay by reducing levels of uric acid. Some people swear by them, and a small study conducted many years ago found that eating cherries may indeed lower uric acid levels. An easier way to get the benefits of cherries is to take 1000 mg daily of cherry fruit extract tablets (available at health-food shops). Strawberries, blueberries, celery and celery seed extracts may have a similar beneficial effect.

The growing child

Healthy growth is an important issue during the first decade of a child's life. At various stages of development, or if diet is inadequate, nutritional supplements may be beneficial. Consult your doctor or health visitor for further advice.

THE FIRST SIX MONTHS

■ Breast milk supplies all the nutrients a full-term baby needs, as well as antibodies to protect against bacteria and viruses in the first few weeks of life.

■ If a breastfeeding mother had an adequate intake of vitamins during her pregnancy, her baby should not require supplements during the first six months.

■ Premature babies have higher nutritional demands, and breast milk may need supplementation with pre-term formula milk to make up for any deficiencies. Consult your doctor.

■ If the pre-term formula milk does not contain vitamins, supplement preparations can be given in the form of drops.

■ After discharge from hospital, premature babies can continue to take pre-term formula milk and vitamin drops.

■ As an alternative to human breast milk, formula milk is designed to meet all the nutritional needs of full-term bottle-fed babies in the first few months of life – but take care not to exceed the scoop recommendations, which could make it too concentrated for your baby's digestive system.

■ The digestive system and kidneys are unable to deal with solid foods until babies are at least four months old, so weaning from milk to soft and puréed adult food is advised at between four and six months.

FROM SIX MONTHS TO FIVE YEARS

■ Breastfed babies should be given vitamin A and D supplements from the age of six months, because breast milk is low in these nutrients.

■ Bottle-fed babies need to drink 500 ml a day of formula milk to reach the right vitamin levels. If your baby takes less, it is advisable to supplement with vitamin A and D drops.

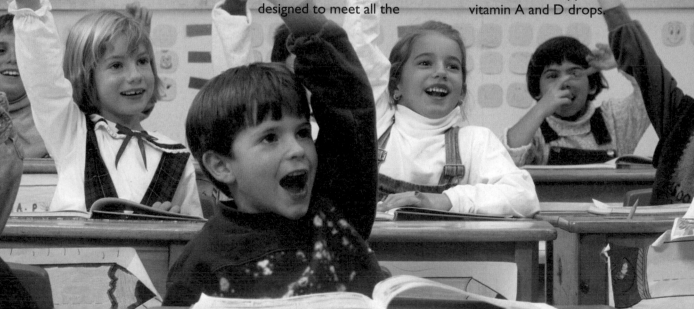

- Follow-on formulas are available for infants over the age of six months.
- Cow's milk can be introduced when a baby is a year old. Use full-fat milk, rather than skimmed or semi-skimmed, as it is higher in vitamins A and D and because babies need the additional energy from the fat.
- Soya milk is a useful substitute for infants allergic to cow's milk. For babies, use a soya-based infant formula milk.
- After one year, soya milk can be introduced as part of a mixed diet, and should be accompanied by supplementary calcium and magnesium and vitamins A, C and D.
- Most children aged from one to five years can benefit from a daily vitamin drop preparation containing 200 mcg vitamin A, 7 mcg vitamin D and 20 mg vitamin C.

SCHOOL-AGE CHILDREN

- Young children have high nutrient requirements in relation to their body size. The five nutrients often lacking in this age group are vitamins C and D, calcium, iron and zinc. A children's multivitamin and multimineral supplement should remedy any deficiencies.
- Even a mild deficiency of vitamin C can lower resistance to infection. It is not stored in the body, so children who do not eat at least two portions of fruit and vegetables daily may benefit from a supplement.
- Vitamin D helps to maintain bone and muscle health. It is created by the action of

sunlight on skin, and also partly provided by animal products in the diet. Vegetarians are especially at risk if they have little exposure to sunlight.
- Calcium, found particularly in dairy products, ensures healthy bone formation. Children under five who are allergic to milk-based products should take a calcium supplement.
- Iron deficiency is the most common nutritional disorder in the UK. A 1995 survey found that, of children aged 1½ to 2½ years, one in eight were anaemic and 28% had low iron stores; about 80% of preschool children did not meet their RNI target for iron.
- Iron deficiency leads to anaemia, common in infants over six months. Iron can be highly toxic if administered inappropriately, or at the wrong dosage, so routine supplementation is not recommended for children. Consult your doctor.
- Most preschool children fail to meet their RNI target for zinc. One reason for this is the popularity of white meats such as chicken over red meats, which are richer in zinc. Children's multivitamin and multimineral preparations contain adequate levels of zinc.

NUTRIENT	1-3 YEARS	4-6 YEARS	7-10 YEARS
SUPPLEMENT REQUIREMENTS FOR GROWING CHILDREN *(Measurement per day)*			
Vitamin C	30 mg	30 mg	30 mg
Vitamin D	7 mcg	*Enough provided by exposure to sunlight*	
Calcium	350 mg	450 mg	550 mg
Iron	6.9 mg	6.1 mg	8.7 mg
Zinc	5 mg	6.5 mg	7 mg

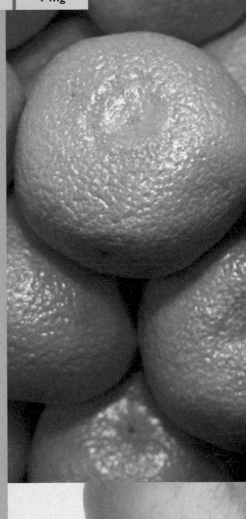

Gum disease

If you have not had gum problems yet, the chances are that you will: three out of four adults over 35 experience tender, swollen or bleeding gums at some point in their lives. But there are plenty of things you can do to relieve pain, heal the gums and preserve your teeth.

Symptoms

- *Gums that bleed after teeth-cleaning.*
- *Red, swollen and tender gums.*
- *Toothache.*
- *Chronic bad breath or a bad taste in the mouth.*
- *Loose or missing teeth.*

SEE YOUR DENTIST ...

- **If you experience red swollen gums or loose teeth. It may save your teeth.**

REMINDER: If you have a medical condition, consult your doctor before taking supplements.

What it is

There are two main types of gum disease: gingivitis and periodontitis. Gingivitis – marked by tender, inflamed gums – occurs when bacteria in the mouth form a thin, sticky film called plaque that coats the teeth and gums. If ignored, plaque will turn into tartar, a hard mineral shell that erodes gum tissue. Over time this will lead to the more serious – and harder to treat – condition known as periodontitis. In advanced periodontal disease the gums recede in places and pockets form around the teeth, which allows bacteria to eat away at the bone anchoring the teeth. Bleeding gums can occasionally be a mark of a more serious disease, so do not ignore symptoms.

What causes it

Poor oral hygiene – including inadequate teeth-cleaning, flossing or rinsing – is the leading cause of gum disease. Other precipitating factors include a high-sugar diet, a very severe lack of vitamin C or other nutrients, and smoking (the chemicals in tobacco smoke harm gums and teeth). Certain medications can make gum disease worse because in some instances they inhibit the production of saliva, which helps to wash away bacteria and sugars. Genetic factors appear to make some people susceptible to gum disease. Women seem to be more prone to gum problems during pregnancy and menopause because of hormonal changes. Diabetes and other chronic diseases that can lower resistance to infection also increase the risk.

How supplements can help

Various supplements, used together, can help to heal sore and bleeding gums. Many factors can be involved in the health of the gums, so the first step should be to take an 'A to Z' multivitamin and mineral formulation

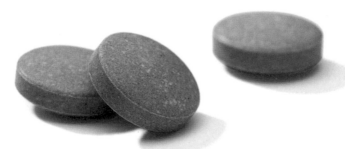

Chewable vitamin C tablets are a convenient way to get this superstar antioxidant, but rinse your mouth after chewing one to prevent damage to tooth enamel.

Vitamin C/ flavonoids	**Dosage:** 1000 mg vitamin C and 500 mg flavonoids twice a day. **Advice:** reduce vitamin C dose if diarrhoea develops.
Vitamin E	**Dosage:** 250 mg twice a day. **Caution:** consult your doctor if you take anticoagulant drugs. **Advice:** pierce the capsule and rub the oil on the gums before swallowing; alternate with folic acid treatment every other day.
Coenzyme Q$_{10}$	**Dosage:** 50 mg once a day. **Advice:** for most efficient absorption, take with food.
Folic acid liquid	**Dosage:** dip cotton wool in liquid; apply to gum line. **Advice:** follow up with vitamin C powder; alternate with vitamin E gum treatment every other day.
Vitamin C powder	**Dosage:** using ½ teaspoon powder, brush along gum line every other day. **Advice:** alternate with vitamin E treatment every other day.

Some dosages may be supplied by supplements you are already taking – see page 195.

regularly. One or more of the recommended supplements can be added to it. Benefits should be noticed within two weeks. People at high risk of gum disease can also take them on a long-term preventative basis.

When taken on a daily basis, antioxidants such as **vitamin C**, **flavonoids** and **coenzyme Q$_{10}$** both protect gum tissue against cell damage and speed healing. They also boost immunity, helping to keep gum-attacking bacteria in check. Studies of coenzyme Q$_{10}$, for example, show that it reduces the depth of pockets formed around the teeth; this stabilises the teeth and aids in shortening the recovery period after dental surgery. Other studies suggest that vitamin C and flavonoids may strengthen connective tissue in the gums and decrease inflammation, and that they are most effective when used together.

In addition, various topical therapies may reduce gum inflammation and bleeding. When taking a **vitamin E** capsule, pierce it with a knife or scissors and rub the oil on the inflamed tissue to soothe the area and promote quicker healing. On alternate days, apply **folic acid liquid** to the gums with a cotton-wool pad. Then, with a very soft toothbrush, gently brush along the gum line with **vitamin C powder**. These topical treatments should be carried out twice a day, after regular cleaning.

What else you can do

☑ Floss at least once a day and clean twice with a soft-bristle brush, using a toothpaste containing fluoride. Also brush the tongue, which collects the same bacteria as those that stick to teeth. Talk to your dental hygienist if you are not sure that you are flossing or cleaning correctly.

☑ Avoid sweets and sticky carbohydrates or clean teeth as soon as you can after eating them; such foods can gather in gum spaces and pockets, particularly in older people, who tend to have more exposed roots.

☑ See a dental hygienist at least once a year for professional tooth 'care' – or more often if you are prone to plaque build-up or have a problem that needs special attention.

Maintaining healthy gums with natural supplements and good dental care may produce more than just an appealing smile. Studies reveal a possible link between the most common type of bacteria causing dental plaque and the development of heart disease. This link is still under investigation, but one theory is that the gum bacteria can enter the bloodstream and promote blood clots or damage the heart muscle.

DID YOU KNOW?

Fluoridation of drinking water dramatically cuts the risk of tooth loss. The trace mineral fluoride interacts with tooth enamel and hardens it, making it 50% to 70% less susceptible to decay.

FACTS & TIPS

■ Natural toothpastes and mouthwashes containing the herb bloodroot supply an antibacterial substance called sanguinarine that helps to reduce the accumulation of dental plaque – the first step in gum disease.

■ Commission E, a German panel of health experts that reviews herbal supplements, recognises chamomile as an effective gargle or mouth-wash for the treatment of gingivitis. Make a chamomile tea using 2 or 3 teaspoons of herb per cup of hot water. Steep for 10 minutes, strain and cool. Use as a daily mouthwash or gargle. Dried sage tea, made in the same way, is also very effective.

Haemorrhoids

More than 50% of people in the UK will develop haemorrhoids during their lives, yet many are not aware that they have them, because haemorrhoids often have few symptoms. When they flare up, natural remedies may have more to offer than conventional treatments.

Symptoms

- *Streaks of blood on lavatory paper.*
- *Bloody, painful bowel movements.*
- *Itching in the anal area.*
- *Painful bump on or near the anus.*
- *Discharge of mucus from the anus.*

SEE YOUR DOCTOR ...

- If you notice blood-streaked lavatory paper for the first time – it is probably haemorrhoids, but anal bleeding can have other causes.

- If bleeding is not related to a bowel movement, even when you have haemorrhoids.

- If blood is dark, not bright red.

- If there is a throbbing pain in the anal area – this may be a blood clot in the haemorrhoid.

- If haemorrhoids have been diagnosed and daily bleeding is severe – you may be at risk of iron deficiency anaemia.

REMINDER: If you have a medical condition, consult your doctor before taking supplements.

What they are

Haemorrhoids (also known as piles) are essentially enlarged (varicose) veins in the anus or rectum. Veins are vessels that return deoxygenated blood to the heart, but sometimes the laws of gravity slow down this process in the lower half of the body. Blood can pool in the veins, stretching and weakening them. The veins in the rectum and anus are particularly susceptible – not only are they in the lower body but also, unlike other veins, they lack valves to prevent the backward flow of blood. (Weak or faulty valves contribute to varicose veins in the legs.)

There are two types of haemorrhoid. The internal ones develop inside the rectum; they sometimes cause bleeding after a bowel movement but otherwise may have no symptoms. Large haemorrhoids have a tendency to prolapse, or fall out of the anus, on defecation, and may have to be pushed back. External haemorrhoids occur around the anal opening. They can be extremely painful but are often 'self-curing'. The pain is usually caused by the fact that the blood has clotted and so cut off the blood suppy to the haemorrhoids; as a result they may simply shrivel up and disappear of their own accord.

What causes them

Straining during a bowel movement is a primary cause of haemorrhoids, because it puts excess pressure on the veins in the anus and rectum. Being overweight or pregnant also weakens these veins. Researchers disagree about whether constipation directly causes haemorrhoids, but people who are constipated often strain to defecate, so at the very least this problem makes haemorrhoids worse. Studies show that frequent diarrhoea also increases the likelihood of haemorrhoids.

In addition, long periods of standing or sitting can lead to the development of haemorrhoids. The muscles that help to propel blood

Ground flaxseeds, taken with water, can compensate for lack of fibre in the diet.

SUPPLEMENT RECOMMENDATIONS

Vitamin C/ flavonoids	**Dosage:** 500 mg vitamin C and 250 mg flavonoids twice a day. **Advice:** reduce vitamin C dose if diarrhoea develops.
Butcher's broom	**Dosage:** 150 mg extract three times a day. **Advice:** standardised to contain 9%-11% ruscogenin.
Zinc	**Dosage:** 15 mg a day. **Advice:** if you take a zinc supplement for more than a month, use one that includes 2 mg copper.
Psyllium	**Dosage:** 1 tablespoon powder in water or juice each day. **Advice:** be sure to drink extra water throughout the day.
Flaxseeds	**Dosage:** 1 tablespoon ground flaxseeds in large glass of water each day. **Advice:** drink at least 8 glasses of water a day.
St John's wort ointment	**Dosage:** apply three or four times a day, as needed. **Advice:** very beneficial when used after a bowel movement.

Note: consider using supplements in blue first; those in black may also be beneficial. Some dosages may be supplied by supplements you are already taking – see page 195.

through the veins lose tone with age, so it is not surprising that haemorrhoids are more common in older people. The tendency to develop haemorrhoids also seems to run in families.

How supplements can help

The recommended supplements are intended to be used in conjunction with a high-fibre diet and regular exercise. Fibre is valuable in bulking up and softening the stool, which makes it easier to pass. Exercise is important in toning the muscles that surround the veins and promotes regular bowel movements.

Unlike over-the-counter ointments, the recommended vitamins and herbs will aid in strengthening the veins and minimising irritation as they heal. In combination, try **vitamin C**, **flavonoids** and the herb **butcher's broom** to help to tone and shrink the veins. **Zinc** plays a role in wound healing; copper is needed with long-term use of zinc, because zinc interferes with copper absorption. If you do not get enough fibre in your diet, or if you believe that you need more, take **psyllium** or **flaxseeds**. Both are effective in easing defecation. When haemorrhoids are painful, apply **St John's wort ointment** (or witch hazel) several times a day, especially after bowel movements. This ointment is also useful in shrinking swollen tissues.

What else you can do

☑ Increase fibre by eating lots of fruit, vegetables, grains and legumes.
☑ Drink at least eight glasses of water a day. Fluid is important in preventing the constipation associated with haemorrhoids.
☑ Remember to breathe normally when lifting weights or heavy objects, or during a bowel movement. Holding your breath increases pressure in the abdomen, which can damage the veins.

DID YOU KNOW?

Overzealous cleaning of the anal area may be counter-productive in dealing with haemorrhoids. Efficient but gentle hygiene is important. Use moistened lavatory paper or special wipes to clean after a bowel movement.

FACTS & TIPS

■ If you have haemorrhoids, make sure that your diet includes plenty of citrus fruits, berries, cherries and onions. They are good sources of fibre and also contain flavonoids, which may help to strengthen the veins.

■ A poultice made from elderberry soothes swollen veins and may relieve the pain of haemorrhoids. Grind up a small amount of the herb and mix it with enough warm water to make a paste. Spread the paste between two or three layers of gauze. Place the poultice against the anal opening and leave it in place for a few hours.

■ Using vitamin E capsules as suppositories can be very helpful in the treatment of haemorrhoids.

Hair problems

Most hair problems, from dandruff and balding to brittleness and greying, are either signs of a poor diet or a genetic predisposition, or simply part of the ageing process. Even if the causes are beyond your control, a few simple remedies can encourage a healthier head of hair.

Symptoms

- *Crusting, flaking or irritation of the scalp.*
- *Increased loss of hair when washing or combing.*
- *Changes in hair colour, texture or growth patterns.*

What they are

Hair is a non-living tissue made up mainly of a fibrous protein called keratin – the same material found in your finger and toenails. The health of your hair requires a plentiful supply of nutrient-rich blood to nourish the hair follicles in the scalp, from which new hair sprouts. On average, hair grows about half an inch a month. It is not unusual for people to shed up to a hundred hairs a day – fortunately, when one falls out another usually grows in its place. Problems can arise when hair becomes dry or brittle, stops growing back, or becomes flecked with dandruff caused by excess flaking and shedding of skin on the scalp.

What causes them

Stress, a poor diet and hormonal changes can all contribute to hair loss. Problems can also result from unhealthy environmental circumstances, genetic factors, immune system disorders, an underactive thyroid gland, specific nutritional deficiencies or medical treatment such as chemotherapy, which often causes hair loss in cancer patients.

How supplements can help

The recommended supplements, which can be taken at the same time as a multivitamin and multimineral formulation, encourage stronger and healthier hair growth by nourishing the roots. There is no miracle remedy that guarantees a luxurious head of hair, but you may notice some improvement within six months, when new hair has had time to grow.

Supplements containing essential fatty acids, such as **fish oils**, flaxseed oil and **evening primrose oil**, provide various benefits. Fish oils are rich in omega-3 fatty acids – without them, hair is often dry and lifeless. Omega-3 fats also have a moisturising effect, and can reduce itching and flaking dandruff, which makes them a useful treatment for eczema and psoriasis of the scalp.

Vitamins and minerals may also slow down hair loss. **Zinc** boosts thyroid function, and may be especially beneficial for brittle or thinning hair which is the result of an underactive thyroid. Zinc needs to be taken with

Biotin and other B vitamins condition the hair from within.

SUPPLEMENT RECOMMENDATIONS

Fish oils	**Dosage:** 2 teaspoons to provide 2 grams omega-3 fatty acids a day. **Caution:** consult your doctor if you take anticoagulant drugs. **Advice:** vegetarians can substitute 1 tablespoon of flaxseed oil.
Evening primrose oil	**Dosage:** 1000 mg three times a day. **Advice:** alternatively, take 1000 mg borage oil once a day.
Zinc	**Dosage:** 15 mg a day. **Advice:** if you take a zinc supplement for more than a month, use one that includes 2 mg copper.
Biotin	**Dosage:** 900 mcg a day. **Advice:** can combat excessive oiliness and flaking; take with vitamin B complex.
Vitamin B complex	**Dosage:** 1 tablet twice a day with food. **Advice:** look for a B-50 complex with 50 mcg vitamin B_{12} and biotin, 400 mcg folic acid and 50 mg all other B vitamins.
Selenium	**Dosage:** 200 mcg once a day. **Caution:** do not exceed a total of 200 mcg from supplements; higher doses may be toxic.

Note: consider using supplements in blue first; those in black may also be beneficial. Some dosages may be supplied by supplements you are already taking – see page 195.

copper to maintain a proper mineral balance in the body. Copper also serves another useful purpose: it is an essential ingredient in melanin, the pigment that colours hair and skin, and may reverse the greying process, in which copper deficiency is a contributing factor. Taking **biotin** and **vitamin B complex** should strengthen the hair, condition the scalp and prevent excessive hair loss. Biotin may also restore lost hair, but only if the loss has been caused by a biotin deficiency.

Selenium is also likely to encourage healthy hair growth. It protects cells against environmental and dietary toxins.

What else you can do

☑ Eat sensibly. Avoid faddish diets that may deprive you of essential nutrients.

☑ Wash your hair with a mild shampoo. Gently towel it dry and apply a conditioner. Avoid harsh chemicals, such as chlorine in swimming pools, and high heat from hair dryers or curling tongs.

☑ Protect your hair and scalp from the sun by wearing a hat.

☑ Perform a weekly scalp massage to stimulate blood flow and relieve stress, which can contribute to hair loss.

Hay fever and other allergies

For millions of people the simple act of opening a window, vacuuming the carpet or stroking a cat provokes sniffles and sneezes. The cause of the symptoms is not pollen, dust or cat hair, however, but an overactive immune system.

Symptoms

- Red, itchy or puffy eyes, sometimes surrounded by dark circles.
- Sneezing.
- Swollen nasal passages.
- Runny nose with a clear discharge.
- Irritated throat.
- Fatigue.

SEE YOUR DOCTOR ...

- If you experience wheezing or difficulty breathing – it may be a sign of an asthma attack, requiring immediate treatment.

- If you develop a headache or fever that gets worse when you bend forwards, or your nasal discharge turns yellow or green – it may be a sinus infection.

- If allergy symptoms interfere with daily activities, and natural supplements do not help.

REMINDER: If you have a medical condition, consult your doctor before taking supplements.

Nettle supplements ease allergy symptoms by reducing nasal inflammation.

What they are

'Allergic rhinitis' is the medical term for the nasal symptoms caused by allergies to airborne particles. The condition can be an occasional inconvenience or a severe problem that interferes with every aspect of daily life. If you notice symptoms during warm weather you may have the seasonal allergies commonly known as hay fever, triggered by tree or grass pollen during late spring and early summer. If you have symptoms all year round – perennial allergies – the most likely culprits are animal fur, household dust mites or mould. These irritants all produce the same symptoms. People who suffer from allergic rhinitis often have a low level of resistance to colds, flu, sinus infections and other respiratory illnesses. In some families, allergic rhinitis may be an inherited condition.

What causes them

When bacteria, viruses or other substances enter the body, the immune system tries to destroy those that might cause illness but ignores harmless particles such as pollen. In allergic individuals the immune system cannot tell the difference between threatening and benign material; as a result, innocuous particles trigger the release of a naturally occurring substance called histamine and other inflammatory compounds in the area where the irritant entered the body – the nose, throat or eyes.

No one knows why the immune system overreacts in this way, but some researchers think that poor nutrition and air pollution may weaken the system. This is why a multivitamin and multimineral formulation should be taken in addition to the supplements listed in the chart.

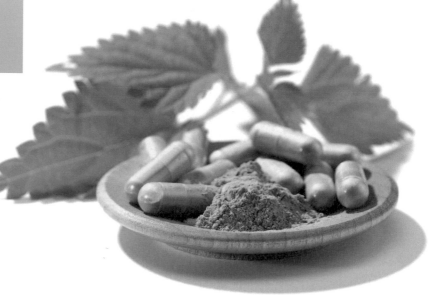

SUPPLEMENT RECOMMENDATIONS	
Quercetin	**Dosage:** 500 mg twice a day. **Advice:** take 20 minutes before meals; often sold in combination with vitamin C.
Nettle leaf	**Dosage:** 250 mg three times a day on an empty stomach. **Advice:** standardised to contain at least 1% plant silica.
Vitamin C	**Dosage:** 500 mg twice a day. **Advice:** reduce dose if diarrhoea develops.
Pantothenic acid	**Dosage:** 100 mg twice a day. **Advice:** take with meals.
Fish oils	**Dosage:** 2 teaspoons a day. **Caution:** consult your doctor if you take anticoagulant drugs.

Note: consider using supplements in blue first; those in black may also be beneficial. Some dosages may be supplied by supplements you are already taking – see page 195.

How supplements can help

For seasonal allergies, take all the supplements in the chart from early spring onwards. In place of over-the-counter drugs, try the flavonoid **quercetin**. Drugs simply block the effect of histamine, but quercetin inhibits its release – without any side effects. Combining it with the herb **nettle leaf** can combat sneezing, itching and swollen nasal passages.

Vitamin C is the main antioxidant in the cells of the respiratory passages. It supports the immune system, and may also have anti-inflammatory and antihistamine effects. The B vitamin **pantothenic acid** should reduce nasal congestion. You may want to take these three nutrients throughout the allergy season, even if you opt for traditional drugs for specific symptom relief.

When taken long term, omega-3 fatty acids from **fish oils** (or flaxseed oil) may help to reduce inflammatory symptoms. Inflammation can also be reduced by tea made from herbs such as chamomile, plantain, sage, eyebright and elderflower, used singly or mixed together. Add 200 ml of boiling water to about 10 grams of dried herbs, infuse for 10 minutes before straining, and drink twice a day. For extra benefit add liquorice tincture to the tea (1 teaspoon per cup).

What else you can do

☑ Stay indoors with the windows closed when pollen counts are high.
☑ If possible, remove carpets from your home and, for furnishings, use loose covers that can be washed.
☑ Encase mattresses and pillows in allergy-proof covers and wash bedding weekly in very hot water. Dust mites collect on these items.
☑ Clean damp areas to prevent the growth of mould.

Headache and migraine

Almost all of us suffer from headaches at some time, and about 6% of headaches can be called migraines. Some supplements may be as effective as, or even superior to, conventional medicine in preventing and treating these conditions.

Symptoms

Tension headache

- Continuous pain in one part of the head or all over it.

- Sore areas in neck and upper back.

- Dizziness and feeling light-headed.

Cluster headache

- Intense throbbing on one side of the head occurring several times a day over a period of up to several months.

Migraine

- Intense, throbbing pain, first near one eye or temple, then throughout one or both sides of the head.

- Nausea and vomiting.

- Painful aversion to light.

- Early warning signs include visual disturbances such as flashing lights or wavy lines; tingling sensations, dizziness and tinnitus; sweating, chills, fatigue; swelling of the face; irritability.

What they are

Tension causes about 90% of headaches. Severe headaches that recur are known as cluster headaches. A migraine is a severe, throbbing pain that usually begins on one side of the head but may affect the whole head; attacks can last for hours or days and may be preceded by warning signs.

What causes them

Most headaches are brought about by muscular tension. Although the precise causes of migraine are unknown, it is thought to be sparked by spasms in the arteries that supply blood to the brain. This may be linked to a low level of the brain chemical serotonin. Migraines run in families, and women are more susceptible than men.

A variety of triggers can bring on cluster headaches or migraines, such as certain foods, stress, lack of sleep, changes in the weather or bright light. Fluctuations in blood sugar levels, liver problems, dental pain, hormonal swings, environmental chemicals and exposure to cigarette smoke are other possible causes.

How supplements can help

Supplements can prevent symptoms from appearing, but prescription medication will probably be needed to combat a severe headache that has already begun. Anyone who suffers recurring headaches or migraines should take **magnesium** and **calcium** long term to maintain healthy blood vessels and reduce muscular tension. Low levels of magnesium are common in people who have migraines. **Feverfew** can reduce the intensity and frequency of headaches and migraines when taken over

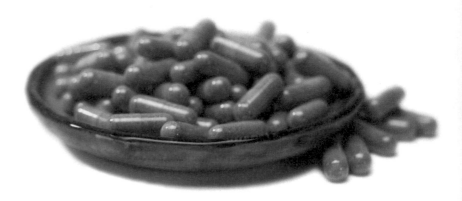

Feverfew supplements may prevent migraine attacks.

SUPPLEMENT RECOMMENDATIONS

Magnesium/calcium	**Dosage:** 200 mg magnesium and 500 mg calcium twice a day. **Advice:** take with food; may be sold as a single supplement.
Feverfew	**Dosage:** 250 mg extract every morning. **Caution:** do not use during pregnancy. **Advice:** standardised to contain at least 0.4% parthenolide.
5-HTP	**Dosage:** 100 mg 3 times a day. **Advice:** consult your doctor if you are taking a prescription antidepressant.
Riboflavin	**Dosage:** 40 mg every morning. **Comments:** best used for chronic migraines.
Chamomile	**Dosage:** up to three cups of tea a day. **Comments:** capsules and tinctures also available.
Valerian	**Dosage:** 250 mg extract twice a day. **Advice:** use products with standardised extract containing 0.8% valeric (or valerenic) acid.
Chasteberry	**Dosage:** ½ teaspoon of tincture twice a day in water, or 225 mg powdered extract in tablet or capsule form twice a day. **Advice:** use extract standardised to contain 0.5% agnuside.
Dandelion	**Dosage to strengthen the liver:** 500 mg of powdered root extract three times a day; **for constipation:** one cup of tea three times a day.

Note: consider using supplements in blue first; those in black may also be beneficial. Some dosages may be supplied by supplements you are already taking – see page 195.

FACTS & TIPS

■ Certain foods and drinks – especially those containing compounds known as amines – are notorious migraine triggers. If you are a migraine sufferer, try to avoid mature cheeses, onions, pickles, nuts, cured meats, red wine, beer, sour cream, freshly baked yeast products, citrus fruits, tomatoes, caffeinated drinks and eggs. Although chocolate is often thought to be a migraine trigger, new studies indicate that it may not be.

■ Eating fish rich in omega-3 fatty acids, such as salmon and tuna, may help to avoid migraines. Omega-3s seem to alter blood chemicals, reducing the risk of blood vessel spasms linked with migraines.

DID YOU KNOW?
Treating headaches with aspirin or other non-prescription painkillers can, in time, interfere with the body's natural ability to fight pain.

several months. **5-HTP**, a form of the amino acid tryptophan and a basic building block of serotonin, may prevent symptoms as effectively as drugs; minor side effects, mainly nausea, tend to disappear in about two weeks, but several months of therapy may be needed.

If your headaches or migraines are frequent, the B vitamin **riboflavin** may be more effective than feverfew or 5-HTP. Riboflavin in high doses seems to raise energy reserves in brain cells. Try drinking **chamomile** tea as a general nerve tonic, to ease stress and relieve pain. **Valerian**, which improves circulation and relieves anxiety, muscle tension and pain, can also be useful. **Chasteberry** treats a range of menstrual complaints, including headaches. **Dandelion** root can help if symptoms are related to constipation (by acting as a mild laxative) or to liver function.

If none of these remedies works, consider adding vitamin C and pantothenic acid. Both boost the production of hormones that assist the body in dealing with the adverse effects of stress.

What else you can do

☑ Identify and eliminate your headache or migraine triggers.
☑ Try biofeedback or relaxation training to cope with stress.
☑ Drink six to eight glasses of water a day and exercise regularly.
☑ Practise deep breathing, which increases oxygen supply to the brain.
☑ Try to eat five or more portions of fruit and vegetables every day.

Heart disease prevention

Lifestyle and dietary strategies can help you to avoid many diseases, but they are probably most effective in preventing heart disease. Recent research confirms that certain nutrients can do much to promote a healthy heart.

Symptoms

- In the early stages, heart disease has no symptoms. Warning signs include high blood cholesterol levels and high blood pressure.

- In the advanced stages: chest, arm or jaw pain (especially after physical activity), palpitations and shortness of breath.

SEE YOUR DOCTOR ...

- To have your blood pressure checked every two years and have a cholesterol check every five years – more often if the levels are high.

- If you have any symptoms of heart disease.

- If you suffer unexplained dizziness, weakness or faintness.

- If you experience skipping or extra heartbeats or other irregularities with any frequency.

- If you have squeezing or crushing chest pain, together with light-headedness, nausea or shortness of breath: this may be a sign of a heart attack – get emergency help immediately.

REMINDER: If you have a medical condition, consult your doctor before taking supplements.

What it is

Heart disease is actually a build-up of fatty deposits (plaque) within the walls of the arteries, a process known as atherosclerosis. As plaque deposits grow they hinder the flow of blood, which carries vital oxygen and nutrients throughout the body. The tiny arteries that thread through the heart and nourish it with blood are particularly susceptible to plaque accumulation – blockages in this area can result in a heart attack.

What causes it

A primary cause of atherosclerosis is high blood cholesterol levels. About three-quarters of the cholesterol in the blood is carried by proteins known as low density lipoproteins (LDL). LDL or 'bad' cholesterol sticks to artery walls and accumulates as plaque. High blood pressure, obesity, smoking, lack of exercise and stress all contribute to plaque build-up and reduce the elasticity of the arteries. In middle age, men have a higher risk of heart disease than women because the female hormone oestrogen is thought to have a heart-protective effect. After the menopause, women are as susceptible as men.

How supplements can help

Supplements are not a substitute for a healthy lifestyle, nor do they target any one risk factor, such as high cholesterol, but people who already have heart disease may benefit from using them. With the exception of vitamin E and fish oils, which may interact with anticoagulant drugs, they are safe to use in combination with prescription drugs for heart disease.

The first four supplements are antioxidants, which inactivate cell-damaging free radicals (unstable oxygen molecules). Each one has a different function, so take them together. **Vitamin E** prevents the first step in the development of plaque – the oxidisation of LDL cholesterol. **Vitamin C** helps to recycle vitamin E and keeps the

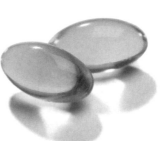

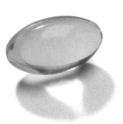

Vitamin E protects cell membranes and helps to prevent atherosclerosis.

Vitamin E	**Dosage:** 250 mg a day. **Caution:** consult your doctor if you take anticoagulant drugs.
Vitamin C	**Dosage:** 500 mg twice a day. **Advice:** reduce dose if diarrhoea develops.
Carotenoids	**Dosage:** 1 capsule mixed carotenoids twice a day with food. **Advice:** each capsule should supply 15 grams mixed carotenoids.
Grape seed extract	**Dosage:** 100 mg twice a day. **Advice:** standardised to contain 92%-95% proanthocyanidins.
Vitamin B$_{12}$/folic acid	**Dosage:** 50-1000 mcg vitamin B$_{12}$ and 400 mcg folic acid a day. **Advice:** sometimes sold as a single supplement.
Vitamin B$_6$	**Dosage:** 50 mg a day. **Advice:** 200 mg vitamin B$_6$ daily over a long period can cause nerve damage; do not exceed the recommended dose.
Fish oils	**Dosage:** 2 teaspoons a day. **Caution:** consult your doctor if you take anticoagulant drugs. **Advice:** vegetarians can substitute 1 tablespoon of flaxseed oil.
Magnesium	**Dosage:** 400 mg a day. **Caution:** do not take if you have kidney disease.

Some dosages may be supplied by supplements you are already taking – see page 195.

see page 195.

arteries flexible. The antioxidant **carotenoids** beta-carotene and lycopene should be taken in a mixed supplement for a proper balance. **Grape seed extract** contains oligomeric proanthocyanidin complexes (OPCs) – flavonoids thought to have many times the antioxidant power of vitamins C and E.

In addition to antioxidants, **folic acid** is an important supplement for reducing homocysteine, an amino acid by-product linked to an increased risk of heart disease. **Vitamins B$_{12}$ and B$_6$** also help to lower homocysteine levels, and vitamin B$_6$ is thought to keep the arteries pliable as well. The omega-3 fatty acids in **fish oils** (or flaxseed oil) help to keep levels of triglyceride, a blood fat related to cholesterol, in check, and the mineral **magnesium** stabilises heart rhythm.

Garlic and artichoke are useful supplements, as they help to lower blood cholesterol. Other herbs that help to protect the heart include hawthorn, ginkgo biloba and psyllium.

What else you can do

☑ Maintain a low-fat diet, especially cutting back on saturated fats.
☑ Eat at least five portions of fruit and vegetables a day, and two portions of oily fish a week.
☑ Eat plenty of soluble fibre to control cholesterol.
☑ Exercise for 30 minutes a day. Activity strengthens the heart, raises the level of less fatty HDL or 'good' cholesterol, and helps weight loss.
☑ Do not smoke – nothing makes up for the damage it does to the heart.

Excess iron may contribute to heart disease in older people. In a recent study, for every 50 mg monthly increase in iron above 250 mg (from food and supplements) the risk of heart disease rose one and a half times in men and three and a half times in women over 60. Older people should not take high dose iron supplements without asking the doctors.

Some of the heart-protective benefits of vitamins C and E may be immediate, according to a recent study. High-fat meals seem to inhibit the ability of the arteries to expand, but when 20 study participants took 1000 mg of vitamin C and 500 mg of vitamin E before eating a high-fat meal, the arteries worked normally. Low-fat meals had no discernible effect on the arteries, and vitamins provided no additional benefits.

DID YOU KNOW?
Many studies indicate that one or two glasses of wine or beer a day may lower the risk of heart disease. The antioxidant flavonoids in red wine (or purple grape juice) are helpful.

FACTS & TIPS
■ Heart attacks are relatively rare in countries where olive oil is consumed liberally – even where the normal diets contain quite a high amount of fat overall. Use olive oil in place of other fats whenever possible.

High blood pressure

The serious health problems caused by high blood pressure and its lack of visible symptoms have given it a reputation as a silent killer. Studies show that lifestyle changes and supplements may sometimes be viable alternatives to prescription drugs.

Symptoms

- *There are often no symptoms, even when blood pressure is in the danger zone. Some people complain of headaches and tinnitus when blood pressure is very high, but usually the condition is discovered during a medical examination.*

SEE YOUR DOCTOR ...

- If your blood pressure remains high (140/90) after two months of treatment with supplements.

Routine blood pressure screening is recommended for everyone, on the following schedule:

- Every two years, if you are generally healthy and have normal blood pressure.

- Every year if you are over-weight or sedentary or have a family history of high blood pressure, or if your blood pressure is 130 to 139 systolic or 85 to 89 diastolic.

- On the schedule your doctor outlines for you if you have high blood pressure.

REMINDER: If you have a medical condition, consult your doctor before taking supplements.

What it is

Blood pressure is the force exerted by the blood on the arteries and veins as it circulates through the body, and is controlled by a complex regulatory system involving the heart, blood vessels, brain, kidneys and adrenal glands. It is normal for blood pressure to fluctuate – even from minute to minute – but in some people it remains chronically high, a condition known medically as hypertension.

Blood pressure is recorded using two numbers. Systolic pressure (the top number in a reading) is the pressure when the heart contracts and forces blood through the arteries; diastolic pressure (the bottom number) reflects the pressure when the heart relaxes. Normal blood pressure is 120 (systolic) over 80 (diastolic) or lower. Hypertension is defined as blood pressure averaging 140/90 or higher in at least two separate measurements.

What causes it

In 90% of people with hypertension the cause is not known. Factors known to increase the risk include a high-sodium diet, obesity, smoking and a family history of high blood pressure. Men are twice as likely to suffer from hypertension as women.

How supplements can help

If you have mild hypertension (140 to 159 systolic and 90 to 99 diastolic), start making lifestyle changes and take calcium and magnesium. If your blood pressure is higher, see your doctor before using supplements. If you already take medication for high blood pressure, do not reduce your dose without your doctor's advice.

In some studies **calcium** has been shown to lower blood pressure; it is also involved in muscle contraction, so is good for the heart and blood vessels. **Magnesium** relaxes the muscles that control blood

The mineral calcium controls nerve impulses that cause muscles to contract.

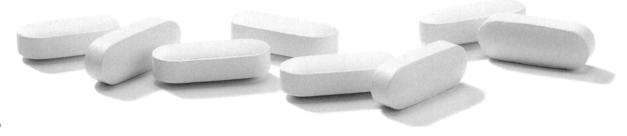

Calcium/ magnesium	**Dosage:** 1000 mg calcium and 400 mg magnesium a day. **Caution:** do not take magnesium if you have kidney disease.
Vitamin C	**Dosage:** 500 mg twice a day. **Advice:** reduce dose if diarrhoea develops.
Fish oils	**Dosage:** 2 teaspoons to provide 2 g omega-3 fatty acids a day. **Caution:** consult your doctor if you take anticoagulant drugs. **Advice:** vegetarians can substitute 1 tablespoon of flaxseed oil.
Hawthorn	**Dosage:** 100-150 mg extract three times a day. **Advice:** standardised to contain at least 1.8% vitexin.
Garlic	**Dosage:** dried concentrate equivalent to 4 grams of fresh garlic a day. **Advice:** use garlic in your cooking, too.
Coenzyme Q_{10}	**Dosage:** 50 mg twice a day. **Advice:** for most efficient absorption, take with food.

Note: consider using supplements in blue first; those in black may also be beneficial. Some dosages may be supplied by supplements you are already taking – see page 195.

vessels, allowing blood to flow more freely, and helps to maintain a balance between potassium and sodium in the blood, which has a positive effect on blood pressure. The mineral potassium is also effective in reducing blood pressure, but potassium supplements are almost never necessary – eating more fruit and vegetables raises potassium levels sufficiently in most people.

If your blood pressure has not dropped after a month, continue taking calcium and magnesium, maintain your lifestyle changes, and begin **vitamin C** and **hawthorn**. Both supplements widen blood vessels; hawthorn helps to moderate the heart rate as well. **Garlic**, also thought to lower blood pressure, can be added to this regimen. Essential fatty acids can be taken in addition in the form of **fish oils** (or flaxseed oil), to encourage good circulation. Relaxing lime flower tea, a general circulatory tonic, may be useful in cases of nervous hypertension.

If there is little improvement after two months, add **coenzyme Q_{10}**; more than a third of people with high blood pressure are thought to have an inadequate supply of this substance. If your blood pressure still does not respond, you may need prescription drugs.

What else you can do

☑ Lose weight. Even a few extra pounds can raise blood pressure.
☑ Walk or take some other form of aerobic exercise regularly.
☑ Eat plenty of fruit, vegetables and low-fat dairy products; reduce fat and salt intake. A new study indicates that this type of diet may be an alternative to prescription drugs for mild hypertension.

Vitamin C helps to lower blood pressure by widening blood vessels. In a preliminary study, 3000 mg of intravenous vitamin C relaxed blood vessels in 17 people with hypertension. Scientists speculate that constricted arteries may be partly caused by the type of cell damage that vitamin C corrects. More research is needed to find out whether supplements produce the same results.

Some researchers believe that a deficiency of vitamin D might contribute to high blood pressure. One scientist from the University of Alabama has noticed that hypertension is less common in areas where there is more daylight (the sun triggers vitamin D production in the body) and thinks that the vitamin may affect the hormones involved in blood pressure. If this is proved, vitamin D supplements may be recommended in some cases of hypertension.

FACTS & TIPS

■ A recent international forum on heart disease recommended lowering the accepted measurements indicating hypertension from 140/90 to 130/85 to prevent more heart attacks, strokes and complications such as kidney disease.

■ Consensus Action on Salt and Hypertension (CASH), a UK pressure group, says that, if official recommendations to cut salt levels in processed foods by 30% were adopted, the incidence of strokes would fall by 16% and heart attacks by 22%.

High cholesterol

A high level of cholesterol in your blood increases the risk of a heart attack and possibly a stroke. Along with dietary changes, vitamins C and E and some effective herbal compounds can help to control your cholesterol level and reduce this risk.

Symptoms

- *High cholesterol usually has no clear symptoms, but it is a risk factor for other disorders with discernible symptoms, such as angina.*

- *When levels are very high, cholesterol may appear as yellow nodules beneath the skin of the elbows or knees, or under the eyes.*

SEE YOUR DOCTOR ...

- **To have your cholesterol levels measured once every five years – more often if your total cholesterol level is 5.6 millimoles per litre or higher.**

- **If home remedies do not lower your total cholesterol sufficiently within two or three months – you may need to take prescription drugs. Conventional drugs reduce heart attack risk by up to 25%.**

REMINDER: If you have a medical condition, consult your doctor before taking supplements.

What it is

Cholesterol is a fat-like substance circulating in the blood. The body needs a certain amount to maintain cell membranes and perform other vital functions, but high levels lead to blocked arteries, which can cause a heart attack. Cholesterol is carried in the blood by two types of protein: low density lipoproteins (LDL), which carry three-quarters of the cholesterol, and high density lipoproteins (HDL). Total blood cholesterol is measured, and separate measurements are taken of LDL ('bad') cholesterol and HDL ('good') cholesterol. High LDL and total cholesterol levels increase the risk of a heart attack, as does a low level of HDL (below 0.9 millimoles per litre). Doctors recommend keeping total cholesterol below 5.6 millimoles per litre, ideally around 5.2 millimoles per litre, and your HDL level as high as possible.

What causes it

High cholesterol levels are often linked to a diet rich in the saturated fat found in animal foods such as beef, butter and whole-fat dairy products and in the coconut oil, palm oil and hydrogenated oils used in processed foods. This theory is no longer widely accepted – cholesterol from food is poorly absorbed, and levels of blood cholesterol are affected mainly by the manufacture of cholesterol in the body – but the body's production of cholesterol is certainly stimulated by high intakes of saturated fat. Excess weight, smoking and lack of exercise also contribute to high cholesterol levels; genetic predisposition may also be a factor.

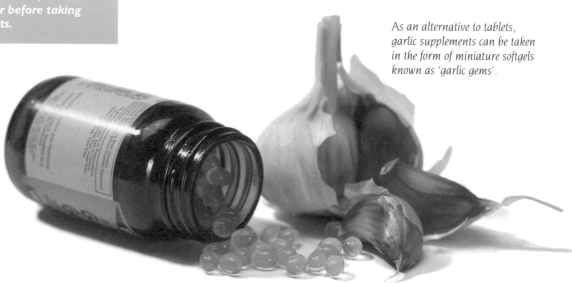

As an alternative to tablets, garlic supplements can be taken in the form of miniature softgels known as 'garlic gems'.

Vitamin E	**Dosage:** 250 mg twice a day. **Caution:** consult your doctor if you take anticoagulant drugs.
Vitamin C	**Dosage:** 500 mg twice a day. **Advice:** reduce dose if diarrhoea develops.
Garlic	**Dosage:** 400-600 mg dried concentrate a day. **Advice:** tablets should be enteric coated; each tablet should provide 4000 mcg allicin potential.
Chromium	**Dosage:** 200 mcg once a day. **Advice:** use easily absorbed forms, such as GTF chromium or chromium picolinate.
Beta-sitosterol	**Dosage:** 300 mg twice a day. **Advice:** long-term use may be necessary.
Artichoke	**Dosage:** Two to six 320 mg capsules daily. **Advice:** standardised to contain 15% cynarin.
Psyllium	**Dosage:** 1 tablespoon of powder dissolved in water or juice twice a day. **Advice:** drink eight glasses of water a day; psyllium may have a laxative effect.

Note: consider using supplements in blue first; the one in black may also be beneficial. Some dosages may be supplied by supplements you are already taking – see page 195.

How supplements can help

Several natural remedies can help to control cholesterol levels. Begin by taking **vitamins E** and **C** and **garlic** together. These are safe for long-term use, even if you are taking a cholesterol-lowering prescription drug. Vitamin E does not lower your cholesterol directly, but raises levels of HDL cholesterol and prevents the first step in the build-up of coronary plaque: the bombardment of LDL cholesterol by free radicals (unstable oxygen molecules). Vitamin C boosts the effectiveness of vitamin E, and is also thought to increase the level of protective HDL cholesterol.

Studies have produced conflicting evidence about the power of garlic to lower cholesterol levels, but on balance they are favourable; many nutritional practitioners believe that it has a positive effect. **Chromium** helps to reduce 'bad' cholesterol and raise 'good' cholesterol in those with diets high in refined foods. Diets lacking in cholesterol-reducing soluble fibre can benefit from the herb **psyllium**, or from oat bran, which has a similar action. **Beta-sitosterol** can be taken to reduce the absorption of cholesterol from food and from bile discharged by the liver into the intestine. **Artichoke** extract may prove to be an effective alternative to cholesterol-lowering medications.

What else you can do

☑ Improve your diet by reducing saturated fats. Substitute oily fish for meat, eat high-fibre foods (grains, vegetables and fruit), include soya protein (available as tofu and soya milk) and use olive oil and mono-unsaturated spreads in place of butter.

☑ Take regular exercise to raise your HDL level.

Clinical studies have indicated that a substance called tocotrienol, extracted from rice bran, can lower levels of cholesterol. Used as a dietary supplement, tocotrienol-rich rice bran oil reduces levels of total cholesterol and LDL cholesterol.

⁓

A new study shows that most people with high cholesterol can achieve a 10% drop in cholesterol levels when they combine a low-fat diet with 5 grams of psyllium taken twice a day. The effect of psyllium is more pronounced in people with higher cholesterol levels.

DID YOU KNOW?

Margarines that lower LDL cholesterol contain plant sterols, extracted from soya beans or pine bark, that reduce the re-absorption of cholesterol from liver bile that has been released into the gut.

FACTS & TIPS

■ A recent American study found that drinking three glasses of orange juice a day raises blood levels of 'good' HDL cholesterol. The reasons for this effect are not known.

■ Home cholesterol tests are convenient and can give you results in a matter of minutes, but are not always reliable and do not measure HDL levels. It is wiser to have your cholesterol level confirmed by a doctor.

HIV/AIDS

New drugs have brought renewed hope in the battle against HIV infection and AIDS, yet discussions about the role of alternative therapies for both conditions remain heated. Research suggests that a number of supplements can serve as vital additions to conventional treatment.

Symptoms

- *Many people infected with HIV have no symptoms.*

- *Persistent fatigue; joint or muscle pain; recurring or prolonged fever, possibly with chills or night sweats.*

- *Frequent sore throats, swollen glands, coughs, colds, cold sores, yeast infections or other types of infection.*

- *Loss of appetite and weight; frequent diarrhoea.*

- *Unusual rashes or skin discoloration, especially purplish markings (Kaposi's sarcoma).*

SEE YOUR DOCTOR ...

- **If you experience any of the symptoms listed above.**

- **If you suspect that you may have been exposed to HIV, the virus that causes AIDS.**

- **If you have been diagnosed with HIV, and symptoms suddenly become worse.**

REMINDER: If you have a medical condition, consult your doctor before taking supplements.

What they are

The human immunodeficiency virus (HIV) causes acquired immune deficiency syndrome (AIDS). Following initial infection with the virus, years may pass before the immune system is damaged to the extent that AIDS-related illnesses arise. AIDS develops when the body can no longer fight off diseases such as pneumonia, fungal or parasitic infestations and certain cancers. So far there is no vaccine against or cure for HIV or AIDS.

What causes them

Once HIV has infected the body it is carried in body fluids such as blood, semen, vaginal secretions and breast milk. It spreads when others come into contact with these fluids, particularly through sexual intercourse or exposure to contaminated blood (the latter can happen among drug users who share needles). Nevertheless, the virus is hard to transmit because it dies very quickly outside the host's body. It does not spread through air or water or travel easily from person to person, for example, through coughing or sharing drinking cups, as many other viruses do.

How supplements can help

The recommended supplements are all aimed at boosting immunity, and should be taken with a multivitamin and multimineral supplement. They can be used in combination with conventional AIDS drugs, and should be continued long term. Benefits may be felt within a month.

Antioxidant therapy – especially large doses of **vitamin C** – shows promise in slowing the disease and strengthening the immune system. Vitamin C appears to fight viruses and fungal infections, and also has anti-inflammatory properties. The nutrient **coenzyme Q$_{10}$** plays a vital role in energy production and may improve stamina in people with AIDS; it also has an antioxidant effect. Other useful antioxidants include **vitamin E** and alpha-lipoic acid.

Low blood levels of **carotenoids** are a feature of HIV – encourage healthy levels by taking a mixed supplement. **Zinc** is crucial to the

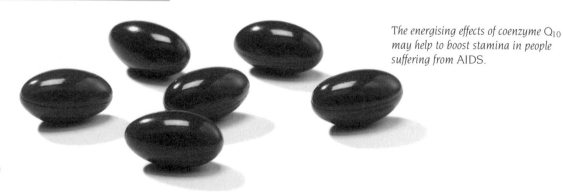

The energising effects of coenzyme Q$_{10}$ may help to boost stamina in people suffering from AIDS.

Vitamin C/ vitamin E	**Dosage:** 500 mg vitamin C twice a day; 250 mg vitamin E daily. **Advice:** vitamin C helps to boost the effects of vitamin E.
Coenzyme Q₁₀	**Dosage:** 30 mg three times a day. **Advice:** for effective absorption, take with food.
Carotenoids	**Dosage:** 15 mg twice a day. **Caution:** make sure that you use natural beta-carotene, not the synthetic version.
Zinc	**Dosage:** 25 mg a day. **Advice:** if you take a zinc supplement for more than a month, use one that includes 2 mg copper.
NAC/amino acid complex	**Dosage:** 500 mg NAC three times a day; for amino acids, follow the directions on the bottle. **Advice:** take both on an empty stomach, but at different times.
Turmeric/ bromelain	**Dosage:** 400 mg turmeric and 500 mg bromelain three times a day. **Caution:** consult your doctor if you take anticoagulant drugs. **Advice:** bromelain to provide 6000 GDU or 9000 MCU daily.
Fish oils	**Dosage:** two teaspoons to provide 2 grams omega-3 fatty acids a day. **Advice:** vegetarians can substitute 1 tablespoon of flaxseed oil. **Caution:** consult your doctor if you take anticoagulant drugs.
Reishi/maitake mushrooms	**Dosage:** 500 mg reishi and 200 mg maitake three times a day. **Caution:** avoid reishi if you take anticoagulant drugs.

Some dosages may be supplied by supplements you are already taking – see page 195.

see page 195.

healthy functioning of the immune system and may help to maintain body weight. Do not exceed the recommended dose – excessive intake may impair immunity. Zinc can be beneficial in fighting pneumonia and fungal infections in the later stages of AIDS. It depletes the body's copper stores, so take both minerals together.

The amino acid **NAC** (N-acetylcysteine), balanced with a mixed **amino acid complex**, acts as an antioxidant, stimulates the immune system, assists in repairing body tissues and fights weight loss. Most notably, NAC seems to interfere with the replication of all viruses, including HIV. The herb **turmeric** (taken with **bromelain** for better absorption) may also block HIV reproduction. **Fish oils** (or flaxseed oil) improve immune function. Some studies suggest that extracts of **reishi** and **maitake** and other Japanese mushrooms can stimulate immunity and improve survival rates in those with certain AIDS-related cancers.

Other supplements that may be helpful are anti-viral garlic and St John's wort, probiotics and glutamine for healthy digestion, and liquorice to support the function of the adrenal glands.

What else you can do

- ☑ Exercise regularly and stop smoking.
- ☑ Reduce stress. Meditation, yoga or a support group may help.

Preliminary research indicates that certain supplements may one day be added to the arsenal of substances known to improve the outlook for people with HIV:

Low levels of vitamin B₁₂ are known to precede progression of the disease. Further studies are required to determine whether B₁₂ supplements could delay its progression.

Test-tube studies suggest that the trace mineral selenium may help to suppress the replication of the AIDS virus.

A recent study in Tanzania showed that multivitamins improved the health of HIV-positive mothers and reduced the numbers of foetal deaths, low birth weights and seriously premature births.

FACTS & TIPS

■ Doctors disagree over the effectiveness of immune-boosting herbs such as astragalus, cat's claw, echinacea, goldenseal and pau d'arco in treating people with HIV and AIDS. Most practitioners who prescribe them suggest taking one herb for two or three weeks, then substituting another. This rotation is important because the body may develop a tolerance for any herb when it is consumed over a long period.

■ Healthy eating will complement the benefits of supplements and AIDS drugs. Consider a vegetarian diet. Avoid alcohol, caffeine, junk foods and sugar. Eating a wide variety of foods in small amounts throughout the day will help to conserve energy.

Impotence

For one man in four over the age of 50 – and for some much younger men too – a sustainable erection can be elusive. In most cases the cause of what doctors call 'erectile dysfunction' is physical and correctable, often by making some surprisingly simple changes.

Symptoms

- A *persistent inability to attain or maintain an erection sufficient for sexual intercourse.*

SEE YOUR DOCTOR ...

- **If you are consistently unable to achieve or maintain an erection – your doctor can help to determine, and correct, the underlying cause.**

- **If stress or new medication is having a detrimental effect on your sexual performance.**

REMINDER: If you have a medical condition, consult your doctor before taking supplements.

What it is

Impotence is the sustained inability to achieve or maintain an erection. An erection occurs when blood vessels in the penis fill with blood, stiffening the organ. The process is sparked by sexual stimulation, which causes nerves in the brain and spine to send signals to arteries in the penis, telling them to expand. Most men experience occasional problems maintaining an erection; this is not a cause for concern.

What causes it

The main cause of impotence is poor circulation and impaired blood flow through the penis – often as a result of atherosclerosis, a hardening of the arteries. Other possible reasons include diabetes, hormonal imbalances, nerve disorders, prostate disease or the side effects of medication. Only one in ten cases has a purely psychological cause.

Because erections occur involuntarily during sleep, it is possible to determine whether the problem is physical or psychological by trying the 'postage stamp test'. Encircle the penis with a strip of stamps, sticking them end to end. If night-time erections occur, the stamps will be torn in the morning, and the cause is probably psychological. This type of impotence is usually stress-related and often temporary.

How supplements can help

A number of supplements, when taken together, may improve blood flow to the penis. **Vitamin C** plays a role in keeping blood vessels supple, helping them to expand and allow more blood to pass through. Omega-3 fatty acids from **fish oils** (or flaxseed oil) also improve blood flow; in the long term they can lower cholesterol and prevent blood vessels from narrowing. **Ginkgo biloba**, which increases blood flow in the brain, seems to have a similar effect on the penis. Ultrasound examinations of 60 impotent men who took

Panax ginseng boosts levels of sex hormones in men, which may remedy some cases of impotence.

Vitamin C	**Dosage:** 500 mg twice a day. **Advice:** reduce dose if diarrhoea develops.
Fish oils	**Dosage:** 2 teaspoons to provide 2 grams omega-3 fatty acids a day. **Caution:** consult your doctor if you take anticoagulant drugs. **Advice:** vegetarians can substitute 1 tablespoon of flaxseed oil.
Ginkgo biloba	**Dosage:** 80 mg extract three times a day. **Advice:** standardised to contain at least 24% flavone glycosides.
Panax ginseng	**Dosage:** 100-250 mg extract twice a day. **Advice:** standardised to contain at least 7% ginsenosides; alternate with Siberian ginseng every two weeks.
Siberian ginseng	**Dosage:** 100-300 mg standardised extract twice a day. **Advice:** alternate with Panax ginseng every two weeks.
Muira puama	**Dosage:** as a tea, 1 teaspoon of dried herb per cup of hot water each morning. **Advice:** may be hard to find; also available as a tincture.
Damiana	**Dosage:** as a tea, 1 teaspoon of dried herb per cup of hot water, three times a day. **Advice:** can be taken in addition to other herbs.

Note: consider using supplements in blue first; those in black may also be beneficial. Some dosages may be supplied by supplements you are already taking – see page 195.

ginkgo biloba showed improved penile blood circulation after six weeks, and after six months 50% of the patients had regained potency. All of these supplements should be used long term (for at least six months) for best results, though benefits may be noticed within a month. Because they have other positive effects on the body they can also become part of a general nutritional maintenance routine.

Other supplements may help when impotence is not related to blood flow. Studies in animals have shown that both **Panax** and **Siberian ginseng** boost testosterone levels and increase mating behaviour; they may produce similar effects in humans. If those are ineffective, try a tea made of the herb **Muira puama** (also known as potency wood), long used in Brazil as an aphrodisiac. **Damiana**, which originates from Mexico, is also said to be an aphrodisiac. It is often used in European herbal medicine but has not been clinically investigated.

What else you can do

☑ Exercise regularly to improve blood flow throughout the body, boost energy and reduce stress.
☑ Limit alcohol intake and do not smoke: both can aggravate impotence.
☑ Consider counselling if stress or anxiety is contributing to the problem.
☑ Ask your doctor for information about the prescription drug Viagra (sildenafil). The manufacturer has not tested Viagra to check its compatibility with herbal treatments, but there have been no reports of drug-supplement interactions so far.

Indigestion

In many cases digestive problems can be prevented by making some simple changes to your diet and lifestyle. But if, like millions of people, you experience the unpleasant and sometimes embarrassing symptoms of indigestion, natural remedies can provide quick relief.

Symptoms

- A *burning sensation behind the breastbone lasting from a few minutes to several hours.*

- A *burning sensation in the throat, or regurgitation of a hot, sour fluid into the back of the throat.*

- *Wind or belching; stomach bloating or rumbling.*

- *Nausea or vomiting.*

- *Abdominal pain; discomfort that worsens when lying down.*

SEE YOUR DOCTOR ...

- If you have pain twice a week or more – it may indicate a peptic ulcer or a disorder of the liver or gall bladder.

- If food is hard to swallow or sticks in your oesophagus.

- If you are vomiting or passing black stools.

- If you are over 45 and are suffering from persistent symptoms.

- If your chest pain is crushing rather than burning or is accompanied by shortness of breath, dizziness, sweating or pain that radiates to your arm or jaw. It may be a heart attack – get medical help immediately.

REMINDER: *If you have a medical condition, consult your doctor before taking supplements.*

What it is

Indigestion, also called dyspepsia, can involve a range of unpleasant symptoms that occur after eating, from bloating, stomach rumbling and abdominal cramps to wind, nausea and vomiting. For many sufferers it is heartburn that causes most distress. To digest food, the stomach (which has a protective mucous lining) produces more than a litre of hydrochloric acid a day. If acid moves up the delicate tissue of the oesophagus, the tube running from the throat to the stomach (which lacks a protective coating), it produces a burning sensation called heartburn, or gastroesophageal reflux. If the oesophagus becomes inflamed it can cause a severe chest pain indistinguishable from angina.

What causes it

Stomach acid usually stays where it belongs, thanks to the action of the lower oesophageal sphincter, a muscle that relaxes only to admit food into the stomach and then shuts tightly. But sometimes it does not close properly, which allows the contents of the stomach to flow back into the oesophagus and causes heartburn. Being overweight, pregnant or a smoker weakens the sphincter. Smoking also dries up saliva, which neutralises acid in the oesophagus and washes it down into the stomach. Certain foods, drinks (such as chocolate, peppermint, orange juice and coffee) and drugs cause the lower oesophageal sphincter to relax.

Clothes that are tight around the waist put added pressure on the abdomen, forcing the stomach contents upwards. Overeating stimulates prolonged acid production to digest the extra food. Stress or anxiety can disrupt the action of the stomach and intestinal muscles necessary for digestion. Talking when eating, or chewing with your mouth open, can cause air to be swallowed, which leads to bloating and indigestion.

Once mixed with saliva, chewable liquorice tablets are very effective for relieving heartburn.

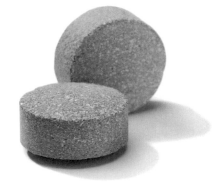
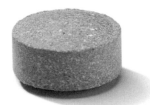

SUPPLEMENT RECOMMENDATIONS

Calcium carbonate	**Dosage:** 250-500 mg three times a day. **Advice:** chewable tablets provide the quickest relief.
Liquorice (DGL)	**Dosage:** two deglycyrrhinised (DGL) chewable tablets (380 mg) three or four times a day between meals, as needed. **Caution:** avoid if you are pregnant.
Aloe vera juice	**Dosage:** ½ cup juice three times a day between meals. **Advice:** containing 98% aloe vera and no aloin or aloe-emodin.
Gamma-oryzanol	**Dosage:** 150 mg three times a day on an empty stomach. **Advice:** also known as rice bran oil.
Choline	**Dosage:** 500 mg three times a day. **Advice:** for chronic heartburn, combine with pantothenic acid and thiamin for a month to see if symptoms abate.
Pantothenic acid	**Dosage:** 100 mg twice a day. **Advice:** for chronic heartburn, combine with choline and thiamin for a month to see if symptoms abate.
Thiamin	**Dosage:** 100 mg a day, taken first thing in the morning. **Advice:** also called vitamin B_1; for chronic heartburn, combine with pantothenic acid and choline for a month to see if symptoms abate.

Note: consider using supplements in blue first; those in black may also be beneficial. Some dosages may be supplied by supplements you are already taking – see page 195.

How supplements can help

Try each single or combination supplement in turn to see which works best for you. All can be used with prescription or over-the-counter indigestion drugs. **Calcium carbonate** is used in antacid tablets and is a good choice for occasional reflux. Deglycyrrhinised **liquorice (DGL)** helps to repair the mucous lining of the stomach and can bring relief. **Aloe vera juice** soothes an irritated oesophagus.

To enhance the digestive process – which will particularly benefit people with chronic indigestion – take **gamma-oryzanol**, a rice bran oil extract. The supplement appears to affect the central nervous system's control of digestion. Alternatively, use the B vitamins **choline**, **pantothenic acid** and **thiamin** in combination for a month. If your symptoms do not diminish, consult your doctor. Chamomile has traditionally been used to soothe digestive upsets; it also acts as a relaxant and relieves cramps.

What else you can do

☑ Eat little and often to minimise production of stomach acid.
☑ Avoid fatty foods and overeating. Limit alcohol, which can increase stomach acid, and give up coffee, which acts as an irritant.
☑ Eat your last meal or snack at least three hours before going to bed and avoid lying down too soon after a meal.
☑ Use gravity to help to prevent reflux by sleeping with the head of your bed elevated by about six inches.

Infertility, female

Being unable to conceive can be frustrating and stressful. Conventional infertility treatments often have side effects, and pose financial and ethical dilemmas. For some women, herbal and nutritional supplements may be an effective alternative.

Symptoms

- *Inability to conceive over a period of six months to a year.*

- *In some women, absence of menstruation, or infrequent or irregular menstruation.*

- *In some women, chlamydia, endometriosis or pelvic inflammatory disease.*

SEE YOUR DOCTOR ...

- **If you suspect that you are infertile – your doctor can assess the problem and help to uncover any underlying causes. Your partner may also need to be examined, because one or both of you may have fertility problems.**

REMINDER: If you have a medical condition, consult your doctor before taking supplements.

The essential fatty acids in fish oils are important for the healthy functioning of the uterus.

What it is

A woman may be infertile if she has not become pregnant within a year in which she has had regular unprotected sexual intercourse during the most fertile time of her menstrual cycle (five days before and on the day of ovulation). Doctors recommend that women over 35 wait only six months before seeking help, because fertility declines with age. About 15% of couples have problems conceiving. In a third of those cases, both the man and the woman have fertility problems. In the remainder, the problem is equally likely to affect either partner.

What causes it

In normal ovulation an egg is released from a woman's ovary in the middle of her menstrual cycle. The egg then travels from the ovary through the fallopian tubes, where it can be fertilised by sperm if the woman has sexual intercourse. Infertility occurs in some women because they ovulate irregularly or do not ovulate at all; in others, the fallopian tubes may be scarred or obstructed. A medical evaluation is necessary to pinpoint the cause of infertility, but women whose periods are irregular or absent are probably not ovulating normally. In some cases, despite extensive testing, no cause can be found.

Irregular ovulation becomes more frequent as a woman enters her late 30s. Hormonal imbalances caused by a variety of factors – weight problems or excess exercise – can also inhibit or prevent ovulation. Medical conditions such as chlamydia, endometriosis and pelvic inflammatory disease can result in scarring and physical obstructions.

How supplements can help

Most of the supplements in the chart can be used in combination with a multivitamin and multimineral formulation, regardless of the cause of infertility; they can also be combined with conventional treatments. It may take three to six months to notice the effects. Do not hesitate to consult a fertility specialist if these treatments are not working for you.

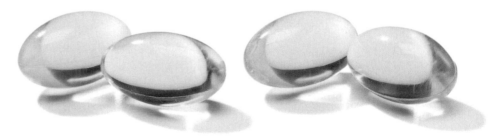

Vitamin B complex	**Dosage:** one tablet each morning with food. **Advice:** look for a B-50 complex with 50 mcg vitamin B_{12} biotin, 400 mcg folic acid and 50 mg all other B vitamins.
Vitamin E	**Dosage:** 250 mg twice a day. **Caution:** consult your doctor if you take anticoagulant drugs.
Zinc	**Dosage:** 25 mg a day. **Advice:** if you take a zinc supplement for more than a month, use one that contains 2 mg copper.
Fish oils	**Dosage:** 2 teaspoons to provide 2 g omega-3 fatty acids a day. **Caution:** consult your doctor if you take anticoagulant drugs. **Advice:** vegetarians can substitute 1 tablespoon of flaxseed oil.
Chasteberry/ false unicorn root	**Dosage:** ½ teaspoon of tincture of each, twice a day. **Caution:** if you find out that you are pregnant, stop taking chasteberry and false unicorn root immediately.

Some dosages may be supplied by supplements you are already taking – see page 195.

The **B complex** vitamins help to maintain a healthy reproductive system. If you become pregnant they will play an essential role in early foetal development: folic acid, in particular, can prevent birth defects. **Vitamin E** is a powerful antioxidant, and reduces levels of free radicals (unstable molecules) which can interfere with the normal functioning of the ovaries and uterus. **Zinc** is necessary for proper cell division – you will need to supplement your copper levels while taking a high dosage of zinc. Omega-3 fatty acids from **fish oils** (or flaxseed oil) support healthy ovarian and uterine function.

If the infertility may be a result of irregular ovulation, try a blend of **chasteberry** (also called vitex) and **false unicorn root** to stimulate the process. Chasteberry has been shown to affect levels of two female hormones – progesterone and prolactin. Low progesterone or high prolactin levels can inhibit ovulation – chasteberry enhances the production of progesterone and suppresses that of prolactin.

What else you can do

☑ Ensure that your diet includes whole grain cereals and oily fish, and at least five portions of fruit and vegetables a day.
☑ Do not smoke. Cigarette smoke reduces fertility and can seriously affect your baby's health and development if you do get pregnant.
☑ Lose weight if you are too heavy, gain it if you are underweight.
☑ Exercise moderately. Strenuous exercise can interfere with ovulation.
☑ Avoid drinking alcohol, or keep your intake to the minimum; drink no more than two cups of caffeinated coffee a day.

Women who drink more than half a cup of black or green tea a day may double their chances of becoming pregnant, according to a recent study. Researchers investigated the effect of caffeine consumption on the fertility of 187 women. Although in this study coffee and caffeine did not seem to affect fertility, researchers could not conclusively rule out a negative impact. They noted that the benefits of tea may be related to some compound in the brew, or it may be that tea drinkers simply have better health habits than coffee drinkers.

FACTS & TIPS

■ Many women use home tests to determine exactly when they are ovulating, but once ovulation does occur, the window of opportunity for conception may already have passed. A study of 221 healthy women aged 25 to 35 found that the peak time for conception is five days before and on the day of ovulation. Intercourse at other times is unlikely to cause pregnancy.

Infertility, male

In every case of infertility there is a 50% chance that the source of the problem lies with the male partner. In certain cases surgery or other medical treatments may be necessary, but safe and gentle natural therapies can often provide the solution.

Symptoms

- *Unsuccessful attempts to cause conception over the period of a year.*

- *In some men, chlamydia or another reproductive-tract infection, which may have left scar tissue blocking the exit of the sperm.*

SEE YOUR DOCTOR ...

- **If you suspect that you are infertile – your doctor can assess the problem and help to uncover any underlying causes. Your partner may also need to be examined, because one or both of you may have fertility problems.**

REMINDER: If you have a medical condition, consult your doctor before taking supplements.

What it is

Doctors recognise infertility as a problem if a man's partner does not become pregnant after a year of unprotected sex with him during the most fertile time of her menstrual cycle. Researchers do not know exactly how many sperm a man needs to be fertile, but they know that the higher the sperm count is, the greater the chances are of conception.

What causes it

Some cases of infertility in men are linked to anatomical defects or scar tissue from a long-healed infection in the reproductive tract, but most of the time the precise cause cannot be identified. Many infertile men have low sperm counts caused by low levels of testosterone, a hormone that stimulates the testes to manufacture sperm. But the number of sperm produced is not the only determinant of fertility; a high percentage of the sperm must be healthy and motile (active), and because sperm are fragile they are easily damaged by naturally occurring unstable molecules called free radicals. Numerous factors can affect levels of both testosterone and free radicals, such as drinking, smoking, poor nutrition and even stress. Some prescription drugs can alter sperm motility and may make conception difficult.

How supplements can help

Surgery is usually the best way to correct anatomical defects, but, for many infertile men, supplements are worth trying. They provide benefits at any age – fertility in men is not age-dependent, unlike female fertility, which declines rapidly after the age of 35. A study of 240 couples undergoing in vitro fertilisation found that sperm collected from men in their sixties was just as lively as that collected from men in their thirties. You will need to take supplements for several months to experience the benefits, and they should be taken in combination with a general multivitamin and multimineral supplement.

Taken together, **vitamin C**, **vitamin E** and mixed **carotenoids** provide a powerful medley of antioxidants that sweep up the cell-damaging free radicals and protect sperm. Vitamin C also increases sperm motility,

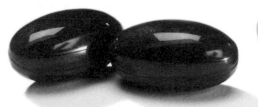

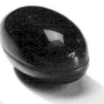

Carotenoid supplements contain a rich blend of sperm-protecting antioxidants.

Vitamin C	**Dosage:** 500 mg twice a day. **Advice:** reduce dose if diarrhoea develops.
Vitamin E	**Dosage:** 250 mg twice a day. **Caution:** consult your doctor if you take anticoagulant drugs.
Carotenoids	**Dosage:** 1 capsule mixed carotenoids twice a day with food. **Advice:** each capsule should supply 15 mg mixed carotenoids.
Zinc	**Dosage:** 25 mg a day. **Advice:** if you take a zinc supplement for more than a month, use one that contains 2 mg copper.
Fish oils	**Dosage:** 2 teaspoons to provide 2 g omega-3 fatty acids a day. **Caution:** consult your doctor if you take anticoagulant drugs. **Advice:** vegetarians can substitute 1 tablespoon flaxseed oil.
Vitamin B$_{12}$	**Dosage:** 1000 mcg once a day. **Advice:** take in the morning, preferably with 400 mg folic acid (a high intake of one can mask a deficiency in the other).
Panax ginseng	**Dosage:** 100-250 mg extract twice a day; rotate with Siberian ginseng. **Advice:** standardised to contain at least 7% ginsenosides.
Siberian ginseng	**Dosage:** 100-300 mg extract twice daily; rotate with Panax ginseng. **Advice:** standardised to contain at least 0.8% eleutherosides.

Some dosages may be supplied by supplements you are already taking – see page 195.

partly by preventing it from clumping together; this vitamin may be especially important for smokers, who tend to have a deficiency of it. **Zinc** plays a crucial role in male reproduction, increasing testosterone production and raising the sperm count. A high dosage of zinc inhibits the body's absorption of copper, which should be taken in combination with it. Omega-3 fatty acids from **fish oils** (or flaxseed oil) encourage healthy sperm and the reproductive tissue. **Vitamin B$_{12}$** is essential to the process of cell division: a deficiency may cause reduced sperm count and motility.

These supplements can be combined with herbal therapies. **Panax ginseng** stimulates testosterone production and sperm formation. Rotate it every three weeks with **Siberian ginseng**, which is also thought to raise the sperm count.

What else you can do

☑ Ensure that your diet includes whole-grain cereals and oily fish, and at least five portions of fruit and vegetables a day.
☑ Avoid alcohol.
☑ Stop smoking.
☑ Try yoga, meditation and other stress-reducing relaxation techniques.
☑ Increase your consumption of soya products (tofu and soya milk, for example) which are high in plant sterols that benefit the health of the prostate gland and improve semen quality.

Inflammatory bowel disease

Painful inflammation of the intestines is characteristic of this chronic condition, which encompasses several related disorders. Symptoms can be eased by dietary changes, vitamin supplements and soothing herbs.

Symptoms

- *At first, constipation and the frequent urge to defecate, with the passage of only small amounts of blood or mucus.*

- *Later, intermittent flare-ups including chronic diarrhoea with rectal bleeding, abdominal pain, a slight fever and general malaise, including arthritis, blurred vision, mouth sores, painful joints, poor appetite, low energy and weight loss.*

- *A severe attack can cause nausea, vomiting, dehydration, heavy sweating, high fever and heart palpitations.*

SEE YOUR DOCTOR ...

- If you have black or bloody stools or suffer from painful, mucus-filled diarrhoea.

- If symptoms suddenly worsen.

- If you have a swollen abdomen or severe pain (especially on the lower-right side) — it may be a sign of appendicitis.

- If severe abdominal pain accompanies a fever with a temperature over 38°C.

REMINDER: *If you have a medical condition, consult your doctor before taking supplements.*

What it is

Inflammatory bowel disease (IBD) is a general term applied to several related disorders, such as Crohn's disease and ulcerative colitis, that often first strike between the ages of 20 and 40. Typically, all or part of the digestive tract becomes chronically inflamed, and begins to develop small erosions or ulcers. Bouts of inflammation are followed by periods of remission lasting for weeks or years. After a decade, sufferers have an increased risk of colo-rectal cancer.

What causes it

Doctors are not sure why people develop IBD, although heredity is thought to play a part — more than a third of IBD sufferers know another family member afflicted with the disease. The condition may be triggered by a bacterium or virus, or by a malfunctioning immune system. Stress, anxiety and sensitivity to certain foods can contribute to flare-ups.

How supplements can help

IBD usually causes a decreased ability to absorb nutrients from food, so a daily high-potency multivitamin is essential. Additional supplements, taken together, may also be beneficial, especially during flare-ups.

Many people with IBD are deficient in B_{12}, folic acid and other B vitamins. Taking **vitamin B complex** replaces lost vitamins and restores proper digestion. **Magnesium** should also be taken, as deficiencies are common among IBD sufferers. **Liquorice (DGL)** has healing properties, as does the anti-inflammatory **vitamin E**. Once symptoms improve, vitamin E can be continued long term, in combination with a high-potency antioxidant such as grape seed extract (100 mg once or twice a day) or quercetin (400 mg a day). Vitamin C (500 mg twice a day) augments the antioxidant benefits of grape seed extract or quercetin.

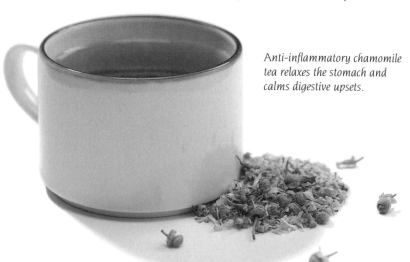

Anti-inflammatory chamomile tea relaxes the stomach and calms digestive upsets.

SUPPLEMENT RECOMMENDATIONS

Vitamin B complex	**Dosage:** one tablet twice a day for flare-ups; then reduce to one tablet each morning for maintenance; take with food. **Advice:** look for a B-50 complex with 50 mcg vitamin B_{12} and biotin, 400 mcg folic acid and 50 mg all other B vitamins.
Magnesium	**Dosage:** 300 mg once a day. **Caution:** do not take magnesium if you have kidney disease.
Vitamin E	**Dosage:** 250 mg twice a day for flare-ups or maintenance. **Caution:** consult your doctor if you take anticoagulant drugs.
Fish oils	**Dosage:** 2 teaspoons to provide 2 g omega-3 fatty acids a day. **Caution:** consult your doctor if you take anticoagulant drugs. **Advice:** vegetarians can substitute 1 tablespoon of flaxseed oil.
Probiotics	**Dosage:** two capsules three times a day on an empty stomach, or two or three pots of bioyoghurt a day. **Advice:** buy acidophilus or bifidus cultures, or a mixture of the two.
Zinc	**Dosage:** 25 mg a day. **Advice:** if you take a zinc supplement for more than a month, use one that includes 2 mg copper.
Liquorice (DGL)	**Dosage:** chew two tablets (380 mg) three times a day, between meals. **Advice:** take during flare-ups; use deglycyrrhizinated (DGL) form only (glycyrrhizin, a key component of liquorice, raises blood pressure).
Chamomile	**Dosage:** one cup of tea up to three times a day. **Advice:** use 2 teaspoons of dried herb per cup.

Note: consider using supplements in blue first; those in black may also be beneficial. Some dosages may be supplied by supplements you are already taking – see page 195.

Other supplements which are also of value when taken on a regular basis include omega-3 fatty acids from **fish oils** (or flaxseed oil), which reduce inflammation and protect and repair the digestive tract, and **probiotics**, which help to restore the normal balance of healthy bacteria in the intestines. **Zinc** supplementation is important – IBD often causes a deficiency. Take this with extra copper, as zinc inhibits its absorption. **Chamomile** tea, a traditional remedy for digestive complaints, may calm some symptoms, and supplements of the amino acid glutamine may have a similar soothing effect.

What else you can do

☑ Determine if certain foods trigger flare-ups and eliminate them from your diet.
☑ Apply a hot-water bottle to the abdomen to prevent cramps.
☑ Minimise stress with yoga, meditation and regular exercise.

RECENT FINDINGS

Italian researchers recently found that fish oils reduce the frequency of intestinal attacks in people with Crohn's disease. Among patients in remission who still had signs of inflammation, only 28% of those taking enteric-coated fish oil capsules relapsed, in contrast with 69% of those taking a placebo.

Nicotine patches may aid remission in cases of ulcerative colitis, according to a small study in America. Of 31 patients who used high-dose nicotine skin patches for four weeks, 12 felt significantly better; only 3 of 33 who wore placebo patches showed improvements. But common side effects included dizziness, nausea and skin rashes, and additional research is needed.

DID YOU KNOW?
More than 50% of people affected by Crohn's disease benefit from a medically supervised exclusion diet which identifies food sensitivities.

FACTS & TIPS

■ The anti-inflammatory drug sulfasalazine, commonly prescribed for IBD, depletes folic acid. If you take this drug, ask your doctor about using a folic acid supplement.

■ Teas made from flaxseed, marshmallow, meadowsweet or slippery elm soothe the intestines. Use 1 or 2 teaspoons per cup, steep for 15 minutes, then strain.

Insect bites and stings

If you go out walking, picnicking or gardening on a summer's afternoon, you can often pay a price for enjoying the open air in the form of insect bites and stings. Fortunately, nature also provides antidotes to the itching and swelling that result.

Symptoms

- *Burning, itching, redness and swelling of the affected area.*

- *Circular red rash, which may develop a few days after a bite.*

- *An allergic reaction (or a non-allergic reaction to multiple stings), including rapid swelling of the eyes, tongue, lips and throat; nausea; irregular heartbeat and difficulty breathing.*

SEE YOUR DOCTOR ...

- **If you receive multiple insect bites or stings. Even if you are not allergic, these can be dangerous.**

- **If you develop a raised, circular red rash, or the area appears ulcerated or infected.**

- **If you experience breathing difficulties, a fever, intense pain or stiffness.**

- **If you have an allergic reaction to an insect bite – get emergency help straightaway. (If you are allergic, carry an emergency kit, available on prescription.)**

REMINDER: If you have a medical condition, consult your doctor before taking supplements.

What they are

During the summer months, and in some climates all year round, people are often bitten by mosquitoes, flies or ticks and stung by ants, bees, wasps or hornets. Insect bites and stings can be itchy and painful, and, although they are not usually serious, some cases may need medical attention. If you are bitten by a tick while abroad, seek medical advice (particularly if a circular red rash develops); in some countries these blood-sucking insects can be carriers of diseases.

If you belong to the minority of people (approximately one in 50) who develop an allergic reaction to the venom of bees or other insects, seek medical treatment immediately if you are bitten or stung.

What causes them

Insect venom contains toxins that cause burning, swelling and itching at the site of the bite or sting. Although mosquitoes, horse flies and ticks bite to get blood for nourishment, wasps and bees are likely to attack only when threatened, though bees may sting if they mistake you for a flower. Your chances of getting stung increase if you wave your arms wildly when a bee or wasp buzzes around you, or if you wear bright colours or perfume, or eat sweet, sticky foods outdoors. There is also a good chance of being bitten by ants if you sit down too close to a nest: woodland and moorland ants are particularly likely to attack.

How supplements can help

Before taking any supplements, remove the sting, if there is one, and wash the area with soap and water. The first remedy to try is **bromelain**, a protein-digesting enzyme obtained from pineapple, which can reduce swelling; use until symptoms subside. Topical treatments can ease pain and itching, and also help the skin to heal: **lavender oil** soothes itching;

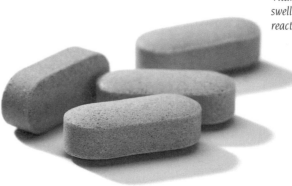

Vitamin C reduces the swelling caused by the body's reaction to insect stings.

Bromelain	**Dosage:** 500 mg three times a day, on an empty stomach, until symptoms subside. **Advice:** should provide 6000 GDU or 9000 MCU daily.
Lavender oil	**Dosage:** apply a few drops to the skin several times a day, or as needed. **Advice:** use 1 or 2 drops every 15 minutes if necessary.
Calendula cream	**Dosage:** rub a small amount into the skin several times a day, or as needed. **Advice:** standardised to contain at least 2% calendula.
Vitamin C	**Dosage:** 500 mg twice a day. **Advice:** reduce dose if diarrhoea develops.
Quercetin	**Dosage:** 500 mg three times a day, 20 minutes before meals. **Advice:** works well in combination with bromelain.
Tea tree oil	**Dosage:** apply 1 drop to the skin several times a day, or as needed. **Advice:** discontinue use if skin irritation develops.

Note: consider using supplements in blue first; the one in black may also be beneficial. Some dosages may be supplied by supplements you are already taking – see page 195.

calendula cream, made from a flower in the marigold family, mitigates swelling and itching, and has an antiseptic effect which helps to prevent infection; and **tea tree oil** can be substituted for calendula.

If you have been stung by a bee or a similar insect, you may need to take additional supplements to control the swelling and relieve pain. **Vitamin C** and the flavonoid **quercetin** are antihistamines – they inhibit the release of histamine, an inflammatory compound produced by the body in response to insect venom. Begin taking both supplements as soon as possible after a sting and continue until the symptoms subside.

Tinctures of echinacea, marigold, myrrh or St John's wort applied directly to the skin may also help to alleviate the effects of bites.

What else you can do

☑ Use insect repellent before leaving home. Citronella oil and tea tree oil are good natural repellents – rub them directly onto the skin.

☑ Do not wear aftershave, hair spray, perfume or sweet-smelling creams – the scent will attract insects.

☑ Do not try to swat insects. If insects swarm nearby, walk away calmly or lie down and cover your head.

FACTS & TIPS

■ Although most essential oils should not be applied directly to the skin, lavender oil is an exception. Rub it into the affected area, but keep it well away from the eyes.

■ For quick relief for a bite or sting, apply bromelain topically in place of lavender oil. Open two capsules and mix the powder with just enough water to make a paste. Smooth it onto the affected area.

Insomnia

About 15% of people in the UK are affected by insomnia at any one time. While you are trying to identify the cause – which may be anything from anxiety to an uncomfortable bed – a variety of safe, natural remedies can help you to drift off to sleep without the risk of side effects.

Symptoms

- *Difficulty falling asleep.*
- *Inability to stay asleep.*
- *Repeatedly waking up too early.*

SEE YOUR DOCTOR ...

- **If insomnia lasts a month or more with no obvious cause.**

- **If sleeping problems follow a traumatic event, such as the loss of a job or a loved one.**

- **If you feel tired most of the time and frequently doze off during the day.**

- **If you are so tired that you cannot function normally.**

REMINDER: If you have a medical condition, consult your doctor before taking supplements.

What it is

Many people think of insomnia as an inability to fall asleep. It also encompasses an inability to stay asleep and/or repeatedly waking up earlier than planned. Sleep problems that last a couple of nights or a few weeks are often related to stress or excitement, but in some cases insomnia can become chronic, lasting for months or even years.

What causes it

Insomnia is considered a symptom of many underlying and often hard-to-recognise conditions or situations. Dietary and lifestyle factors, a major illness, medication, physical pain and even a bad mattress can all contribute to sleeplessness. For most people, tension, anxiety and depression lie at the root of insomnia. Discovering the basic cause or causes of your sleep problems may take some detective work, but it is ultimately the best way to bring about a cure.

How supplements can help

The supplements listed should provide immediate relief from insomnia. Unless otherwise stated, most can be used together, and should be taken about 45 minutes before retiring. First, try one remedy at a time to see whether it works for you.

Numerous studies have found that **valerian** – one of the most researched of all herbal supplements – is an effective sleep aid. It works better for some people when combined with other sedating

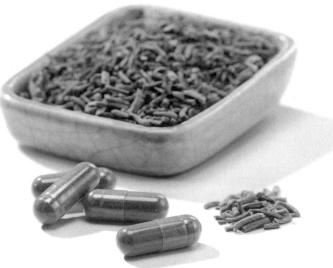

Teas or capsules containing the dried roots of the sedative herb valerian relieve tension and induce natural sleep.

Valerian	**Dosage:** 250-500 mg extract. **Advice:** take before going to bed – start with the lower dose and increase as needed; use as an alternative to 5-HTP.
Calcium/ magnesium	**Dosage:** 500 mg calcium and 250 mg magnesium. **Advice:** take before going to bed, with food; sometimes sold as a single supplement.
Vitamin B$_6$/ niacin	**Dosage:** 50 mg B$_6$ and 500 mg nicotinamide (niacin). **Advice:** take together before going to bed.
Chamomile	**Dosage:** 2 teaspoons of dried herb in a cup of tea. **Advice:** mild enough to use each evening with other sedating supplements.
5-HTP	**Dosage:** 100 mg before going to bed. **Advice:** especially useful when combined with B$_6$ or magnesium; an alternative to herbal extracts such as valerian.

Note: consider using supplements in blue first; those in black may also be beneficial. Some dosages may be supplied by supplements you are already taking – see page 195.

More than 200 scientific studies have found valerian effective against insomnia. A group of Swiss researchers recently reported that people who took the herb fell asleep faster and stayed asleep longer than those given a placebo.

A 16-week study of 43 healthy adults (aged 50 to 76) with moderate sleep problems, published in the *Journal of the American Medical Association*, concluded that up to 40 minutes of vigorous walking four times a week helped participants not only to fall asleep but also to sleep soundly through the night.

DID YOU KNOW?
One reason why many people feel tired after Christmas lunch is that turkey is especially rich in the amino acid tryptophan, a natural sleep inducer.

FACTS & TIPS

■ Avoid taking natural sleep aids alongside conventional sedative drugs; excessive drowsiness may result.

■ Avoid stimulating herbs that keep you awake, such as ginseng, guarana, kola nut and ginger.

■ Health authorities in Germany and other countries recognise chamomile, valerian and other herbal sedatives as medications. They are often prescribed by doctors and covered by health insurance.

herbs such as **chamomile** and passionflower. These herbs, taken as capsules, tablets, teas or tinctures, promote relaxation and reduce stress, making it easier to fall asleep.

In some instances a nutrient deficiency, particularly a lack of **calcium**, **magnesium** or **vitamin B$_6$**, can lead to sleep problems; replenishing these nutrients often eases the problem. The B vitamin **niacin**, taken with B$_6$, helps to ease anxiety (niacin should be bought in the form of nicotinamide). It may be helpful to try magnesium or B$_6$ along with **5-HTP** (5-hydroxytryptophan) – a derivative of the amino acid tryptophan, which raises levels of the sleep-inducing chemical, serotonin. 5-HTP is a good alternative to herbal remedies.

Other plants still commonly used to aid sleep include Californian poppy, hops, lemon balm, lime flowers, vervain and wild lettuce. Add 200 ml of boiling water to about 10 grams of your chosen dried herb or a mixture of the herbs, infuse for 10 minutes and strain. Drink before retiring. Tablets of St John's wort may also be helpful for some people.

What else you can do

☑ Stick to a regular sleep schedule, even at weekends.
☑ Use your bed only for sleeping, not for reading or watching television.
☑ Exercise regularly (though not in the evening) to help reduce stress.
☑ Avoid alcohol, caffeine and tobacco.
☑ Try meditation, during the day and before retiring.
☑ Before going to bed have a leisurely hot bath containing 10 drops of lavender oil.
☑ Have a bedtime drink of hot milk sweetened with honey.
☑ Try sleeping on a pillow filled with relaxing herbs.

Irritable bowel syndrome

Though 20% of adults suffer a few symptoms of irritable bowel syndrome, tests often find no physical abnormalities. Many of those who resign themselves to living with the discomfort find that natural remedies bring welcome relief.

Symptoms

- Constipation, diarrhoea or alternating bouts of each (usually after meals) for several months.

- Abdominal cramping, often relieved by a bowel movement.

- Mucus in the stools.

- Intestinal gas and bloating.

SEE YOUR DOCTOR ...

- If you have abdominal pain accompanied by any changes in defecation patterns or stool consistency.

- If the abdominal pain is continuous, or severe and accompanied by a fever.

- If there is blood in your stools.

- If you lose weight without intending to do so.

REMINDER: If you have a medical condition, consult your doctor before taking supplements.

What it is

Food is propelled through the digestive tract by rhythmic contractions of the intestinal muscles – a process known as peristalsis. In irritable bowel syndrome (IBS) the muscles go into spasm and the contractions become uncoordinated. This disturbance can cause the contents of the intestines to move too fast or too slowly, leading to abdominal pain and diarrhoea or constipation.

What causes it

Over the years researchers have proposed many causes for IBS, none of which has been proved. The list of suspects includes bacterial, parasitic or viral infections, the overuse of antibiotics, lactose intolerance or adverse reactions to foods such as wheat or broccoli. Some researchers believe that people with IBS have highly sensitive smooth muscle tissue, not only in the gastrointestinal tract but also elsewhere in the body. Others believe that the condition results from inflammation in the lining of the intestine. One underlying factor in almost all cases of IBS is stress, which aggravates the symptoms. Because no one is sure exactly what undermines healthy bowel function, doctors tend to diagnose IBS by eliminating other ailments with similar symptoms, such as diverticular disorders or inflammatory bowel disease.

How supplements can help

Natural supplements are effective in controlling many of the symptoms of IBS. Those listed here can be combined with one another or with conventional drugs. **Peppermint oil** capsules – enteric-coated to ensure that the oil passes through the stomach into the intestine before being released – are very effective in calming the spasms that cause abdominal

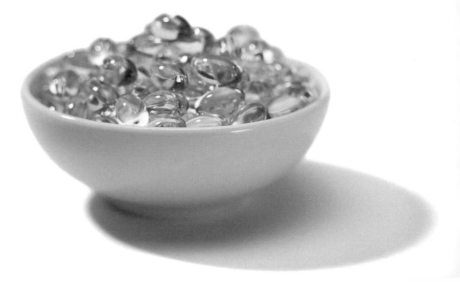

The oil from the leaf and stem of the peppermint plant – in capsule or liquid form – helps to prevent intestinal spasms.

SUPPLEMENT RECOMMENDATIONS

Peppermint oil — **Dosage:** 1 or 2 capsules three times a day between meals.
Advice: buy enteric-coated capsules with 0.2 ml of oil each; start at the lower dose and increase if necessary.

Psyllium — **Dosage:** 1-3 tablespoons of powder dissolved in water or juice a day.
Advice: drink eight glasses of water throughout the day.

Probiotics — **Dosage:** 2 capsules three times a day on an empty stomach, or two or three pots of bioyoghurt a day.
Advice: buy acidophilus or bifidus cultures, or a mixture of the two.

FOS — **Dosage:** 2000 mg a day.
Advice: take in combination with probiotics; not effective for IBS when used alone.

Some dosages may be supplied by supplements you are already taking – see page 195.

pain, and also soothe other symptoms. In a study of 110 people with IBS the capsules reduced abdominal pain in 79% of those taking them. Virtually no adverse reactions were seen.

Psyllium, a type of dietary fibre, eases IBS symptoms for many people – although not for all. In most cases, it works to correct constipation, and is useful in combating diarrhoea because it absorbs water in the intestine and adds bulk to the stool (bulk also seems to lessen the severity of spasms). Drink extra water when using psyllium. If you find that it aggravates your symptoms, stop taking it.

Probiotics are cultures of the 'friendly' bacteria that normally inhabit the intestine. They help to digest food and prevent the unchecked growth of harmful bacteria. **FOS** (fructo-oligosaccharides) – indigestible carbohydrates that feed the friendly bacteria – are sometimes added to probiotic supplements, but can also be bought separately.

Other useful herbs which can be used to make soothing teas include marshmallow, slippery elm and agrimony – an astringent which stimulates digestive secretions. Supplements of glutamine, an amino acid, can also calm inflamed tissue.

What else you can do

☑ Add more high-fibre foods, such as fruit, vegetables, grains and beans, to your diet, but do this gradually to minimise bloating and wind. Eating plenty of these foods may eliminate the need for psyllium.

☑ Eat smaller, more frequent meals. Limit your intake of alcohol, caffeine and foods high in fat.

☑ Take control of stress. Relaxation techniques or biofeedback may help.

☑ Exercise for at least 20 minutes a day to keep the bowels moving normally and reduce stress.

☑ With the help of your doctor, try an elimination diet: stop eating foods that you think may cause you problems, and add them back one at a time over several weeks to identify which, if any, cause symptoms.

FACTS & TIPS

■ Lactose intolerance (a sensitivity to the sugars in milk products) may trigger IBS symptoms. The ability to digest lactose often declines with age because of a decrease in the amount of the enzyme lactase in the small intestine. To find out if this is your problem, drink a small glass of skimmed milk on an empty stomach. If you notice wind, diarrhoea, pain or bloating within four hours, repeat the test with soya milk – if no symptoms occur, you are probably sensitive to dairy products.

Kidney disorders

Our kidneys rid the body of waste and can become overloaded by toxins or drugs, or as a result of certain disorders. Kidney stones and infections are potentially very serious and need medical attention – supplements may help to prevent their occurrence.

Symptoms

- *Fluid retention.*
- *Nausea or vomiting.*
- *Loss of appetite.*
- *Pain between the upper back and the lower abdomen and groin.*
- *Pus or blood in urine.*

What they are

Kidney stones are caused by an accumulation of mineral salts which become crystallised in the urinary tract, and vary in size from tiny specks to lumps big enough to block the urinary flow. Calcium oxalate stones are the most common. Three other types are formed by uric acid, the amino acid cystine, and struvite (consisting of phosphates).

Kidney diseases include inflammation of the organs' filtering units (known as glomerulonephritis, or Bright's disease) or kidney infection (pyelonephritis) – both serious conditions. Glomerulonephritis may result in the loss of blood protein in the urine; it may be associated with high blood pressure and water retention in the tissues. Only one good kidney is needed for optimal health, so kidney disease is not normally life-threatening, but kidney failure is a very serious condition.

What causes them

A typical Western diet high in refined foods and animal protein is a major cause of kidney stones, although a hereditary predisposition, depressed immunity or the poor functioning of calcium-regulating glands may be implicated. Refined carbohydrates and sugar increase insulin production, which causes the excretion of higher levels of calcium. When the intake of fluid is inadequate, excessive sweating or dehydration can also cause concentrated urine in which urinary salts can become solidified.

Uric acid stones form when not enough urine is excreted or when there is too much uric acid in the blood. They are often linked with gout. Stones composed of the amino acid cystine are brought about by a rare congenital defect. Struvite stones are caused by infection – often in the urinary tract. It is critical to have the type of stone identified before it can be decided which natural therapy is the most appropriate.

The disease glomerulonephritis is caused by an immunological reaction to infection. The kidneys can become infected when the flow of urine further down the urinary tract becomes blocked and the infectious

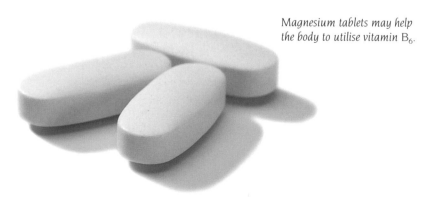

Magnesium tablets may help the body to utilise vitamin B$_6$.

Magnesium	**Dosage:** 400 mg daily. **Caution:** do not take in cases of kidney failure.
Vitamin B$_6$	**Dosage:** 50 mg twice daily. **Advice:** when taken with magnesium it can decrease oxalate excretion.
Dandelion leaf	**Dosage:** drink two pints of dandelion leaf tea daily. **Advice:** stimulates excretion of uric acid.
Vitamin C	**Dosage:** 500 mg twice a day. **Advice:** reduce dose if diarrhoea develops.
Vitamin E	**Dosage:** 250 mg a day. **Caution:** consult your doctor if you take anticoagulant drugs.
Ginkgo biloba	**Dosage:** 80 mg extract three times a day. **Advice:** standardised to contain 24% ginkgo flavone glycosides.
Cranberry	**Dosage:** 400 mg extract twice a day. **Advice:** alternatively, drink 500 ml of unsweetened juice a day.

Some dosages may be supplied by supplements you are already taking – see page 195.

agents spread back from the bladder. Problems can also arise from drug use, diabetes or shock, which can all cause protein in the urine. High blood pressure can be a cause or a result of kidney disease.

How supplements can help

Patients given **magnesium** and **vitamin B$_6$** have been found to excrete much lower amounts of oxalate, and these supplements may be useful in preventing and healing oxalate stones. If uric acid stones are being formed, **dandelion leaf** tea may promote urinary excretion of uric acid. The toxic free radicals generated in glomerulonephritis are reduced by **vitamin C**, **vitamin E** and **ginkgo biloba** – powerful antioxidants which can improve kidney health. Gingko biloba is anti-inflammatory and can boost blood supply to the kidneys by helping to prevent atherosclerosis. **Cranberry** prevents adhesion of bacteria to the linings of the urinary tract and may help in reducing infections. Extract of artichoke has been shown to have a cleansing and detoxifying effect. A study in Japan showed that spirulina can decrease toxicity in the kidneys caused by certain drugs.

What else you can do

☑ To avoid calcium oxalate stones: omit foods containing oxalic acid such as spinach, rhubarb, chocolate, peanuts and strawberries; reduce consumption of protein-rich animal products; increase consumption of leafy vegetables (other than spinach), as vitamin K may be protective.
☑ To avoid uric acid stones: reduce foods rich in purines, which are metabolised to uric acid, including red meats, seafood and asparagus.
☑ To avoid struvite stones: antibiotic therapy may be necessary, but the infections that cause them can be reduced by cranberry extract or juice, and by herbal teas such as corn silk, elderflower and marshmallow leaf, used singly or in combination.

Kidney stones are often caused by excess calcium, so patients are traditionally recommended to decrease their intake of milk, but research by Washington State University shows that milk and milk products may actually help to prevent the formation of kidney stones.

DID YOU KNOW?
Kidney stones are ten times more common in the UK today than they were at the beginning of the 20th century.

FACTS & TIPS

■ Bacteria may play a key role in the formation of kidney stones. Finnish research shows that instead of accounting for between 10% and 15% of cases, as was previously thought, bacteria may be responsible for as many as 90%. Antibiotics may therefore offer a useful treatment for stones.

■ Once kidney stones have formed there is a 20-50% chance that they will recur. A vegetarian, high-fibre diet that includes a minimal amount of animal proteins and processed foods may help to prevent recurrence.

■ Diabetic kidney disease, known as nephropathy, makes up 42% of new cases of advanced kidney disease in the UK. It is also the fastest growing cause of kidney dialysis and transplantation, accounting for over 100,000 cases a year.

Later life

It is never too late to benefit from adopting a healthier lifestyle, and, whatever your age, nutritional supplements have a positive role to play in maintaining the body in good condition.

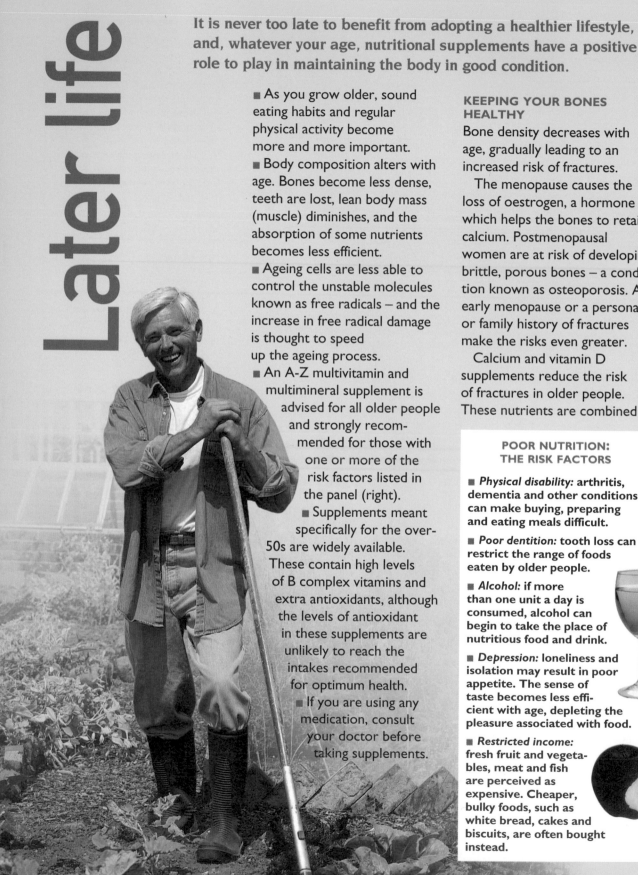

■ As you grow older, sound eating habits and regular physical activity become more and more important.

■ Body composition alters with age. Bones become less dense, teeth are lost, lean body mass (muscle) diminishes, and the absorption of some nutrients becomes less efficient.

■ Ageing cells are less able to control the unstable molecules known as free radicals – and the increase in free radical damage is thought to speed up the ageing process.

■ An A-Z multivitamin and multimineral supplement is advised for all older people and strongly recommended for those with one or more of the risk factors listed in the panel (right).

■ Supplements meant specifically for the over-50s are widely available. These contain high levels of B complex vitamins and extra antioxidants, although the levels of antioxidant in these supplements are unlikely to reach the intakes recommended for optimum health.

■ If you are using any medication, consult your doctor before taking supplements.

KEEPING YOUR BONES HEALTHY

Bone density decreases with age, gradually leading to an increased risk of fractures.

The menopause causes the loss of oestrogen, a hormone which helps the bones to retain calcium. Postmenopausal women are at risk of developing brittle, porous bones – a condition known as osteoporosis. An early menopause or a personal or family history of fractures make the risks even greater.

Calcium and vitamin D supplements reduce the risk of fractures in older people. These nutrients are combined

POOR NUTRITION: THE RISK FACTORS

■ *Physical disability:* arthritis, dementia and other conditions can make buying, preparing and eating meals difficult.

■ *Poor dentition:* tooth loss can restrict the range of foods eaten by older people.

■ *Alcohol:* if more than one unit a day is consumed, alcohol can begin to take the place of nutritious food and drink.

■ *Depression:* loneliness and isolation may result in poor appetite. The sense of taste becomes less efficient with age, depleting the pleasure associated with food.

■ *Restricted income:* fresh fruit and vegetables, meat and fish are perceived as expensive. Cheaper, bulky foods, such as white bread, cakes and biscuits, are often bought instead.

with magnesium in 'bone formula' preparations. Regular weight-bearing exercise also helps to maintain bone mass.

HEALTHY DIET CHECKLIST
To maintain good health as you grow older, include the following foods in your diet:
■ Fruit and vegetables for fibre, phytochemicals and vitamins.
■ Wholegrain products such as wholemeal bread for energy.
■ Meat, lentils, fortified breakfast cereals and well-cooked eggs for iron.
■ Dairy foods for calcium.
■ Foods rich in vitamin D, such as canned sardines and pilchards, margarines fortified with vitamin D, and evaporated or dried milk.
■ Two portions a week of oily fish such as sardines and mackerel, for essential fatty acids.
■ To avoid dehydration and prevent constipation, drink plenty of fluids.

THE ROLE OF VITAMINS AND MINERALS
The vitamins and minerals that play a particularly important part in maintaining the good health of older people are described below, and recommended daily intakes are given in the table.

ANTIOXIDANT VITAMINS
Vitamins C and E and beta-carotene 'mop up' unstable free radicals which damage body cells. A high intake is thought to help prevent heart disease, cancer and cataracts. Vitamin E also improves immune function.

NUTRIENTS FOR HEALTHY AGEING
Except for vitamin D, Reference Nutrient Intake (RNI) values for the over-50s are the same as for the under-50s. Higher intakes may be needed in older people because of a reduced absorption of nutrients.

ANTIOXIDANT VITAMINS
Daily RNIs
■ *Vitamin C:* 40 mg
■ *Vitamin E:* No RNI; Safe Intake about 10 mg, depending on intake of polyunsaturated fats.
Recommended optimum levels
■ *Vitamin C:* 200 mg
■ *Vitamin E:* 100 mg
■ *Mixed caretonoids:* 15 mg

ANTIOXIDANT MINERALS
Daily RNIs
■ *Zinc:* men 9.5 mg; women 7 mg
■ *Selenium:* men 75 mcg; women 60 mcg
Recommended optimum levels
■ *Zinc:* 15 mg
■ *Selenium:* 75 mcg
■ *Mixed caretonoids:* 15 mg

CALCIUM
Daily RNI
700 mg

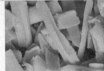

VITAMIN D
Daily RNI
10 mcg for over-65s

B VITAMINS
Daily RNIs
■ B_2: men 1.3 mcg; women 1.1mg
■ B_6: men 1.4 mg; women 1.2 mg
■ B_{12}: 1.5 mcg
■ *Folic acid:* 200 mcg
Recommended optimum levels
■ *As RNIs*

ANTIOXIDANT MINERALS
Institutionalised elderly people are at risk of zinc deficiency, which can depress the immune system and prolong wound healing. Dietary intake of selenium has been shown to be insufficient in all age groups. Selenium helps to protect all the body's tissues against free radical damage, and maintains healthy skin, hair and eyesight.

CALCIUM
Because calcium builds bones, intake should be maintained above the recommended levels throughout life to ensure good skeletal health later in life.

B VITAMINS
Vitamin B_{12} maintains the protective outer covering of the nerves, and low levels can lead to neurological problems.

The body uses folic acid for blood formation and cell metabolism. Low levels of folic acid, vitamin B_6 or B_{12} increase the risk of heart disease. Metabolism of folic acid can be affected by anti-inflammatories and diuretics, and people on these medications for long periods should take a daily supplement. Depression in the elderly, often associated with a lack of folic acid, can be helped by a daily supplement.

VITAMIN D
Vitamin D helps the body to absorb calcium and phosphorus, minerals required for bone formation. It is produced when the skin is exposed to the sun — a process that becomes less efficient with age. Older people also spend less time in the sunshine than the young.

Liver disorders

Early diagnosis of a liver disorder can save your life. Though some hepatitis viruses cause an acute but temporary flu-like illness, others can produce a chronic, persistent liver infection. Natural therapies aim to protect the liver and boost the immune system.

Symptoms

- Fatigue and weakness; a general feeling of poor health.

- Temperature.

- Nausea and vomiting; loss of appetite; weight loss.

- Aching muscles or joints.

- Abdominal discomfort, pain, or swelling.

- Jaundice (yellowish tinge of skin and whites of eyes).

- Dark urine and pale stools.

SEE YOUR DOCTOR ...

- If you think you have been exposed to hepatitis, either through contaminated food or water or by sexual contact with an infected person.

- If you develop lingering flu-like symptoms. During its acute phase, viral hepatitis so closely resembles flu that it is often misdiagnosed.

- If you develop jaundice or other symptoms of hepatitis.

REMINDER: If you have a medical condition, consult your doctor before taking supplements.

What they are

Among the numerous functions of the liver are the metabolism of carbohydrates, fats and proteins, the elimination of toxins and the storage of certain nutrients. The most common disorder to affect this vital organ is hepatitis, or inflammation of the liver. Of the two forms of hepatitis, acute and chronic, the first is easier to treat. Hepatitis can be caused by any of six viruses known as A, B, C, D, E and G. Hepatitis A, the most common form, is highly contagious, and produces acute flu-like symptoms, but usually causes no long-lasting damage. Hepatitis B and C can linger for years, often causing few or no symptoms, but in some cases leading to irreversible liver scarring (cirrhosis) or liver cancer. The types D, E and G are rare.

All forms of hepatitis impair the liver's ability to process proteins and carbohydrates, to secrete fat-digesting bile and to rid the body of toxins and waste – but the chronic forms are the most dangerous, because they may ultimately lead to liver failure.

What causes them

Whether contracted through contaminated food or water (type A) or through blood transfusions, infected hypodermic needles or sexual intercourse (types B and C), hepatitis is most often caused by a viral infection. It can also be caused by certain medications, toxic chemicals or years of alcohol abuse. Rarely, an autoimmune dysfunction – in which the immune system attacks the body's own tissues – is to blame. Sometimes no cause can be determined.

How supplements can help

The recommended supplements should be used together, along with conventional drugs, until symptoms of acute hepatitis subside. Benefits may be noticed within a week. For chronic disease, take them long term.

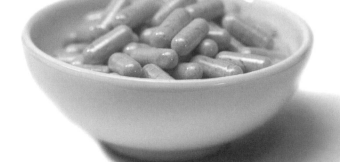

Capsules of the liver-protecting herb milk thistle help to improve the function of this key organ.

Vitamin C and **vitamin E** are powerful antioxidants that act together to help to protect liver cells against damage from free radicals; **alpha-lipoic acid** also provides antioxidant protection, and may enhance the potency of these vitamins. The action of antioxidant vitamins may be augmented by drinking at least four cups of green tea every day. Not only does the herb **milk thistle** protect the liver, it also promotes the growth of new liver cells and improves liver function.

Other liver-protecting herbs are **liquorice**, which contains antiviral and antioxidant compounds, and **dandelion root**. Dandelion works well as part of a liver-detoxifying formula called a **lipotropic combination** (which also includes the B vitamins choline and inositol, as well as milk thistle) – a blend thought to speed the flow of bile and cell-damaging toxins away from the liver. Optimal liver function is dependent upon adequate magnesium intake. People on diets high in refined foods, which tend to be low in magnesium, may benefit from a magnesium supplement (250 mg daily).

What else you can do

☑ Be cautious about what you eat and drink when travelling in areas of poor sanitation and high disease rates: eat only cooked foods, drink bottled water, and be wary of medical or dental treatment in such areas.

☑ Don't drink alcohol, especially during, and for a month after, an acute illness, or until your doctor says your liver function tests are normal.

☑ Ensure that disposable or sterilised needles are used if you undergo acupuncture, body piercing, tattooing or similar procedures.

Lupus

A butterfly-shaped facial rash may be the first sign of this autoimmune disease in which the immune system mistakenly attacks healthy cells. Various forms of therapy can help to ease symptoms, delay the progression of this disease and boost overall health.

Symptoms

- Joint pain and inflammation, skin rashes, a fever, fatigue, chest pain or cough, hair loss, strong tendency to sunburn, blurred vision and swollen glands.

- There are many other symptoms, because lupus can affect almost any part of the body. Symptoms typically first appear between the ages of 15 and 35. Proper diagnosis may be difficult.

SEE YOUR DOCTOR ...

- If you experience any lingering unexplained illness, especially if symptoms include a fever, joint pain, weight loss, rashes or breathing difficulties. Seek an accurate diagnosis, which may take some persistence, as soon as possible.

REMINDER: If you have a medical condition, consult your doctor before taking supplements.

What it is

A chronic inflammatory disease marked by flare-ups and remissions, lupus has been called the 'great impostor' because it can cause such a wide array of symptoms in almost any part of the body, including the skin, joints, heart, brain and kidneys. Women are affected eight to ten times more frequently than men.

What causes it

When lupus strikes, the immune system goes awry and produces abnormal cells that travel through the body, attacking healthy tissues. It is not clear what causes the condition, although heredity, sex hormones or infections may play a role. A variety of stimuli – including sunlight, childbirth, stress and drugs – may trigger an attack.

How supplements can help

A wide array of supplements, taken together on a long-term basis, may relieve symptoms, slow down the progression of the disease and lessen the need for conventional drugs, which frequently have serious side effects. All the supplements can be used with conventional prescription drugs for lupus, but because it is a serious disease they should be taken only under medical supervision. Benefits may be noticed within a month.

Vitamin B complex works throughout the body to maintain the health of skin, mucous membranes, blood, nerves and joints. Along with **vitamins C** and **E** and **selenium** – all antioxidants – B-complex vitamins can speed up healing and help to protect the heart and blood vessels, joints, skin and other areas that can be damaged by the inflammatory process of lupus. Vitamin E may be particularly effective for skin and joint problems. Omega-3 fatty acids (from **fish oils**,

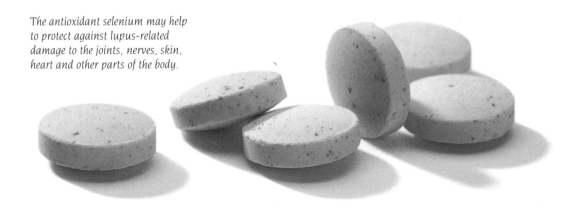

The antioxidant selenium may help to protect against lupus-related damage to the joints, nerves, skin, heart and other parts of the body.

SUPPLEMENT RECOMMENDATIONS

Vitamin B complex	**Dosage:** one tablet each morning with food. **Advice:** look for a B-50 complex with 50 mcg vitamin B_{12} and biotin, 400 mcg folic acid and 50 mg all other B vitamins.
Vitamin C/ vitamin E	**Dosage:** 500 mg vitamin C twice a day; 250 mg vitamin E daily. **Advice:** vitamin C helps to boost the effects of vitamin E.
Fish oils	**Dosage:** 2 teaspoons to supply 2 grams of omega-3 fatty acids a day. **Caution:** consult your doctor if you take anticoagulant drugs. **Advice:** vegetarians can substitute 1 tablespoon of flaxseed oil.
Evening primrose oil	**Dosage:** 1000 mg three times a day. **Advice:** you can substitute 1000 mg borage oil once a day.
Selenium	**Dosage:** 200 mcg a day. **Caution:** do not exceed the recommended dose; higher doses may be toxic.
Zinc	**Dosage:** 25 mg a day. **Advice:** if you take a zinc supplement for more than a month, choose one that includes 2 mg copper.

Note: consider using supplements in blue first; those in black may also be beneficial. Some dosages may be supplied by supplements you are already taking – see page 195.

flaxseed oil or **evening primrose oil**) may be beneficial as well. These can limit inflammation in the joints, kidneys, skin and other areas; they may also lower cholesterol levels, which might be elevated. **Zinc** promotes healing and, along with vitamin C, may help to regulate the immune system. Zinc depletes copper stores, so it should be taken with that mineral when used long term.

Herbal practitioners have found that lime flowers, burdock, gotu kola and wild yam can be helpful for relieving the symptoms of lupus; they can be taken singly or in combination. Add 200 ml of boiling water to about 10 grams of dried herb and infuse for ten minutes before straining; drink once or twice a day. When lupus is accompanied by cold hands and feet caused by Raynaud's disease, ginkgo biloba may be helpful; take 80 mg of extract three times a day.

What else you can do

☑ Minimise exposure to sunlight and, when you are out of doors, use high-SPF sunscreens.

☑ Get plenty of rest. Join a support group to help to reduce stress.

RECENT FINDINGS

Preliminary studies indicate a connection between lower-than-average blood levels of three nutrients – vitamins A and E and beta-carotene – and the development, years later, of lupus. Additional studies are needed to determine whether these levels contributed to the onset of lupus or if they were a result of early, undiagnosed disease activity.

DID YOU KNOW?

Lupus sufferers may want to avoid alfalfa (lucerne) in any form – including sprouts, seeds, tablets and tea. It contains a substance called canavanine, which has been linked with flare-ups.

FACTS & TIPS

■ Conventional lupus drugs, including high doses of steroids and cancer drugs, can have side effects as bad as the disease itself, causing weakened bones, cataracts, diabetes and other serious problems. Supplements may allow you to use lower – and therefore safer – doses of such drugs.

Macular degeneration

This condition, caused by the deterioration of part of the retina, is the commonest cause of blindness in people over 50. Getting plenty of antioxidants – potent protectors of the body's cells – appears to be a key factor in preventing the disorder.

Symptoms

- A *blurry, grey or blank spot in the centre of the field of vision; peripheral vision remains sharp in one or both eyes.*

- *Distorted vision, in which straight lines look wavy, printed words seem blurred or objects appear to be the wrong size or shape.*

- *Faded or washed-out colours.*

SEE YOUR DOCTOR ...

- **If you develop any of the above symptoms – if necessary, you will be referred to an ophthalmologist.**

REMINDER: If you have a medical condition, consult your doctor before taking supplements.

What it is

In macular degeneration the macula – the light-sensitive area in the centre of the retina that controls the central visual field and the ability to see colours – breaks down and impairs the eyesight. Although peripheral vision (the ability to see the outside edges of the scene being looked at) remains intact, the centre of the field of vision is blurry, grey or filled with a large blank spot. As a result it may become difficult or impossible to read, drive and watch television – or even to recognise someone's face.

There are two forms of this disorder. In age-related, or 'dry', macular degeneration the macula thins, and bits of debris gather beneath it. The condition develops slowly and accounts for 90% of all cases. In haemorrhagic, or 'wet', macular degeneration new blood vessels grow underneath the retina, pushing up like the roots of a tree cracking the pavement above. These fragile vessels often leak fluid and blood, causing scar tissue to form and central vision to deteriorate rapidly.

What causes it

Damage from free radicals, the unstable oxygen molecules that can harm cells, is probably the leading cause of macular degeneration. A diet high in saturated fats, tobacco smoke and exposure to sunlight can lead to the formation of free radicals in the retina. High blood pressure, heart disease and diabetes may also be contributing factors because they limit blood flow to the eyes.

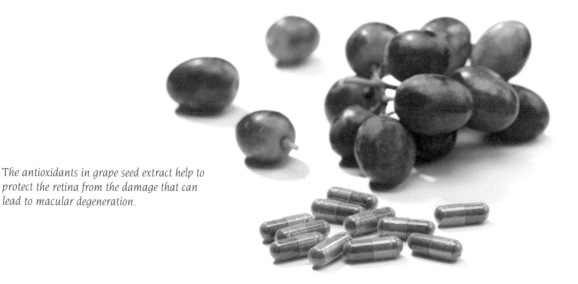

The antioxidants in grape seed extract help to protect the retina from the damage that can lead to macular degeneration.

Vitamin C	**Dosage:** 500 mg twice a day. **Advice:** reduce dosage if diarrhoea develops.
Vitamin E	**Dosage:** 250 mg twice a day. **Caution:** consult your doctor if you take anticoagulant drugs.
Lutein	**Dosage:** 15 mg a day with food. **Advice:** benefits may take six months to two years to develop.
Zinc	**Dosage:** 25 mg a day. **Advice:** if you take a zinc supplement for more than a month, choose one that includes 2 mg copper.
Bilberry	**Dosage:** 80 mg extract three times a day. **Advice:** standardised to contain 25% anthocyanidins.
Grape seed extract	**Dosage:** 100 mg twice a day. **Advice:** standardised to contain 92%-95% proanthocyanidins.
Ginkgo biloba	**Dosage:** 40 mg extract three times a day. **Advice:** standardised to contain at least 24% flavone glycosides.
Selenium	**Dosage:** 200 mcg a day. **Caution:** do not exceed the recommended dose; higher doses may be toxic.

Note: consider using supplements in blue first; those in black may also be beneficial. Some dosages may be supplied by supplements you are already taking – see page 195.

How supplements can help

Working as antioxidants, **vitamin C**, **vitamin E** and different types of **carotenoids** can neutralise the free radicals linked to macular degeneration. The carotenoids lutein and zeaxanthin are especially important as they protect the macula by filtering out the sun's harmful ultraviolet rays. **Zinc** plays a key role in the functioning of the retina as well. Many older people are deficient in this mineral, which some research can slow down the progression of the disorder. You will also need to take extra copper, because zinc inhibits its absorption.

For maximum protection take all these supplements, plus **bilberry**. This herb contains antioxidant compounds and enhances blood flow to the retina. **Grape seed extract** or **ginkgo biloba** can be substituted for it; though neither is as effective as bilberry, grape seed may be a good choice if you have poor night vision, and ginkgo is useful for those who also show signs of memory loss. **Selenium** can be added in an effort to boost the body's overall antioxidant activity.

What else you can do

☑ Wear sunglasses and wide-brimmed hats to protect your eyes.
☑ Stop smoking: it is a major contributor to macular degeneration.
☑ Eat plenty of dark green vegetables (they are high in the carotenoids lutein and zeaxanthin), tomatoes and tomato-rich products (from which lycopene, another carotenoid, is well absorbed).

Drinking a glass of wine a day may prevent macular degeneration. A study of more than 3000 people aged 45 to 74 found that drinking moderate amounts of wine reduced their risk of the eye condition by 19%. Other alcoholic beverages were not associated with a lower risk.

Eating spinach or kale may prevent macular degeneration, because they are very high in lutein and zeaxanthin. In one study, individuals who ate about 600 grams of spinach or kale a day were 43% less likely to develop age-related macular degeneration than people eating little of these leafy green vegetables.

DID YOU KNOW?
People with blue or green eyes need to take special care. They are particularly susceptible to the damage from the sun that can cause macular degeneration.

FACTS & TIPS

■ Macular degeneration rarely occurs in people under 50. However, a quarter of those over 65 and a third of those over 80 show signs of having the condition.

■ People who smoke a packet or more of cigarettes a day are more than twice as likely to develop macular degeneration than those who have never smoked. Even smokers who have given up are 30% more likely to suffer from the disease.

Menopause

Women now have more options to help them deal with menopausal symptoms. Hormone replacement therapy is conventional medicine's answer, but many women find that natural therapies can also provide relief from afflictions such as hot flushes and night sweats.

Symptoms

- Hot flushes.
- Night sweats.
- Menstrual irregularities.
- Vaginal dryness.
- Irritability or mild depression.

What it is

Typically, a woman's ovaries stop releasing eggs in her early 50s, and her menstrual cycle ceases. When she has not had a period for six months she is said to have completed the menopause. Though the menopause is not a disease it can have some unpleasant symptoms. For five to ten years before a woman has her last period she may experience menstrual irregularities, hot flushes and irritability; after the menopause she faces possible vaginal dryness, a decline in bone mass and an increased risk of heart disease.

What causes it

As the ovaries gradually stop manufacturing the hormones oestrogen and progesterone, menopausal symptoms and the risk of heart disease and osteoporosis increase. To address these concerns some women opt for hormone replacement therapy (HRT), but worries about links between long-term HRT and breast cancer, or simply a belief that nature should take its own course, motivate other women to try natural remedies. These therapies are also beneficial for the women who experience menopausal symptoms while still menstruating (a stage called perimenopause); most doctors advise against HRT at this stage.

How supplements can help

If you choose not to take HRT, you may want to use the herbs listed in the chart to control hot flushes and other symptoms. Taking them in some combination should work best. First, try **black cohosh** and **chasteberry**. These herbs help to stabilise hormone levels, reducing hot flushes and lessening depression and vaginal dryness. **Siberian ginseng** is considered a good female tonic and may have other benefits too.

If this combination does not provide relief, add dong quai or liquorice root. Some studies suggest that although it is not helpful for menopausal symptoms when used alone, **dong quai** may boost the effect of other herbs. **Liquorice** has plant-based compounds

Soya isoflavone supplements may help to minimise the side effects of the menopause, especially for women who do not eat soya products regularly.

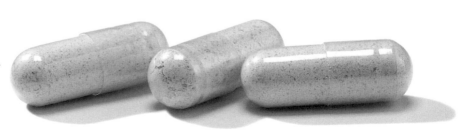

SUPPLEMENT RECOMMENDATIONS

Black cohosh	**Dosage:** 40 mg extract twice a day. **Advice:** standardised to contain 2.5% triterpenes.
Chasteberry	**Dosage:** 100 mg standardised extract once a day. **Advice:** also called vitex; should contain 0.5% agnuside.
Siberian ginseng	**Dosage:** 100-300 mg extract a day. **Advice:** standardised to contain at least 0.8% eleutherosides.
Calcium/ magnesium	**Dosage:** 600 mg calcium and 300 mg magnesium a day. **Advice:** choose a supplement that also contains 10 mcg vitamin D.
Dong quai	**Dosage:** 200 mg, or 30 drops tincture, three times a day. **Advice:** standardised to contain 0.8%-1.1% ligustilide.
Liquorice	**Dosage:** 200 mg standardised extract three times a day. **Caution:** can raise blood pressure; consult your doctor before you take it.
Soya isoflavones	**Dosage:** 50 mg a day. **Advice:** choose products that contain genistein and daidzein.
Vitamin E	**Dosage:** 250 mg twice a day. **Caution:** consult your doctor if you take anticoagulant drugs.

Note: consider using supplements in blue first; those in black may also be beneficial. Some dosages may be supplied by supplements you are already taking – see page 195.

see page 195.

RECENT FINDINGS

In a study of soya's effect on menopausal symptoms, researchers found that women who consumed soya daily experienced less severe hot flushes and night sweats. In addition, they had a 10% drop in total cholesterol, a 12% decrease in LDL 'bad' cholesterol, and a 6-point drop in diastolic blood pressure. Test participants added about 2 tablespoons of soya protein powder to their diets each day for six weeks.

Natural treatments for menopausal symptoms are becoming increasingly popular, following trials showing problems with HRT. A recent 12-week study found that an isoflavone supplement improved five of the commonest menopause symptoms, including libido, hot flushes and, in particular, insomnia.

FACTS & TIPS

■ Vitamin C and flavonoids may reduce the heavy menstrual bleeding that often occurs near the time of the menopause. These nutrients strengthen the capillary walls which weaken just before and during menstruation. Flavonoids may also control hot flushes and mood swings. Some practitioners suggest taking 500 mg of vitamin C along with 250 mg of flavonoids twice a day.

(phytoestrogens) that perform functions similar to those of the oestrogen produced by a woman's body. In addition, some nutrients may be of value in lowering the risk of heart disease and osteoporosis in women after menopause. Studies have shown that soya foods may protect against heart disease; in addition, hot flushes and other menopausal symptoms are rare in countries where soya is a dietary staple. If you dislike the taste of soya foods, consider supplements with **soya isoflavones**, the compounds thought to be partly responsible for the protective effect of soya.

Studies suggest that **vitamin E** aids in protecting against heart disease by preventing LDL 'bad' cholesterol from adhering to artery walls; some women find that high doses of vitamin E also relieve hot flushes. **Calcium** and **magnesium** are essential for strong bones and help to prevent osteoporosis; combine them with vitamin D for proper absorption. (You also might want to take vitamin E, calcium, magnesium and vitamin D even if you are using HRT.)

What else you can do

☑ Avoid alcohol, chocolate, coffee and spicy foods; they can all make hot flushes worse.

☑ Get regular exercise, which can reduce the number of hot flushes and help to prevent heart disease. Light weight-training may help to protect the bones.

☑ Soak in a lukewarm bath for 20 minutes each morning; some women find that this routine prevents hot flushes all day long.

Menstrual disorders

Though most women experience some discomfort (such as a day or two of mild cramps) during their menstrual periods, a number suffer troublesome irregularities that can cause severe pain or major inconvenience each month.

Symptoms

■ *Menstrual cramps or sharp pains in the lower abdomen and back that sometimes shoot down the legs. May be accompanied by nausea, diarrhoea and fatigue.*

■ *Excessive menstrual bleeding.*

■ *Missed or irregular periods.*

SEE YOUR DOCTOR ...

■ If your cramps are incapacitating, last longer than three days or occur between periods.

■ If you need a fresh tampon or sanitary towel every hour.

■ If you have severe cramps for the first time as an adult.

■ If you have severe cramps while taking birth control pills.

■ If you are not pregnant but miss three periods, or your periods are more than 45 days apart.

■ If you bleed between periods (intramenstrual bleeding, or IMB) or after the menopause.

REMINDER: If you have a medical condition, consult your doctor before taking supplements.

What they are

The three most common menstrual disorders are cramp-like pains (dysmenorrhoea), heavy bleeding or prolonged periods (menorrhagia) and irregular or absent periods (amenorrhoea). These conditions usually affect women in times of hormonal change, such as adolescence or the years shortly before the menopause, but they may occur at any time during the reproductive years.

What causes them

Menstrual pains are triggered by prostaglandins – hormone-like substances released during menstruation by cells in the lining of the uterus (endometrium). Women who bleed so heavily that they have to change a tampon or pad every hour or so, and those whose periods last longer than seven days, are considered to have menorrhagia. Though the most common causes of this condition are hormonal or nutritional imbalances, an abnormal growth in the uterus (a fibroid) can induce heavy bleeding. In addition, blood vessels in the uterus tend to be weak and rupture easily. Hormonal imbalances as well as extreme exercise or diet regimens can lead to amenorrhoea.

How supplements can help

The menstrual disorder you experience determines the supplements you should use. All those recommended in the chart can be combined with over-the-counter or prescription drugs. To combat menstrual pains, omega-3 fatty acids (from **fish oils** or flaxseed oil) help to block prostaglandin production. The herb **chasteberry** eases PMS-like symptoms by balancing hormone levels and is quite useful if you also

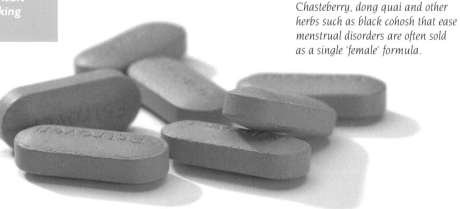

Chasteberry, dong quai and other herbs such as black cohosh that ease menstrual disorders are often sold as a single 'female' formula.

Fish oils	**Dosage:** 2 teaspoons to supply 2 grams of omega-3 fatty acids a day. **Caution:** consult your doctor if you take anticoagulant drugs. **Advice:** vegetarians can substitute 1 tablespoon of flaxseed oil.
Chasteberry	**Dosage:** 100 mg standardised extract, or 40 drops tincture in water, once a day on rising. **Advice:** also called vitex; should contain 0.5% agnuside.
Dong quai	**Dosage:** 200 mg extract, or 30 drops tincture, three times a day. **Advice:** standardised to contain 0.8%-1.1% ligustilide.
Shepherd's purse	**Dosage:** 3 ml (about 60 drops) tincture three times a day. **Advice:** good for heavy periods and spotting between periods.
Iron	**Dosage:** up to 17 mg a day. **Advice:** your doctor may prescribe a higher dose after a blood test.
Vitamin C/ flavonoids	**Dosage:** 500 mg vitamin C and 250 mg flavonoids twice a day. **Advice:** sometimes sold as a single supplement.

Note: consider using supplements in blue first; those in black may also be beneficial. Some dosages may be supplied by supplements you are already taking – see page 195.

RECENT FINDINGS

In a study designed to determine the effect of vitamins on birth defects, women who took a daily multivitamin had more regular menstrual cycles than those given a placebo.

—◊—

Fish oil supplements may lessen menstrual pains. In a study of adolescent girls – prone to painful cramps because of high hormone levels – those who took fish oil supplements needed less painkilling medication to control their cramps than those who did not. Further study is needed to confirm these results.

have breast tenderness; add another herb, **dong quai**, to enhance its benefits, but not if you have heavy bleeding. These three supplements may reduce the need for pain relievers such as ibuprofen.

To help to relieve amenorrhoea, first make sure you are not pregnant. Then try chasteberry and dong quai, along with an 'A to Z' multivitamin and mineral supplement, to restore normal periods. The herbs may correct hormonal imbalances and may regulate the menstrual cycle. However, six months of treatment may be needed before you see any beneficial effect.

To treat menorrhagia, take the herb **shepherd's purse**. Some women may also need extra **iron**, because heavy blood flow depletes stores of this mineral, and, paradoxically, low iron levels may promote abnormal menstrual bleeding. Always check with your doctor before self-treating with iron, however. **Vitamin C** and **flavonoids** strengthen capillaries – the tiniest blood vessels – in the uterus, so they are less likely to rupture and cause additional bleeding.

What else you can do

☑ To relax the uterus and relieve menstrual pains, take a hot bath or use a heated pad.

☑ Exercise – activity releases endorphins, the body's natural painkillers.

FACTS & TIPS

■ Various herbal teas can ease menstrual disorders. To relieve painful cramps, try chamomile or cramp bark tea; for excessive bleeding, sip either shepherd's purse, red raspberry or lady's mantle tea; for missed periods, drink squawvine tea. Use 2 teaspoons of your chosen herb for each 225 ml of hot water, steep for 10 to 15 minutes, strain and drink.

Mouth ulcers

Given their diminutive size, it is hard to fathom how mouth ulcers can hurt as much as they do. Commonsense self-care measures can assist you in avoiding these painful sores, and supplements may help you to reduce their frequency and speed their healing.

Symptoms

- *Small white or yellowish sores surrounded by a red area on the tongue, gums or soft palate, or inside the lips or cheeks.*

- *Burning, itchiness or a tingling feeling before a sore appears.*

- *Raw pain when eating and speaking; strongest during the first few days.*

SEE YOUR DOCTOR ...

- If pain is too severe for you to consume adequate liquids.

- If more than four sores appear throughout your mouth.

- If sores persist longer than two weeks.

- If your temperature is 38.3°C or higher.

- If sores occur more than two or three times a year.

REMINDER: If you have a medical condition, consult your doctor before taking supplements.

What they are

Though they are not serious, mouth ulcers can be so troublesome that they can cause intense pain when talking, kissing, drinking and eating. Affecting women more often than men, these shallow, ulcerated areas appear singly or in small clusters inside the mouth, and range in size from as tiny as a pinhead to as large as a 5p coin. Ulcers emerge rather suddenly and usually go away within one to three weeks. Fortunately it is possible to ease the discomfort they cause.

What causes them

The mouth is often the first organ to show signs of nutrient deficiency owing to the rapid turnover of the cells in its lining. As a result stress may bring on mouth ulcers because it causes the body's immune system to overreact to bacteria normally present in the mouth. Mouth ulcers can also be precipitated by a number of actions, such as irritating the mouth cavity with a rough filling or a jagged or chipped tooth or wearing ill-fitting dentures. Maybe you have accidentally or unconsciously gnawed the inside of your cheek, used a toothbrush with very hard bristles or brushed too vigorously. Occasionally, even eating acidic, spicy or salty foods – tomatoes, citrus fruits, hot peppers, cinnamon, nuts or potato crisps – can be the initiating factor.

Some practitioners believe that recurring mouth ulcers are an allergic reaction to food preservatives – benzoic acid, E210; methylparaben, E218; or sorbic acid, E200, to name a few – or to

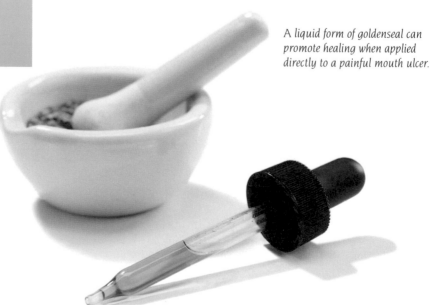

A liquid form of goldenseal can promote healing when applied directly to a painful mouth ulcer.

SUPPLEMENT RECOMMENDATIONS	
Vitamin C/ flavonoids	**Dosage:** 500 mg vitamin C and 250 mg flavonoids three times a day. **Advice:** reduce vitamin C dose if diarrhoea develops.
Vitamin B complex	**Dosage:** one tablet each morning with food. **Advice:** look for a B-50 complex with 50 mcg vitamin B_{12} and biotin, 400 mcg folic acid and 50 mg of all other B vitamins.
Echinacea	**Dosage:** 200 mg extract two or three times a day at the first sign of a sore. **Advice:** begin with higher dose and reduce as sore heals; as a preventative, take 200 mg each morning for three weeks of each month.
Liquorice (DGL)	**Dosage:** chew one or two deglycyrrhizinated liquorice (DGL) tablets (380 mg) three or four times a day. **Advice:** take between meals.
Goldenseal	**Dosage:** apply liquid form to the sore three times a day. **Advice :** wait at least an hour after application before eating.

Note: consider using supplements in blue first; those in black may also be beneficial. Some dosages may be supplied by supplements you are already taking – see page 195.

something in a food. Gluten, the protein found in wheat and some other grains, has been singled out as the most likely offender.

How supplements can help

If you are troubled by mouth ulcers, an 'A to Z' multivitamin and mineral formulation should always be taken. In addition, try one or more of the recommended supplements. First try the immunity-boosting **vitamin C**, which helps to heal the mouth's mucous membranes; **flavonoids** are natural compounds that enhance the effectiveness of this vitamin. People prone to mouth ulcers may be deficient in B vitamins; try a daily **vitamin B complex** if the 'A to Z' formulation with the extra vitamin C seems to be ineffective. **Echinacea** strengthens the immune system, and lower doses of this herb (take 200 mg each morning, three weeks a month) may also stop ulcers forming. Chewable **liquorice (DGL)** tablets coat and protect sores from irritants and help them to heal, and **goldenseal** in liquid form applied directly to the sore also promotes healing.

What else you can do

☑ Keep your mouth clean and healthy by flossing and cleaning your teeth at least twice a day. Be gentle and use a soft-bristled brush.
☑ See your dentist if a tooth problem is irritating your mouth.
☑ Be aware if you're constantly gnawing at the inside of your cheek.
☑ Do not eat spicy foods if you are prone to recurrent mouth ulcers. Avoid coffee and chewing gum, other known irritants.

DID YOU KNOW?
Even the ancient Greeks were plagued by mouth ulcers. It was Hippocrates, called the father of medicine, who in the 4th century BC coined the medical term for them: *aphthous stomatitis.*

FACTS & TIPS
■ It might be supposed that onions, with their strong flavour, would irritate the mouth and cause mouth ulcers, but – on the contrary – eating them regularly might actually prevent these sores. Onions contain sulphur compounds with antiseptic properties, and they are also a leading source of the flavonoid quercetin, which stops the body releasing inflammatory substances in response to allergens.

Multiple sclerosis

Multiple sclerosis can cause fatigue, impair vision and inhibit mobility in previously healthy people. Conventional drugs have limited impact on the disease, prompting interest in the part that supplements might play in slowing down its progress.

Symptoms

- *Early signs mimic those of many other conditions. They include blurred or double vision, tingling in the arms or legs, clumsiness or unsteadiness, and other motor, visual and sensory problems.*

- *The disease's course varies greatly. Depending on its severity, a person with MS may experience severe fatigue, muscle stiffness and tremors, poor coordination, impaired speech, and continence difficulties. Symptoms often come and go.*

SEE YOUR DOCTOR ...

- **If vision or motor skills become impaired with no known cause** – your doctor can rule out other neurological conditions, such as a brain tumour.

- **If you suffer an acute attack.**

REMINDER: If you have a medical condition, consult your doctor before taking supplements.

What it is

Multiple sclerosis (MS) is a progressive and degenerative nerve disorder that most often strikes during young adulthood. The disease follows a highly variable course. In some people damage to the optic nerve or nerves in the brain and spinal cord may lead to difficulty in seeing or walking, slurred speech, loss of bowel or bladder function, clouded thinking and paralysis – but many of those with MS experience long periods of remission and minimal disability.

What causes it

Many experts believe that MS is an autoimmune disorder in which the body's immune system attacks its own nerve tissue. What triggers this reaction is unknown. It may be a virus – perhaps even a common one, such as measles or herpes simplex – that has been dormant for years.

How supplements can help

Supplement therapy should start as soon as possible after MS has been diagnosed. It has several goals: to enhance antioxidant activity and protect nerve cells from the highly reactive molecules called free radicals; to boost the production of fatty acids and other substances that build up nerves; and to decrease nerve inflammation. Start with an 'A to Z' multivitamin and multimineral formulation, then add the supplements listed in the chart. All can be taken together, and with conventional prescription drugs. It may take a month for benefits to be noticed. **Vitamins C** and **E** are valuable in treating MS on account of their antioxidant properties. **Vitamin B complex** and extra **vitamin B$_{12}$** are important as well

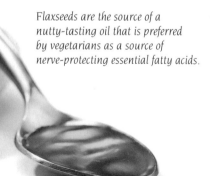

Flaxseeds are the source of a nutty-tasting oil that is preferred by vegetarians as a source of nerve-protecting essential fatty acids.

SUPPLEMENT RECOMMENDATIONS

Vitamin C/ vitamin E	**Dosage:** 500 mg of vitamin C and 250 mg of vitamin E twice a day. **Advice:** vitamin C helps to boost the effects of vitamin E; reduce dose of vitamin C if diarrhoea develops.
Vitamin B complex	**Dosage:** one tablet a day. **Advice:** look for a B-50 complex with 50 mcg vitamin B_{12} and biotin, 400 mcg folic acid and 50 mg all other B vitamins.
Vitamin B_{12}	**Dosage:** 1000 mcg three times a day. **Advice:** best taken as methylcobalamin.
Fish oils	**Dosage:** two teaspoons to supply 2 grams of omega-3 fatty acids a day. **Caution:** consult your doctor if you take anticoagulant drugs. **Advice:** vegetarians can substitute 1 tablespoon of flaxseed oil.
Evening primrose oil	**Dosage:** 1000 mg three times a day. **Advice:** can substitute 1000 mg borage oil once a day.
Ginkgo biloba	**Dosage:** 40 mg extract three times a day. **Advice:** standardised to contain at least 24% flavone glycosides.

Note: consider using supplements in blue first; the one in black may also be beneficial. Some dosages may be supplied by supplements you are already taking – see page 195.

because they play a role in maintaining nerve structure and function. Some studies show that MS patients have low levels of vitamin B_{12}, or have problems processing it efficiently. It is also important to get extra essential fatty acids from omega-3 fats in **fish oils** (or flaxseed oil) and **evening primrose oil**; they reduce inflammation and, over time, help to build healthy nerves.

The herb **ginkgo biloba** may be beneficial because it acts as an antioxidant and improves blood flow to the nervous system. Other supplements worth trying are St John's wort (300 mg extract three times a day), black cohosh, oats, ginseng and ginger, all of which have been used by herbal practitioners with some success.

What else you can do

☑ Sensible exposure to sunlight many benefit MS sufferers, but avoid becoming overheated. Sunbathing, heavy exertion and very hot baths can all make symptoms worse.

☑ Ask your doctor about nutritional therapies. Some special diets have been developed that may slow down the progress of MS.

☑ Exercise gently to improve muscle strength and flexibility – but not during an attack.

☑ If your full-time work schedule is physically demanding, investigate part-time work or working from home.

Muscle aches and pains

Although they are not serious, muscle cramps and the muscle soreness that results from physical overexertion can be very uncomfortable. The weekend gardener is just as likely to be affected as the world-class athlete.

Symptoms

- *Sudden tightening of the muscles during physical activity.*

- *Soreness and stiffness in the muscles after activity, often not beginning until 24 to 48 hours later.*

- *Muscle spasms occurring at night, usually in the calf muscle.*

- *A muscle that feels hard to the touch, called a knot.*

- *In severe cases, visible twitching of the affected muscle.*

SEE YOUR DOCTOR ...

- **If tightness or cramping occurs in the chest muscle – this may be a sign of a heart attack.**

- **If pain causes numbness or radiates down arms or legs.**

- **If muscle aches and pains begin to occur frequently.**

- **If night-time calf cramps are interfering with sleep.**

REMINDER: If you have a medical condition, consult your doctor before taking supplements.

What they are

There are two common types of muscle pain. The first is soreness and stiffness that develop as the result of overdoing some physical activity – whether running a marathon, digging in the garden or simply carrying a heavy bag of groceries. This kind of pain, which doctors call delayed-onset muscle soreness (DOMS), typically begins a day or two after the activity and can last up to a week.

The second type of muscle pain, when a muscle suddenly contracts and cannot relax, is known as a cramp. Cramps are most common in the thigh, calf or foot, and can strike at any time, even during sleep.

What causes them

Even if you are physically fit, any unaccustomed strenuous activity may cause muscle soreness. For example, a dedicated jogger who helps a friend to move furniture will probably be rewarded with aching arms and shoulders. Most doctors think that such pain is a symptom of microscopic tearing of the muscles, which rebuild themselves in a matter of days. Activities that require lengthening a muscle against force – such as running downhill or lowering a weight – are most likely to produce this kind of injury. Almost any kind of exercise or activity involves this type of movement.

Muscle cramps are not the result of injury, but no one knows exactly why they occur. The cause may be an imbalance in the minerals that govern muscle contraction and relaxation – calcium, magnesium, potassium and sodium – or a lack of fluid. Exercising too strenuously during the day may lead to calf cramps painful enough to wake you from a sound sleep, as can wearing high heels, or sleeping with your toes pointed or with bedding wrapped too tightly around your legs.

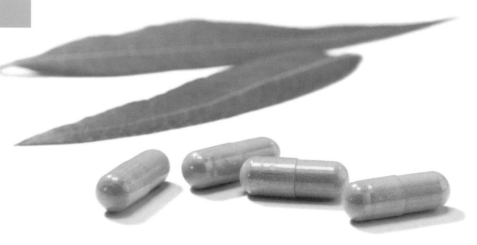

The white willow tree yields a herbal pain reliever that is helpful for muscle aches.

Calcium/ magnesium	**Dosage:** 500 mg calcium and 200 mg magnesium twice a day. **Advice:** take with food; sometimes sold as a single supplement.
Vitamin E	**Dosage:** 250 mg a day. **Caution:** consult your doctor if you take anticoagulant drugs.
Bromelain	**Dosage:** 500 mg three times a day on an empty stomach. **Advice:** should provide 6000 GDU or 9000 MCU daily.
White willow bark	**Dosage:** one or two capsules three times a day as needed for pain (follow instructions on the packet). **Advice:** standardised to contain 15% salicin.
Valerian	**Dosage:** 250-500 mg standardised extract at bedtime. **Advice:** start with the lower dose and increase as needed.

Note: consider using supplements in blue first; the one in black may also be beneficial. Some dosages may be supplied by supplements you are already taking – see page 195.

How supplements can help

To balance the minerals needed for proper muscle contraction, take supplements of **calcium** and **magnesium** on a routine basis. (Most people get enough sodium in their diet, but many do not get enough potassium. This is best obtained by eating plenty of fruit and vegetables, rather than from supplements.) Add **vitamin E** daily if you are prone to exercise-related cramps or night-time calf cramps.

For soreness, consider the herbs **bromelain** and **white willow bark**, which have the same benefits as, and can be substituted for, over-the-counter pain medications such as aspirin or ibuprofen; in fact they are gentler on your system and help the muscles to heal themselves. Bromelain (an enzyme derived from pineapple) has an anti-inflammatory effect on the muscles and helps excess fluid to drain from the site of a muscle injury.

The herb white willow bark, often referred to as 'nature's aspirin', is an effective pain reliever. **Valerian** is a natural sleep aid that can be useful if soreness interferes with sleep. Take these supplements in any combination until the soreness goes away. Black cohosh may be helpful for reducing general muscular aches and pains; add yarrow if cold or flu symptoms are suspected as the cause. Arnica cream, applied topically, may be helpful if the discomfort has been caused by too much physical activity.

What else you can do

☑ Eat plenty of fruit and vegetables for potassium and antioxidants, and whole-grain cereals, nuts and seeds for magnesium.

☑ Drink plenty of fluids before, during and after exercise.

☑ Warm up before exercise and stretch afterwards to help muscles relax.

☑ If pain is severe, apply ice to sore muscles to reduce inflammation.

DID YOU KNOW?

Pregnant women should take care during exercise because they are at high risk of muscle cramps. The metabolic needs of the developing baby affect the normal balance of body fluids, making cramps more likely.

FACTS & TIPS

■ A herbal oil massage can soothe muscle soreness. Blend 1 tablespoon of a neutral oil, such as almond oil, with a few drops of any of the following botanical oils: marjoram, basil, rosemary, eucalyptus, ginger, lavender, peppermint or wintergreen. Gently rub the oil mixture into sore muscles.

■ To ease a cramp in your calf muscle, stand up, put your full weight on the affected leg and bend the knee slightly. Another way to obtain relief is to flex your foot, grab your toes and the ball of your foot, then gently pull towards your knee as you lie down. Massage your calf at the same time to relax the muscle.

■ Stretching exercises can reduce the risk of muscle soreness following demanding physical activity. Stand about a metre from a wall, step one foot forward and lean against the wall with your forearms. Keeping your back heel on the ground, hold the stretch for 15 to 20 seconds to loosen the calf. Repeat with the other foot.

Nail problems

Nails protect both the fingertips and the toes, are very helpful when peeling off price tags – and are sometimes regarded as a sign of beauty. They can even provide clues about your overall health and any underlying diseases. Good nutrition is the key to nail vitality.

Symptoms

- *Dry, brittle nails that split and grow slowly could be caused by nutritional deficiencies.*

- *Thick, yellowed nails (often the toenails) may be harbouring a fungus. Debris collecting under the nail may cause it to peel away from the nail bed below.*

- *Changes in nail colour, shape or texture may indicate an underlying illness.*

SEE YOUR DOCTOR ...

- **Nail irregularities may signal a more serious medical disorder; for example, white streaks running the length of the nail may indicate heart disease, while a bluish tint under the nails (rather than a healthy pink) could be a sign of asthma or emphysema.**

REMINDER: If you have a medical condition, consult your doctor before taking supplements.

What they are

Composed mainly of a fibrous protein called keratin, nails are one of the body's strongest tissues, but they can grow more slowly than normal, become weakened or break for a number of reasons. One of the most common problems is a fungal infection.

What causes them

Nutrition plays a key role in nail growth and appearance. An insufficient intake of the B vitamins, for example, can produce ridges in the nails, and a lack of calcium can cause dryness and brittleness. Too little vitamin C or folic acid may be partly responsible for the development of hangnails. In addition, nails can change colour when the blood does not get enough oxygen as a consequence of an underlying illness (such as asthma), and white flecks under the nails may be caused by a lack of zinc. In addition, exposure to chemicals can dry nails out, which makes them weak and brittle.

The fungus that causes athlete's foot may infect toenails as well. It thrives in sweaty shoes and socks and can enter any tiny breaks in nails caused by strenuous physical activities such as jogging.

How supplements can help

Various supplements can be used as general nail strengtheners. About eight weeks of therapy may be required before results are noticed. **Biotin** and other **B vitamins**, taken together with **vitamins C** and **E**, have a synergistic effect that helps the body to build keratin and other proteins that it needs to make nails strong. As well as strengthening the skeleton,

Timed-release capsules of vitamin C help to build strong, healthy nails.

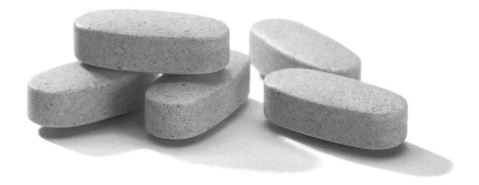

Biotin	**Dosage:** 900 mcg a day for eight weeks. **Advice:** take with meals.
Vitamin B complex	**Dosage:** one tablet each morning with food. **Advice:** look for a B-50 complex with 50 mcg vitamin B_{12} and biotin, 400 mcg folic acid and 50 mg all other B vitamins.
Vitamin C/ vitamin E	**Dosage:** 500 mg vitamin C twice a day; 250 mg vitamin E daily. **Advice:** vitamin C helps to boost the effects of vitamin E; reduce vitamin C dose if diarrhoea develops.
Bone-building formula	**Dosage:** follow instructions on the packet. **Advice:** supplement should provide at least 600 mg calcium, 250 mg magnesium and 5 mcg vitamin D a day.
Fish oils	**Dosage:** 2 teaspoons to provide 2 g of omega-fatty acids a day. **Caution:** consult your doctor if you take anticoagulant drugs. **Advice:** vegetarians can substitute 1 tablespoon of flaxseed oil.
Evening primrose oil	**Dosage:** 1000 mg three times a day. **Advice:** can substitute 1000 mg borage oil once a day.
Tea tree oil	**Dosage:** for fungal infections, rub on affected nails twice a day. **Caution:** tea tree oil should never be ingested. **Advice:** use pure tea tree oil.

Note: consider using supplements in blue first; the one in black may also be beneficial. Some dosages may be supplied by supplements you are already taking – see page 195.

a **bone-building formula** supplies calcium and other minerals that benefit the nails. **Fish oils** (or flaxseed oil) and **evening primrose oil** are rich in two different types of essential fatty acids, both of which nourish nails and prevent them from cracking. If you have white flecks under your nails try taking extra zinc (15 mg daily, preferably with added copper). Extra silicon is prescribed for weak nails by some practitioners, but the efficacy of this treatment lacks clinical evidence.

Nails infected with a fungus, unfortunately, are harder to treat. Oral vitamin C, taken with vitamin E, remains a good option, because it boosts immunity and may aid the body in fighting off the infection. In addition, try rubbing **tea tree oil**, garlic oil or calendula ointment on affected nails twice a day for several months.

What else you can do

☑ Do not trim cuticles. They protect nails from fungi and bacteria.

☑ Wear gloves if you're doing household chores or if you are using any type of chemical. Apply petroleum jelly to nails after your hands have been in water.

☑ Keep nails short. Long nails break easily. Soak nails before trimming, to prevent splitting and peeling.

RECENT FINDINGS

In a comparative study, tea tree oil and clotrimazole, a popular antifungal medication, performed equally well in people with nail fungus. After six months of therapy, 60% of people in each treatment group experienced partial or full recovery.

Swiss researchers discovered that people with thin, weak and split nails who took 2500 mcg of biotin daily experienced a 25% increase in nail thickness.

DID YOU KNOW?
Vets have long used biotin to strengthen horses' hooves, which are composed primarily of keratin. Biotin has now been shown to make human nails stronger too.

FACTS & TIPS

■ A daily cup of tea made from oat straw, horsetail or nettle leaf may improve nail health. These herbs are rich in silica and other minerals necessary for nail growth.

■ Tea tree oil is much cheaper and has fewer side effects than prescription antifungal drugs, but like them it does not always work.

■ Despite claims to the contrary, gelatin will not strengthen nails or help them to grow. The protein in gelatin does not contain the right mixture of amino acids needed for nail formation.

Nausea and vomiting

Although they are uncomfortable and unpleasant to experience, nausea and vomiting are natural – possibly lifesaving – reactions to eating something dangerous, or to illness. But occasionally they occur even when there is no risk to health.

Symptoms

- *Sweating and shivering.*
- *Excessive salivation.*
- *Dizziness.*
- *Weakness.*
- *Shortness of breath.*
- *Abdominal pain.*
- *Loss of appetite.*

SEE YOUR DOCTOR ...

- If you become significantly dehydrated.
- If you vomit blood or black grainy-looking matter.
- If you have nausea and a temperature.
- If you suspect that a drug is giving you nausea.
- If morning sickness prevents you from eating properly.

REMINDER: *If you have a medical condition, consult your doctor before taking supplements.*

What they are

Nausea is an overall uncomfortable 'woozy' feeling that is sometimes described as 'coming in waves'. It is often accompanied by sweating, shivering or increased saliva production. Sometimes nausea culminates in what doctors refer to as emesis – most people call it 'being sick'. During this process your stomach muscles relax, and the normal rhythmic contractions that propel food through your small intestine shift into reverse, sending the contents back into the stomach. The stomach then contracts and pushes the contents upwards through the oesophagus. Vomiting is valuable because it enables the body to rid itself of toxic matter – and most people feel much better afterwards.

What causes them

Decaying food (which may contain harmful bacteria), illnesses such as flu, some medications (even those that are helpful in other ways, such as chemotherapy drugs used to treat cancer) and too much alcohol can induce nausea and vomiting. Among other causes of these ailments are overeating or eating rich foods, strong smells (from smoke, perfume or food odours), stress and anxiety, and motion sickness.

In other cases the nerves in the stomach become confused and transmit warning signals to the brain, even when no real threat to health exists. For example, the high levels of hormones released during pregnancy are beneficial but are also thought to be the cause of morning sickness. Elevated hormone levels may be the reason why nausea is one symptom of premenstrual syndrome (PMS).

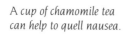

A cup of chamomile tea can help to quell nausea.

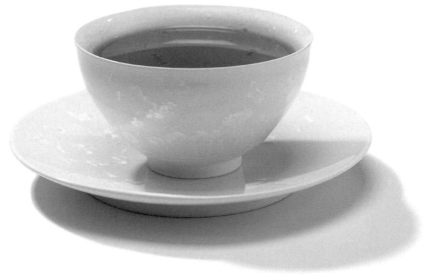

Ginger	**Dosage:** 200 mg extract every four hours as needed. **Advice:** increase dose if necessary; in an emergency take ginger in any form.
Peppermint oil	**Dosage:** one enteric-coated capsule three times a day. **Advice:** each capsule should contain 0.2 ml peppermint oil.
Chamomile	**Dosage:** one cup of tea up to three times a day. **Advice:** infuse 2 teaspoons dried herb in 200 ml boiled water.

Some dosages may be supplied by supplements you are already taking – see page 195.

How supplements can help

When you feel nauseous and have the urge to vomit, there is almost nothing you can do to stop it. If you are suffering from food poisoning it is better not to fight this powerful reflex, because the offending food needs to be purged from your system. But when nausea persists or is the result of pregnancy, motion sickness, stress, essential drugs or strong odours, natural remedies can provide welcome relief.

Your first choice should be **ginger**, in capsule form or as a tea. Its restorative powers spring from its volatile oils, which enhance digestion, soothe irritated membranes and tone the muscles of the digestive tract. In addition, ginger stimulates the liver to produce bile, which helps to digest fats; this action is especially useful in cases of overeating. To combat motion sickness take your first dose of ginger three to four hours before travelling. If you are pregnant you can probably use ginger safely for morning sickness as long as you don't take too much – check with your doctor. If you are trying to relieve the nausea caused by chemotherapy, consult your doctor; avoid ginger if your blood platelet count is low – high doses may interfere with blood clotting.

Peppermint oil or tea helps to ease spasms in the digestive tract, so may be useful for nausea accompanied by intestinal cramping. Peppermint oil is fairly powerful when taken internally, so peppermint tea is probably a better choice for any nausea linked with pregnancy. If ginger and peppermint do not work (and your nausea is not caused by pregnancy) try **chamomile** tea, which balances digestive secretions and soothes the stomach and liver.

What else you can do

☑ To relieve nausea, lie down with a cold cloth on your forehead. Focus on your breathing to prevent yourself from thinking about how you feel.
☑ Avoid exposure to strong, unpleasant odours that can trigger nausea, such as tobacco smoke, chemical preparations, cleaning supplies or perfume.
☑ Do not eat for two hours after vomiting, but drink as much as you can to replenish lost fluids. (Water, juice and noncaffeinated beverages in small sips are best.) If you vomit again, suck ice cubes.

RECENT FINDINGS

A review of studies assessing natural remedies for morning sickness concluded that ginger and vitamin B_6 are effective, but warned that little is known about their effect on the developing baby. In doses of 25 to 50 mg a day, vitamin B_6 is both safe and beneficial. Ginger is safe too, as long as you don't overdo it. A pregnant woman should always consult her doctor before using supplements.

FACTS & TIPS

■ Herbal teas that calm a queasy stomach can do double duty by providing much-needed fluids after vomiting. Try a tea of ginger, chamomile or peppermint; drink three or four cups a day. Or steep $1/8$ teaspoon nutmeg and 1 teaspoon ground cinnamon in very hot water for 10 minutes, strain, then drink. Sweeten with honey, if you wish.

■ Acupressure may halt nausea in its tracks. Place your right thumb on the inside of your left forearm, about two thumb-widths from the crease of your wrist. Press firmly with your thumb for about a minute, then move your thumb half a finger-width closer to the wrist crease. Apply firm pressure for about one minute more. Repeat on the right forearm.

Nervous disorders

The tingling of a foot or hand that 'falls asleep' is caused by temporary nerve compression, but disorders of the nervous system are often chronic and painful. Supplements, combined with a good diet, can do much to promote healthy nerve cells.

Symptoms

- *Numbness, tingling, pain or weakness, usually in the feet, hands or legs.*

- *Loss of feeling in the limbs.*

- *Shooting pain, normally in the legs.*

SEE YOUR DOCTOR ...

- If your bouts of numbness, tingling or weakness are frequent or persistent – they could be signs of an underlying disorder.

- If numbness or tingling comes on suddenly and lasts longer than half an hour. If it is accompanied by weakness, particularly down one side of the body, it could be a stroke – get help immediately.

REMINDER: *If you have a medical condition, consult your doctor before taking supplements.*

What they are

Either of the two main parts of the nervous system can be affected by disorders: the central nervous system, which consists of the brain and spinal cord, or the peripheral nervous system, which communicates with the limbs, skin, intestine, heart and glands. Anxiety and insomnia can be caused by the central nervous system overreacting to stress. The mental dysfunction which characterises Alzheimer's disease is caused by a severe loss of brain nerve cells, as is Parkinson's disease, which damages nerve communication in the brain. Disorders directly connected with the peripheral nervous system include neuralgia, shingles and numbness.

What causes them

Nerves are grouped together and encased in a fatty coating called a myelin sheath. Persistent numbness, tingling or pain can occur if the sheath is damaged, or if the nerves themselves are inflamed, compressed or injured. Nerve cells need proper nourishment and the support of good blood circulation to function properly. A build-up of fatty deposits (known as atherosclerosis) in the minor arteries is the main cause of poor circulation in the peripheral nervous system. This is usually caused by a high-fat diet, high blood pressure, smoking or being overweight.

The numbness and tingling of some nerve disorders has no obvious cause. If a medical condition is identified, it is often progressive nerve damage linked with poor blood sugar control. This is known as diabetic neuropathy, and primarily affects the feet. Numbness and pain in the hands may be carpal tunnel syndrome, which occurs when the middle nerve in the wrist is inflamed or compressed. Numbness and pain running down the thigh and leg may be caused by a herniated disc, or other problem in the spine, in which the main nerve to the legs (the sciatic nerve) is compressed.

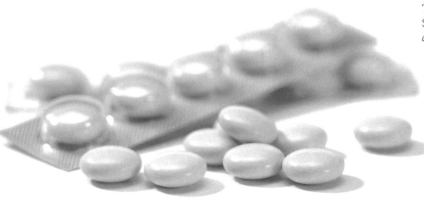

The calming sedative herb St John's wort can ease nerve pain and help to reduce inflammation.

Vitamin B complex	**Dosage:** one tablet twice a day with food. **Advice:** choose a complex with 50 mcg vitamin B$_{12}$ and biotin, 400 mcg folic acid and 50 mg all other B vitamins.
Evening primrose oil	**Dosage:** 1000 mg three times a day. **Advice:** you can substitute 1000 mg borage oil a day.
Vitamin B$_{12}$	**Dosage:** 1000 mcg vitamin B$_{12}$ twice daily **Advice:** take sublingual form for the most efficient absorption.
Fish oils	**Dosage:** 2 teaspoons to supply 2 grams omega-3 fatty acids a day. **Caution:** consult your doctor if you take anticoagulant drugs. **Advice:** vegetarians can substitute 1 tablespoon of flaxseed oil.
Alpha-lipoic acid	**Dosage:** 200 mg twice a day. **Caution:** may affect blood sugar levels; diabetics should use with care.
Magnesium	**Dosage:** 200 mg twice a day. **Advice:** take with food.
Ginkgo biloba	**Dosage for poor circulation:** 120 mg of extract a day in two or three doses. **Dosage to boost blood supply to the brain:** up to 240 mg a day. **Advice:** standardised to contain 24% ginkgo flavone glycosides.
Bilberry	**Dosage:** 100 mg extract twice a day. **Advice:** also eat whole bilberries and blueberries.

Note: consider using supplements in blue first; those in black may also be beneficial. Some dosages may be supplied by supplements you are already taking – see page 195.

How supplements can help

For a healthy nervous system take **vitamin B complex**. Vitamin B$_6$ has an anti-inflammatory effect, which makes it especially important for people suffering from diabetic neuropathy or carpal tunnel syndrome. The gamma-linolenic acid in **evening primrose oil** is also useful for treating diabetic neuropathy. **Vitamin B$_{12}$**, which may be deficient in older people, maintains healthy myelin sheaths, as do the essential fatty acids in **fish oils** (or flaxseed oil) which also ensure proper communication between the brain and nerve cells. **Alpha-lipoic acid** has a powerful antioxidant effect which is thought to protect against nerve damage. **Magnesium** is needed to transmit nerve and muscle impulses – a deficiency can cause nervousness and irritability. **Ginkgo biloba** has a positive effect on the central nervous system: it enhances blood (and therefore oxygen) supply to the brain and also increases the amount of blood reaching the extremities. **Bilberry** also improves circulation. Herbalists use anti-inflammatory herbs such as St John's wort to treat sciatica; this works best in combination with manipulation by an osteopath or chiropractor.

What else you can do

☑ Exercise to increase blood flow to the extremities and nourish nerves.
☑ Inactivity increases nerve discomfort – do not sit still for long periods.
☑ Chilli ointment applied three times a day can ease nerve pain.

A German study of 73 patients with damage to the nerves that control involuntary bodily functions, such as heartbeat, found that alpha-lipoic acid may reverse diabetic nerve damage. Patients were given either 800 mg a day of alpha-lipoic acid or a placebo. After four months the nerve function of those taking alpha-lipoic acid improved, whereas the condition of those in the placebo group worsened. More study is needed to confirm these findings and also to determine whether the same results can be obtained with lower doses.

FACTS & TIPS

■ Fish and nuts are rich in essential acids which may have a healing effect on the nerves. Try to eat these foods at least twice a week for their beneficial effect.

■ Oat extract is well known as a stimulating, strengthening nervine tonic, particularly in disorders associated with depression or exhaustion. It can be taken in the form of a cereal (porridge oats), as a juice made from pressed young plants or as a tincture.

■ A tincture of the herb passiflora alleviates neuralgia and the nerve pain associated with shingles; alternatively, the dried herb can be used to make a calming tea.

Osteoporosis

A progressive condition characterised by a loss of mineral content in the bones, osteoporosis is a major cause of bone fractures, but it can be prevented. The earlier in life you begin to address the problem, the better your chances of avoiding pain and broken bones later on.

Symptoms

- *The first sign can be dramatic: a severe backache or a fracture (often of the spine, hip or wrist).*

- *Other classic symptoms include a gradual loss of height accompanied by the initially subtle development of a stooped posture (dowager's hump).*

- *Dental X-rays may detect early osteoporosis by revealing bone loss in the jaw.*

SEE YOUR DOCTOR ...

- If you suspect that you have fractured a bone.

- If you have sudden severe back pain – this may indicate a spinal compression fracture.

- If you experience significant bone pain (in the spine, ribs or feet) after an injury.

- If you have no symptoms but have significant risk factors – ask your doctor whether you should have a short painless test to measure your bone density.

REMINDER: If you have a medical condition, consult your doctor before taking supplements.

What it is

Osteoporosis, whose name comes from the Latin for 'porous bones', is a progressive condition that diminishes the mass (mineral content) of bones and weakens their structure, thus making them highly susceptible to fracture. The condition affects one in three women and a large number of men. Hormone replacement therapy protects against osteoporosis, but many women decide against its use. Although no single measure is sufficient to prevent the disorder, a combination of supplements and lifestyle changes can be effective in limiting damage.

What causes it

The decline in oestrogen after the menopause is directly related to the dramatic rise of osteoporosis in older women. This hormone assists the body in absorbing calcium and keeps the bones strong. (Older men experience osteoporosis as well, but bone loss is generally less severe because they have denser bones.) Early menopause is another risk factor, as are both lack of regular weight-bearing exercise and a diet low in calcium and other nutrients necessary for optimal bone production. Your risk of osteoporosis is also higher if you are small-boned (white and Asian women tend to be small-boned), underweight or postmenopausal, if you have a family history of osteoporosis, or if you have taken steroids or anticonvulsants for long periods.

How supplements can help

The recommended supplements – when taken for at least six months – can help to strengthen bones. They are safe to use together and with

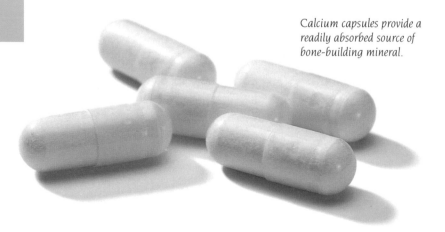

Calcium capsules provide a readily absorbed source of bone-building mineral.

SUPPLEMENT RECOMMENDATIONS

Calcium	**Dosage:** 500 mg twice a day. **Advice:** take with food.
Vitamin D	**Dosage:** 10 mcg twice a day. **Advice:** particularly important during winter, when exposure to sun is limited.
Magnesium	**Dosage:** 200 mg twice a day. **Advice:** take with food.
Boron	**Dosage:** 3 mg a day. **Advice:** reduces calcium loss; may enhance oestrogen's effects.
Vitamin C	**Dosage:** 500 mg twice a day. **Advice:** reduce dose if diarrhoea develops.
Zinc	**Dosage:** 15 mg a day. **Advice:** if you take a zinc supplement for more than a month, use one that contains 2 mg copper.
Manganese	**Dosage:** 2 mg twice a day. **Advice:** involved in bone metabolism.

Some dosages may be supplied by supplements you are already taking – see page 195.

prescription osteoporosis drugs and oestrogen therapy. Bone-building combination products may be a convenient and less expensive way to obtain many of these supplements, but be cautious if you are taking anticoagulant drugs because many supplements contain vitamin K, which can enhance the blood's clotting ability.

Calcium is vital for maintaining bone strength; **vitamin D** ensures that calcium is well absorbed, and the minerals **magnesium** and **boron** help to convert vitamin D into a usable form. Recent research links the antioxidant **vitamin C** to greater bone mass and improved formation of collagen, a protein that strengthens the bones and connective tissue. Also important for mineral absorption and bone health are **zinc**, copper and **manganese**. Adding other key vitamins and minerals, such as silicon, vitamin B_6 and folic acid, provides further protection.

What else you can do

☑ Perform regular weight-bearing exercise (such as walking or lifting weights) in which the legs or other parts of the body meet resistance.
☑ Stop smoking. Giving up the habit will benefit not only the bones but also your general health as well.
☑ Limit your alcohol intake to no more than one or two units a day.
☑ If you are menopausal, consider hormone replacement therapy.
☑ Eat calcium-rich foods such as low-fat dairy products, canned sardines and salmon (include the soft bones).
☑ Eat plenty of fruit and vegetables for vitamins and trace minerals, and plenty of soya products for isoflavones (particularly genistein and daidzein), which have oestrogenic properties.

Parkinson's disease

Although there is still no cure for this slowly progressive brain disorder, advances continue to be made that can greatly improve the quality of life for sufferers. Prompt treatment may help to ease tremors, stiffness and other disabling symptoms.

Symptoms

- *Shaking or trembling limbs and rigid muscles.*
- *Slow and shuffling walk.*
- *Stooped posture.*
- *Drooling, impassive expression and infrequent blinking.*
- *Trouble in swallowing or talking.*
- *Incontinence and constipation.*
- *Anxiety, depression and, in severe cases, confusion and memory loss.*

SEE YOUR DOCTOR ...

- **If you have any symptoms of Parkinson's disease.**

- **If you have been diagnosed with Parkinson's and notice new symptoms – these may be side effects of prescription drugs for Parkinson's disease that can be easily remedied.**

REMINDER: If you have a medical condition, consult your doctor before taking supplements.

What it is

Parkinson's disease, named after the British doctor who identified it in the early 19th century, is the most common degenerative disorder of the nervous system, afflicting 120,000 people in the UK and millions more throughout the world. It usually strikes after the age of 60, although 5% of people diagnosed with the disease in the UK are under 40. It is more common in men than in women. Though symptoms are usually very mild at first, they generally worsen over time.

What causes it

In people suffering from Parkinson's disease, cells in an area of the brain called the basal ganglia gradually die and no longer produce the chemical dopamine, the substance which helps to transmit impulses from nerve to nerve. Lack of dopamine causes the progressive stiffness, shaking and loss of muscle coordination typical of the disorder. Although viral brain infections, antipsychotic drugs and exposure to herbicides or toxins are known to be responsible for a small number of cases, most of the time no underlying cause can be determined.

How supplements can help

Anyone suffering from this serious ailment should be under close medical supervision, and should not take supplements without first discussing their use with his or her doctor.

Taken together with an 'A to Z' multivitamin and multimineral formulation, the supplements listed in the chart can help to temper or slow down the progression of symptoms, particularly if they are taken in the early years of the disease. Results may be noticed within about

Vitamin E is one of several antioxidants that can help to slow down the progression of Parkinson's symptoms.

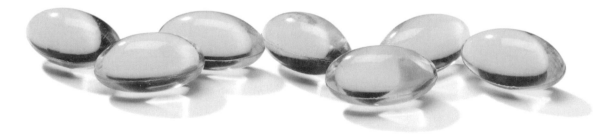

SUPPLEMENT RECOMMENDATIONS

Vitamin B$_6$	**Dosage:** 50 mg a day. **Caution:** people taking the prescription drug levodopa (L-dopa) without its companion drug carbidopa should not take B$_6$.
Coenzyme Q$_{10}$	**Dosage:** 50 mg three times a day. **Advice:** for most efficient absorption, take with food.
NADH	**Dosage:** 5 mg a day. **Advice:** best taken in the morning or between meals.
Vitamin E	**Dosage:** 250 mg a day. **Caution:** consult your doctor if you take anticoagulant drugs.
Vitamin C	**Dosage:** 500 mg twice a day. **Advice:** reduce dose if diarrhoea develops.
Fish oils	**Dosage:** 2 teaspoons to supply 2 grams of omega-3 fatty acids a day. **Caution:** consult your doctor if you take anticoagulant drugs. **Advice:** vegetarians can substitute 1 tablespoon of flaxseed oil.
Ginkgo biloba	**Dosage:** 80 mg extract three times a day. **Advice:** standardised to contain at least 24% flavone glycosides.

Note: consider using supplements in blue first; those in black may also be beneficial. Some dosages may be supplied by supplements you are already taking – see page 195.

eight weeks, but supplements must usually be continued long term. You can try them separately or in combination, but only on the advice of your doctor. Some, such as vitamin B$_6$, can interact adversely with drugs prescribed for the treatment of Parkinson's disease.

Most of the supplements, including **vitamin B$_6$**, work to increase production of the brain chemical dopamine (levels of this B vitamin are often depleted in people with Parkinson's). **Coenzyme Q$_{10}$**, **NADH** (nicotinamide adenine dinucleotide, related to the B vitamin niacin), **vitamin E** and **vitamin C** are all antioxidants that help to protect cells, including the dopamine-producing ones in the brain. Vitamins C and E may be especially effective in those people who have not yet started taking conventional medications for the disease. Omega-3 fatty acids from **fish oils** (or flaxseed oil) have nerve-nourishing effects that can boost dopamine levels; the antioxidant nutrients listed in the chart should be taken with these essential fatty acids. The herb **ginkgo biloba** increases blood circulation in the brain, which helps to ensure that its nerve cells are adequately nourished.

What else you can do

☑ Walk every day and stretch to keep muscles toned and strong.
☑ Keep your mind stimulated with new interests and challenges. Recent studies suggest that daily mental exercise may diminish symptoms.
☑ Counselling may help you to manage stress. Join a local support group.
☑ Ask your doctor to refer you to a physiotherapist and a speech therapist, and to keep you informed about new drug treatments.

RECENT FINDINGS

A Dutch survey of more than 5300 people aged 55 to 95 found that those with high amounts of vitamin E in their diets were less likely to have Parkinson's disease. This provides further evidence of the protective role played by this antioxidant vitamin.

In a study of 80 people with early Parkinson's disease, supplementation with coenzyme Q$_{10}$ appeared to slow down the progressive deterioration of function.

'Gene hunters' at the US National Institutes of Health have identified a rare gene for Parkinson's disease; the discovery may open doors to potential new therapies.

FACTS & TIPS

■ Good dietary sources of vitamin B$_6$, which helps the brain to produce dopamine, include avocados, potatoes, bananas, fish and chicken.

■ While there is still no cure for Parkinson's disease, herbs can help to strengthen the tissues of the brain and balance the chemicals involved in nerve function. By doing so, they may assist the sufferer to cope with the condition and may even delay its progression. Herbs traditionally used (but not clinically tested) for the treatment of Parkinson's disease include black cohosh, cramp bark, ginseng, passion flower and valerian.

Pregnancy

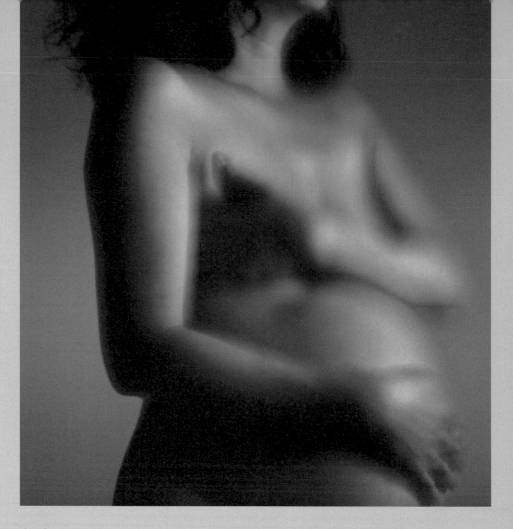

A mother's diet before and during pregnancy influences the size and efficiency of the placenta, through which the baby receives all it needs for growth and development.

If you are pregnant or trying to conceive, consult your doctor before taking supplements. Pregnant women should take special care not to exceed recommended dosages – because some vitamins are stored by the body, high levels can lead to birth defects.

There is increasing evidence to suggest a link between the way a baby grows inside the uterus and its risk of developing heart disease, hypertension, diabetes, obesity or cancer in later life. For example, babies assessed by paediatricians as short or thin at birth are thought by some researchers to have a greater chance of developing coronary heart disease as adults. Babies who do not grow adequately in the uterus also have an increased risk of sickness in early life and even of sudden infant death.

Prenatal supplements containing nutrients in amounts appropriate for pregnancy are now widely available, and can be especially helpful for women with poor or restricted diets.

The relationship between a healthy diet in pregnancy and having a healthy baby may seem complex, but women should take heart. Many thousands give birth to healthy, normal-weight babies each year even if the pregnancy was unplanned.

FOLIC ACID SUPPLEMENTS
Regular supplements of folic acid, or folate (a B vitamin), before and after conception reduce the risk of neural-tube defects such as spina bifida in babies. While a woman is trying to conceive, 400 mcg folic acid should be taken daily, and continued until the 12th week

B GROUP VITAMINS: RNIs FOR PREGNANT AND BREASTFEEDING WOMEN

NOTE: vitamin amounts are given in mg per day *plus 400 mcg folic acid supplement	THIAMIN pork, beans, lentils, breakfast cereals, oranges, fish, cheese	RIBOFLAVIN eggs, yeast extract, fish, milk, yoghurt, breakfast cereals, peas	NIACIN meat and poultry, breakfast cereals, bread, pasta, fish, potatoes	VITAMIN B$_6$ breakfast cereals, milk, meat, nuts, potatoes, mushrooms	VITAMIN B$_{12}$ cheese, milk, meat, fortified soya milk, white fish	FOLIC ACID orange juice, broccoli, black-eyed beans, Brussels sprouts
DURING PREGNANCY	0.9	1.4	13	1.2	1.5	200*
WHILE BREASTFEEDING	1.0	1.6	15	1.2	2.0	260

of pregnancy. Good dietary sources of folate include fortified breakfast cereals, Brussels sprouts, broccoli, oranges and yeast extract.

IRON

Pregnant women produce extra blood to supply the baby and the placenta, and iron is needed to make additional red blood cells. Tannin in tea hinders its absorption; vitamin C greatly increases its uptake.

During pregnancy the body becomes more efficient at iron absorption. For women who enter pregnancy with low iron stores – usually those who eat few iron-rich foods, or who have previously suffered from heavy periods – ferrous iron supplements may be recommended to prevent anaemia. High intakes of iron can cause constipation, and may compromise zinc supplies because the two minerals compete for absorption.

Easily absorbed iron, known as 'haem' iron, is found in animal foods such as kidneys, heart, lean red meat, turkey, chicken and canned fish such as sardines and pilchards. However, liver, although an excellent source of iron, is not recommended in pregnancy because it can contain very high levels of retinol (a form of vitamin A), which may be detrimental to the developing baby.

CALCIUM

A woman's absorption of calcium increases during pregnancy. As long as dietary supplies of the mineral are adequate, supplements are not necessary. The recommended level of 700 mg per day can be met by eating plenty of dairy foods, baked beans and canned sardines with bones.

In the early stages of pregnancy, calcium is mobilised from stores in the bones, to be returned later on. For this reason, adolescent girls who become pregnant should take calcium supplements – their bones have not yet calcified sufficiently to cope with the additional demands of pregnancy, and their bone health may suffer in the long term. A 'bone formula' with a calcium/magnesium ratio of 2:1

ESSENTIAL FATTY ACIDS

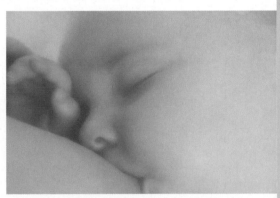

Essential fatty acids (EFAs) are required by the human body from conception to old age. Balanced amounts must come from the omega-6 EFAs (mainly from seed oils) and the omega-3 EFAs (mainly from fish oils).

Western diets tend to be abundant in the former and lacking in the latter; in pregnancy this imbalance can have harmful consequences, such as a predisposition to pre-eclampsia and premature births. The key omega-3 EFAs, eicosapentaenoic acid (EPA) and docosahexaenoic acid (DHA), are crucial for the development of a baby's brain and eyes. They are best obtained by eating oily fish, but fish liver oils (cod or halibut liver oil) must not be taken in pregnancy because they are high in retinol (vitamin A).

is ideal, since magnesium is also important for bone health and is often lacking in the diet.

Breastfeeding mothers need a daily 1250 mg calcium intake to produce breast milk. This can easily be supplied by drinking milk, eating calcium-rich dairy foods or taking 1000 mg a day in a supplement.

MAGNESIUM

This mineral, which is crucial for bone formation, is also present in breast milk. During pregnancy, stores of magnesium in the bones may be removed if dietary intake is inadequate. Lack of magnesium may contribute to pre-eclampsia.

The RNI for magnesium is 250 mg a day, rising to 320 mg during breastfeeding. Food sources include wholegrain cereals, bran-rich breakfast cereals, nuts and beans.

ZINC

Healthy cell growth and development is not possible without zinc. In men, sperm motility is reduced if the seminal fluid is low in zinc, and research has shown that women with diets low in zinc are at increased risk of having premature or low-birth-weight babies.

Pregnant women with an adequate intake of zinc from dietary sources such as meat, nuts, shellfish, beans and milk are unlikely to need supplementation because the body adapts to its extra requirements by increasing absorption from the diet.

If used in pregnancy, supplements should contain at least the RNI of 7 mg zinc a day. The RNI rises to 13 mg a day for the first four months of exclusive breastfeeding. Eating foods that supply your

additional requirements for protein at this time is likely to increase intake sufficiently.

COPPER

This mineral, a constituent of breast milk, is required in bone formation. Dietary sources include dried apricots, meat, nuts, rice, wholemeal pasta and breakfast cereals. The RNI is 1.5 mg a day.

SELENIUM

Bread, Brazil nuts, fish and some grains contain the powerful antioxidant selenium. Extra selenium is not required during pregnancy, but studies have shown that a deficiency may be linked to miscarriage.

Breastfeeding mothers need 75 mcg of selenium a day, which can be obtained either in the diet by eating selenium-rich foods or by taking a

PLANNING FOR A HEALTHY BABY

DIET
Crucial development of the foetus and placenta often takes place before a woman realises she is pregnant, so it is important for a prospective mother to establish a balanced diet before conception (see pages 15-23).

BODY WEIGHT
Underweight women may have too little body fat to produce oestrogen – a hormone essential for normal menstrual cycles – while overweight women may have problems with ovulation. It is advisable to lose excess weight before trying to conceive, because dieting while you are trying for a baby or pregnant could lead to an inadequate supply of essential nutrients. To check whether your weight is within the recommended healthy range, see pages 358-9.

SMOKING
Prospective parents should both give up smoking before trying for a baby. Smoking is associated with

low-birth-weight babies, infant death and complications in pregnancy. No supplement can offset the adverse consequences of smoking while pregnant.

ALCOHOL
Alcohol consumption can decrease fertility in both men and women, so preconceptual intake should be kept to a minimum or avoided. Heavy consumption of alcohol by a pregnant woman can damage a baby, leading to mental retardation or foetal alcohol syndrome, in which the baby is born with an alcohol dependency. Health professionals disagree about whether a small amount of alcohol is permissible during pregnancy. The usual advice is to abstain, or to drink no more than one unit of standard strength alcohol per day (a small glass of wine, half a pint of beer or a single measure of pub spirits). Drinking more than two units a day of alcohol can damage an unborn baby.

multivitamin and multimineral supplement.

VITAMIN A

This vitamin is needed for cell growth, skin and membrane development and a range of metabolic functions. RNI values are 700 mcg for pregnant women and 900 mcg for breastfeeding mothers. These amounts are easily obtained from average diets, and supplementation is not recommended.

Pregnant women should avoid high intakes of vitamin A in the form of retinol, since levels as low as 2800 mcg a day may lead to birth defects.

For this reason, liver and liver products, which can contain very high levels of retinol, are not recommended during pregnancy. Equally, prenatal and pregnancy supplements should not contain retinol – most now contain beta-carotene, which is much safer because it is converted into vitamin A by the body as required.

Fruit and vegetables rich in beta-carotene include mangoes, carrots, sweet potatoes, canteloupe melons, papaya, peaches and dark green vegetables. Vitamin A is also found in milk, butter, cheese, yoghurt, egg yolk and kidneys.

VITAMIN D

During pregnancy and breast-feeding vitamin D is required to assist calcium in the forma-tion of bones and teeth. Most

of our needs are supplied by the action of sunlight on skin; in the diet it is found only in animal products such as oily fish, fortified fat spreads and egg yolk.

Women who habitually cover up their skin for cultural or religious reasons, and whose diet contains no forti-fied products or animal foods, are at risk of a deficiency. For these women, supplements containing 10 mcg vitamin D are recommended during pregnancy and breastfeeding.

VITAMIN C

The RNI for vitamin C, which is essential for tissue growth and repair, is 50 mg a day in pregnancy and 70 mg while breastfeeding. A diet rich in fruit and vegetables will readily supply this daily requirement.

A glass of orange juice provides around 80 mg of vitamin C. In a recent study of almost 700 first-time mothers, low intakes of vitamin C were linked to reduced placental size and low birth weight.

B GROUP VITAMINS

The B complex vitamins are involved in releasing energy from food. The table on page 341 includes the RNI for each key member of this group during pregnancy and breast-feeding, and shows the dietary sources for them.

Vitamin B complex supple-ments may benefit women with poor diet, although pregnancy does not increase require-ments of all the B vitamins.

CARING FOR YOU AND YOUR BABY

MORNING SICKNESS

Among traditional remedies for morning sickness, ginger root seems to be the most enduring and successful. Ginger can be taken in the form of capsules, tablets, tea, ginger ale (check that it includes real ginger) or fresh root ginger.

Pysllium or flaxseed, also called golden linseed, can help to alleviate constipation, which often afflicts pregnant women. Take the seeds or husks with water to bulk out the stools.

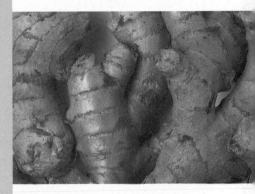

PREPARING FOR THE BIRTH

Some midwives recommend raspberry leaf to strengthen and tone the uterus. It is thought to encourage effective contractions, reducing the duration of labour. It should be taken only after 34 weeks of pregnancy; before this time it could cause miscarriage. Two or three tablets daily containing 400 mg raspberry leaf extract should be taken with meals.

VITAMIN K FOR NEWBORN BABIES

Vitamin K is routinely given at birth to reduce the risk of the life-threatening haemorrhagic disease of the newborn. Intra-muscular injections of vitamin K have long been used, but fears of a possible, though remote, link to leukaemia brought about the use of oral vitamin K. Several oral doses are routinely given to breastfed babies, but many paediatricians still believe that intramuscular injections are more effective.

Premenstrual syndrome

Many women are all too familiar with the symptoms of PMS. Affecting both the body and the emotions, this condition can be difficult to diagnose – except that it starts a week or so before menstruation and then disappears.

Symptoms

- *Irritability, mood swings, anxiety and depression.*
- *Abdominal bloating; swelling of hands and fingers.*
- *Breast pain and tenderness.*
- *Fatigue, lack of energy and insomnia.*
- *Headache and backache; joint and muscle aches.*
- *Constipation and diarrhoea.*
- *Cravings for specific foods, especially carbohydrates.*

SEE YOUR DOCTOR ...

- If PMS is severe and includes deep depression or excessive breast pain.

- If symptoms last all month – other conditions, such as clinical depression or an under-active thyroid, can mimic PMS.

REMINDER: If you have a medical or psychiatric condition, consult your doctor before taking supplements.

What it is

In the week before their periods begin many women experience crying spells, cravings for sweets and outbursts of anger. These, as well as some 200 other symptoms – including fatigue, depression, bloating, headaches and breast pain – characterise the condition known as premenstrual syndrome (PMS). The monthly symptoms vary from woman to woman in number and severity; most women experience only a few of them or are only mildly inconvenienced by them. However, for 5% to 10% of women PMS can be so severe that it interferes with their ability to live a full life.

What causes it

Why some women suffer from PMS and others do not is a mystery. Some experts believe that PMS may stem from an imbalance of the female hormones oestrogen and progesterone during the second half of the menstrual cycle, following ovulation. Too much oestrogen combined with too little progesterone may be connected with changes in the balance of the brain chemicals that control mood and pain; this hormonal irregularity can lead to mood changes and carbohydrate cravings. The imbalances are also associated with increased levels of the hormone prolactin, which results in breast tenderness and prevents the liver from clearing excess oestrogen from the body as efficiently as it should.

Another theory is that PMS symptoms are caused by low levels of serotonin, a brain chemical (neurotransmitter) that sends signals from nerve cell to nerve cell. Although the results of clinical studies examining the connection between serotonin and PMS are inconsistent, many women report that their PMS symptoms improve when they undergo treatment designed to return serotonin levels to normal. Improving the body's production and use of serotonin is particularly helpful in lifting depression.

Chasteberry may help to correct the hormonal imbalances that are thought to contribute to PMS.

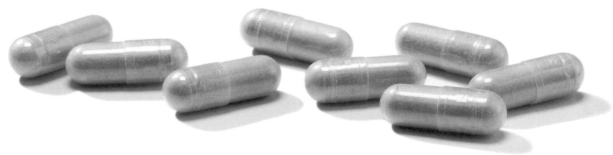

Chasteberry	**Dosage:** 225 mg extract a day when not menstruating. **Advice:** also called vitex; choose a product standardised to contain 0.5% agnuside.
Vitamin B$_6$	**Dosage:** 50 mg a day. **Caution:** doses exceeding 200 mg over a long period can cause nerve damage.
Evening primrose oil	**Dosage:** 1000 mg three times a day. **Advice:** you can substitute 1000 mg borage oil once a day.
Magnesium	**Dosage:** 200 mg once or twice a day. **Advice:** take with food.
St John's wort	**Dosage:** 300 mg extract three times a day. **Advice:** standardised to contain 0.3% hypericin.

Some dosages may be supplied by supplements you are already taking – see page 195.

How supplements can help

A combination of nutritional supplements, taken for part or all of the menstrual cycle, can relieve PMS symptoms. If you usually take conventional medications to deal with the problem, consult your doctor before combining them with supplements.

Chasteberry acts on the pituitary gland in the brain (which controls the production of oestrogen and progesterone in the body) and may be useful in correcting hormonal imbalances. The herb dong quai (200 mg extract three times a day) may enhance chasteberry's effectiveness; combination products with additional herbs such as black cohosh are often available.

Or, instead of chasteberry, try **vitamin B$_6$**, which assists the liver in processing oestrogen, increases progesterone levels and enables the brain to make serotonin. (Some practitioners recommend combining chasteberry and vitamin B$_6$.) The essential fatty acids contained in **evening primrose oil** may help to ease breast tenderness and control carbohydrate cravings. Many women with PMS have been found to be deficient in **magnesium** and may benefit from supplements of it.

Although some books recommend that supplements to alleviate PMS should be taken from the time of ovulation until your period begins, it is much better to take them regularly on a daily basis. If your primary PMS symptom is depression or anxiety, or if the other supplements are not effective, it is worth trying **St John's wort**.

What else you can do

☑ Exercise several times a week to lift your spirits and help your body to release fluids that cause bloating and breast tenderness.
☑ Cut back on caffeine, alcohol and salt, which can contribute to PMS.
☑ Keep a symptom diary; it can give you a sense of control and a better understanding of your physical and emotional feelings, aid in proper diagnosis and help to determine which treatment works for you.

Chasteberry may be a more effective treatment for PMS than vitamin B$_6$, according to a recent German study. Women who took chasteberry had a greater reduction in typical PMS symptoms – breast tenderness, swelling, tension, headache and depression – than those consuming B$_6$. Overall, 36% of those in the chasteberry group were free of symptoms compared with 21% of participants in the vitamin B$_6$ group.

In an American study of 500 women, researchers found that taking 1200 mg of calcium a day reduced PMS symptoms by more than 50%. Compared with women given a placebo, those using calcium showed improvement in mood swings, food cravings, bloating and menstrual pain. The researchers now believe that low calcium levels may contribute to the hormonal imbalance thought to be a factor in PMS.

FACTS & TIPS

■ PMS may have positive aspects. Some researchers have found that women who suffer from PMS are very attuned to their surroundings and have sharp memories, not just in the days or week immediately before their periods but all month long.

Prostate problems

If you are a man over 50 you are more likely than not to have a prostate problem – usually a benign enlargement of the gland. Herbal and nutritional therapies can ease discomfort and may prevent or delay the need for conventional drugs or surgery.

Symptoms

- Frequent, urgent need to urinate, particularly at night.
- Difficulty or hesitancy in urinating; inability to empty the bladder.
- A weak urine stream or dribble.
- Burning during urination, fever, shivering, pain behind the scrotum or painful ejaculation.

SEE YOUR DOCTOR ...

- If you have any symptoms of a prostate condition – a simple examination and PSA blood test can help distinguish a benign prostate disorder from cancer.
- If you have blood in the urine or semen.

REMINDER: If you have a medical condition, consult your doctor before taking supplements.

What they are

These disorders typically cause urinary complaints because they affect the prostate, the walnut-sized gland that is located below the bladder and surrounds the urethra (the tube that transports urine out of the bladder). By far the most common problem is BPH (benign prostatic hyperplasia, or hypertrophy), a noncancerous enlargement of the prostate that occurs in more than half of men aged over 50. BPH can progress for many years, with few or no symptoms at first. It is not a risk factor for developing prostate cancer, but a doctor should evaluate your condition to rule out cancer and prostate inflammation (prostatitis), which are more serious.

What causes them

As men age the prostate typically enlarges. No one is sure why this happens, though male sex hormones may play a role. Depending on the degree of enlargement, the prostate can press against the urethra and impede the flow of urine, causing the symptoms of BPH. Less often, men develop prostatitis, which is usually caused by a bacterial infection that begins elsewhere in the urinary tract, or cancer. In these conditions, swelling of the prostate or growth of a tumour can disrupt urine flow.

How supplements can help

The recommended supplements are most effective for mild to moderate BPH and may take a month or longer to produce results. They can be safely used over a long period, along with any conventional drugs your doctor may have prescribed. See your doctor every six months to check whether they are working. Supplements may also help some cases of mild prostatitis, but prostate infections and cancer require prompt

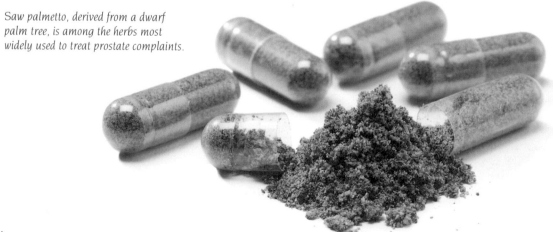

Saw palmetto, derived from a dwarf palm tree, is among the herbs most widely used to treat prostate complaints.

SUPPLEMENT RECOMMENDATIONS

Zinc	**Dosage:** 25 mg a day. **Advice:** if you take a zinc supplement for more than a month, use one that includes 2 mg copper.
Vitamin E	**Dosage:** 250 mg a day. **Caution:** consult your doctor if you take anticoagulant drugs.
Saw palmetto	**Dosage:** 160 mg extract twice a day between meals. **Advice:** standardised for 85%-95% fatty acids and sterols.
Beta-sitosterol	**Dosage:** 20 mg three times a day. **Advice:** also present in saw palmetto and nettle root.
Fish oils	**Dosage:** 2 teaspoons to supply 2 grams of omega-3 fatty acids a day. **Caution:** consult your doctor if you take anticoagulant drugs. **Advice:** vegetarians can substitute 1 tablespoon of flaxseed oil.
Nettle root	**Dosage:** 250 mg extract twice a day. **Advice:** standardised to contain at least 1% plant silica.
Amino acids	**Dosage:** 500 mg each of glycine, alanine and glutamine daily. **Advice:** after one month, add a mixed amino acid complex.

Note: consider using supplements in blue first; those in black may also be beneficial. Some dosages may be supplied by supplements you are already taking – see page 195.

medical intervention. **Zinc**, one of the key nutrients for prostate health, has been shown to reduce the size of the gland and ease BPH symptoms. Zinc interferes with copper absorption, so take copper too. Extra **vitamin E** can aid in preserving prostate health: as an antioxidant it scavenges free radicals, which can damage DNA and lead to cancer.

Herbs may also help to relieve symptoms of BPH and slow down prostate growth. **Saw palmetto**, the best-researched of these, can be very effective, partly by altering hormone levels; it may also be useful in curbing inflammation and swelling in chronic cases of prostatitis. Saw palmetto can be combined with **nettle root**, which may boost its ability to ease symptoms and slow down progression of BPH. One of the active components of both saw palmetto and nettle root is **beta-sitosterol**. This is available in its pure form as a dietary supplement and may be helpful in reducing BPH symptoms. Additional nutrients are recommended. The essential fatty acids in **fish oils** (or flaxseed oil) help to prevent the swelling and inflammation of the prostate in BPH and prostatitis. In addition the **amino acids** glycine, alanine and glutamine, taken together each morning on an empty stomach, may aid in relieving symptoms, but they do not slow prostate growth.

What else you can do

☑ Don't take decongestants or other over-the-counter cold remedies; they can make symptoms worse.

☑ To help to reduce urinary complaints, avoid caffeinated and alcoholic drinks, especially beer. Reduce consumption of liquids in the evening.

Psoriasis

Although this persistent skin condition, which flares up and retreats in cycles, is not life-threatening, it can be extremely painful for some sufferers. There is no known prevention or cure for psoriasis, but nutritional and herbal supplements may help to control it.

Symptoms

- *Patches of raised, inflamed red skin with white flaking scales.*
- *Itching.*
- *Loosened, pitted, discoloured fingernails or toenails.*
- *Cracked or blistered skin, with pain in severe cases.*
- *Joint pain and stiffness.*

What it is

Psoriasis is a noncontagious chronic skin condition characterised by raised, inflamed red patches that are usually covered with whitish or silvery scales. Sufferers typically develop it between the ages of ten and thirty, but it can occur at any time. The rash is usually confined to the scalp, elbows, knees, lower back or buttocks. Fingernails and toenails can become yellow or pitted. Though flare-ups are unsightly, most cases are not itchy or particularly painful, but about 15% of people with psoriasis have such severe and widespread rashes that they suffer great discomfort and may be unable to perform daily activities. In about 5% of cases, joint pain and swelling similar to symptoms of rheumatoid arthritis develop.

What causes it

When someone is suffering from psoriasis, the skin cells in certain parts of the body replicate much faster than normal. Skin cells originate in the deep layers of the skin and usually take about 28 days to come to the surface, where they are sloughed off. However, in areas of skin affected by psoriasis this process takes only eight days – the new cells accumulate so quickly that they never have a chance to mature. As a result, the skin becomes red and inflamed and develops overlapping white scaly patches.

The reason why skin growth is accelerated in certain areas is not known, but the fact that one in three sufferers has a family history of psoriasis has led some practitioners to conclude that there is a genetic aspect to the disorder. Certain stimuli – alcohol, stress, sunburn, cold temperatures, dry air, skin injury, throat infection and some medications – may also trigger the onset of psoriasis or worsen existing lesions.

How supplements can help

All the supplements in the chart may help to control psoriasis flare-ups, and can be taken in combination; most people experience improvement in about a month. In addition, all psoriasis sufferers should take an 'A to Z' multivitamin and mineral formula, which should contain chromium

Studies show that the essential fatty acids in fish oils, available in softgel form, can help to control outbreaks of psoriasis.

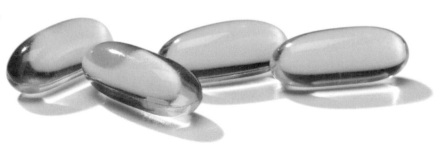

SUPPLEMENT RECOMMENDATIONS

Fish oils	**Dosage:** 2 teaspoons to supply 2 grams omega-3 fatty acids a day. **Caution:** consult you doctor if you take anticoagulant drugs. **Advice:** vegetarians can substitute 1 tablespoon of flaxseed oil.
Vitamin C	**Dosage:** 500 mg twice a day. **Advice:** reduce dose if diarrhoea develops.
Vitamin E	**Dosage:** 400 mg a day. **Caution:** consult your doctor if you take anticoagulant drugs.
Selenium	**Dosage:** 100 mcg a day. **Caution:** toxic in high doses; total daily intake should not exceed 350 mcg.
Zinc	**Dosage:** 25 mg a day. **Advice:** if you take a zinc supplement for more than a month, use one that contains 2 mg copper.
Milk thistle	**Dosage:** 150 mg extract twice a day. **Advice:** standardised to contain at least 70% silymarin.

Note: consider using supplements in blue first; the one in black may also be beneficial. Some dosages may be supplied by supplements you are already taking – see page 195.

see page 195.

(200 mcg) and selenium (75 mcg). Omega-3 essential fatty acids, found in **fish oils** (and flaxseed oil), block the action of arachidonic acid, a substance made by the body that causes inflammation. (Low levels of omega-3s are common in people with psoriasis.) **Vitamin C** and **vitamin E** are powerful antioxidants that may prevent damage to skin cells. When combined with vitamin E, **selenium** has been shown to have an anti-inflammatory effect. **Zinc** is necessary for maintaining healthy skin and nails, and promotes healing. (Extra copper is important because long-term zinc use interferes with copper absorption.) **Milk thistle**, a herb with anti-inflammatory properties, may control the rash and slow down the abnormal skin cell proliferation. For outbreaks, apply a cream containing Oregon grape (10% extract) to skin lesions three times a day to reduce their size and provide relief from pain and itching.

Although they have not been clinically evaluated, several other herbs have been used for many years by medical herbalists for the treatment of psoriasis; they include yellow dock, red clover, burdock, sarsaparilla and Oregon grape.

What else you can do

☑ Get some sun. Just 15 to 30 minutes of sunlight a day may improve psoriasis lesions in three to six weeks. Apply a sunscreen with an SPF of 15 or greater to nonaffected areas to guard against sunburn.

☑ Use a humidifier in the winter. Dry indoor air may cause lesions.

☑ Apply moisturiser all over your body – and especially on lesions – to prevent dry skin and reduce itching. Aloe vera gel is a good choice.

☑ Eat oily fish often (good choices include mackerel, sardines, tuna, salmon and herring) or take your fish oils in capsule form.

Raynaud's disease

Imagine that your fingers quickly become numb when you go outside on a winter's day, or even when you accept a cold drink at a summer picnic. This often happens to people who have Raynaud's disease, a little-understood circulatory disorder.

Symptoms

- *Temporary colour change (first white, then a reddish blue) in the skin of the affected areas in response to cold or stress.*

- *Numbness, tingling or a drop in skin temperature in affected areas.*

- *Gradual changes in skin texture.*

- *In advanced cases, sores on the tips of the fingers.*

SEE YOUR DOCTOR ...

- If small sores develop or the skin becomes very smooth, shiny or tight.

- If episodes impair manual dexterity or sense of touch.

- If symptoms increase in severity or frequency.

REMINDER: If you have a medical condition, consult your doctor before taking supplements.

What it is

First identified in 1862 by Maurice Raynaud, a French physician, Raynaud's disease affects the tiny arteries (arterioles) that deliver blood to the skin of the fingers, toes, nose and ears. In some people, cool temperatures prompt spasms in these blood vessels; this reduces blood flow and deprives the area of oxygen. As a result the skin changes colour and may tingle or go numb. Although it can be annoying and uncomfortable, in most cases Raynaud's disease is not associated with more serious circulatory problems.

What causes it

The cause of Raynaud's is not known. However, some experts believe that the blood vessels of people with the disease overreact to the cold, possibly as the result of an instability in the nerves of the affected areas. More women than men are affected by the disorder.

Raynaud's can either occur on its own or accompany other medical conditions such as migraine headaches, rheumatoid arthritis, lupus, atherosclerosis or an underactive thyroid. (When an underlying cause can be found the disorder is called Raynaud's phenomenon.) Going outside in winter, reaching into a refrigerator, or even entering an air-conditioned room often produces symptoms that can last from minutes to hours. Stress is also a trigger. Raynaud's symptoms may be a side effect of decongestants and some heart or migraine medications.

How supplements can help

Raynaud's disease is often chronic, so these supplements may be most helpful when used over the long term. **Vitamin E** improves blood flow through the arteries. The mineral **magnesium** has many beneficial

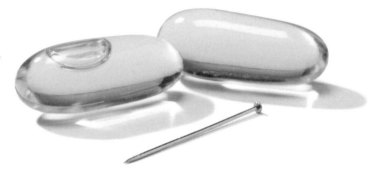

To relieve the symptoms of Raynaud's disease, use a pin to prick open an evening primrose capsule and massage the oil into your fingers or toes.

SUPPLEMENT RECOMMENDATIONS

Vitamin E	**Dosage:** 250 mg a day. **Caution:** consult your doctor if you take anticoagulant drugs.
Magnesium	**Dosage:** 200 mg twice a day. **Advice:** take with food; reduce dose if diarrhoea develops.
Ginkgo biloba	**Dosage:** 40 mg extract three times a day. **Advice:** standardised to contain at least 24% flavone glycosides.
Evening primrose oil	**Dosage:** one or two capsules, applied topically, each day. **Advice:** you can substitute capsules of borage oil.
Fish oils	**Dosage:** 2 teaspoons to supply 2 grams of omega-3 fatty acids a day. **Caution:** consult your doctor if you take anticoagulant drugs. **Advice:** vegetarians can substitute 1 tablespoon of flaxseed oil.

Note: consider using supplements in blue first; those in black may also be beneficial. Some dosages may be supplied by supplements you are already taking – see page 195.

effects on the cardiovascular system. One of these – its ability to relax constricted blood vessels – makes it useful for Raynaud's. An alternative is **ginkgo biloba**, a herb that is especially effective in widening small blood vessels. In one study the gamma-linolenic acid (GLA) in **evening primrose oil** was demonstrated to improve Raynaud's symptoms when massaged into the fingertips. The oil can be used alone or with the other supplements. (Borage oil is a good substitute; it also contains GLA and is generally less expensive.)

If these treatments don't help, try **fish oils**. In a placebo-controlled study of 32 patients with Raynaud's, fish oil supplementation delayed the onset of symptoms by an average of 15 minutes. Other herbs that can be helpful include garlic, hawthorn and ginger; they all help to relax the small blood vessels in the extremities of the body.

What else you can do

☑ Avoid nicotine and caffeine, which cause blood vessels to contract.
☑ Practice biofeedback and other relaxation techniques.
☑ Take precautions to prevent injuring affected areas.
☑ Protect yourself from the cold by wearing mittens – which keep the fingers warmer than gloves – and heavy socks in winter. Use gloves when reaching, even briefly, into a freezer or supermarket frozen food cabinet.
☑ Don't take decongestants, and ask your doctor if any other medications you are taking might trigger your symptoms.

CASE HISTORY
Remedy for Raynaud's

Until a magazine article alerted her to ginkgo biloba, winter was Ann D.'s least favourite season. Even though she wore heavy gloves to combat the cold, her fingers still changed colour – going from healthy pink to deathly white. Her doctor diagnosed that it was Raynaud's disease, but he wasn't optimistic about treating it. 'I could tell that he gave me a prescription just to pacify me,' Ann recalls.

'But then I tried ginkgo,' she says. 'What a finger-saver, especially when I added a little vitamin E every day.' Though she had to wait a month for results, her patience paid off. Today, while remaining wary of excessive cold, she is a champion of supplements, and enjoys sharing her success with others.

'Raynaud's is pretty common,' Ann comments, 'but not many people who have it realise what it is. Those who do often simply suffer. I can truly recommend ginkgo for safe, natural – and very effective – relief.'

Rosacea

The ruddy complexion of many fair-skinned people may not always be a healthy glow but rather a sign of rosacea, a common skin problem. Even though there is no cure, symptoms of this chronic condition can often be controlled and skin damage prevented.

Symptoms

- *Frequent, prolonged redness and flushing of the cheeks, nose, forehead and chin.*

- *Feeling that skin is being pulled tightly across the face.*

- *The appearance of tiny red spots and bumps in the affected area.*

- *Bumpiness, redness and swelling on the nose.*

- *Bloodshot, burning or itchy eyes.*

SEE YOUR DOCTOR ...

- **If you develop any of the symptoms listed above.**

- **If your skin does not promptly return to its normal colour after you blush.**

REMINDER: If you have a medical condition, consult your doctor before taking supplements.

What it is

The first signs of rosacea (rose-AY-shah) are recurrent patches of redness on the cheeks, nose, forehead and chin, and the appearance of tiny blood vessels just under the skin. As the disorder progresses, the skin on the face becomes ruddier and then permanently inflamed; bumps may also form. The eyes may be affected too, and develop burning or itching. In severe rosacea the nose may develop excess tissue.

About one in 20 adults has rosacea, with fair-skinned people at the highest risk. Although women are three times more likely to develop the condition than men, the latter have more severe symptoms. Smokers are vulnerable because nicotine impairs circulation. Without treatment, rosacea may worsen; conventional therapy often includes long-term use of antibiotics.

What causes it

Rosacea occurs when unknown genetic and/or environmental factors cause blood vessels in the skin to lose their elasticity and dilate easily, sometimes permanently. Blood vessel abnormalities are one possible cause. Episodes can be triggered by any stimulus that leads to flushing, including hot or spicy foods or beverages; alcohol or caffeine; stress; weather; vigorous exercise; hormonal changes (especially at menopause); and certain medications (especially nicotinic acid, a form of niacin prescribed for heart disease, and some blood pressure drugs).

How supplements can help

Rosacea is a chronic condition, so supplements should be continued indefinitely; it may be about a month before initial improvements are obvious. Begin with the B vitamins. Then add vitamin C, the minerals and

Fish oils can be effective in reducing inflammation and may help to minimise rosacea flare-ups.

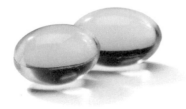
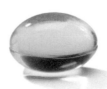
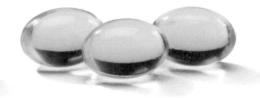

Vitamin B complex	**Dosage:** one tablet each morning with food. **Advice:** look for a B-50 complex with 50 mcg vitamin B_{12} and biotin, 400 mcg folic acid and 50 mg all other B vitamins.
Vitamin C	**Dosage:** 500 mg twice a day. **Advice:** reduce dose if diarrhoea develops.
Zinc	**Dosage:** 25 mg a day. **Caution:** if you take a zinc supplement for more than a month, use one that includes 2 mg copper.
Fish oils	**Dosage:** 2 teaspoons to supply 2 grams of omega-3 fatty acids a day. **Caution:** consult your doctor if you take anticoagulant drugs. **Advice:** vegetarians can substitute 1 tablespoon of flaxseed oil.

Some dosages may be supplied by supplements you are already taking – see page 195.

the essential fatty acids, if necessary. All can be used in addition to the antibiotics that are often prescribed for rosacea.

A deficiency of B vitamins is common in people with rosacea, so **vitamin B complex** is beneficial. As for **vitamin C**, it strengthens the membranes that line the blood vessels and the connective tissue between skin cells. It also minimises the release of histamine, a chemical that widens blood vessels in response to an allergic substance. **Zinc** helps to heal the top layer of the skin (epidermis) and regulates blood levels of vitamin A. (Add copper for long-term use.) And the essential fatty acids in **fish oils** (or flaxseed oil) reduce inflammation, control the cells' use of nutrients and produce hormone-like substances called prostaglandins which stimulate contraction of blood vessels.

What else you can do

☑ Use fragrance-free, greaseless make-up and facial cleansers. Never use astringents on your skin.
☑ Gently blot – never rub – your face dry after washing.
☑ Wear a sunscreen with an SPF of at least 15 when you are outdoors.

A study of 31 patients with rosacea found that 84% tested positive for *Helicobacter pylori*, the organism that causes peptic ulcers. This explains why some rosacea sufferers respond to the antibiotics used to treat these ulcers.

DID YOU KNOW?

Some rosacea sufferers have very high numbers of the tiny skin mites that live in human hair follicles. A breakdown of the immune system is the probable cause. Riboflavin and other B vitamins may help to control mite growth.

FACTS & TIPS

■ To soothe inflamed skin, splash your face with a strong chamomile and marigold (calendula) tea. Pour 500 ml of very hot water over 1 tablespoon of each herb. Cover the infusion and let it sit for 20 minutes, then strain, cool and use it to wash your face.

■ People who wear make-up may be able to conceal persistent redness with a sheer green base applied under a foundation matching their normal skin tone.

■ Men with rosacea may minimise flare-ups by shaving with an electric razor rather than a blade.

Shingles

Remember chicken pox? The virus is still lurking in your nerve cells and can flare up at any time during your adult years, causing the intensely painful blisters known as shingles. The good news is that natural remedies can often help to ease this sometimes lingering condition.

Symptoms

- *Intense burning and tingling in one area of the body, followed after one to three days by a reddening of the skin. May be accompanied by headache and a temperature.*

- *Clusters of bubble-like, fluid-filled blisters that form on an inflamed band of skin – usually on the torso or buttocks but sometimes on the face or arms.*

- *Intense pain and itching around the blisters, which form scabs after 10 days. The pain typically subsides after two or three weeks but sometimes persists for months or years (postherpetic neuralgia).*

SEE YOUR DOCTOR ...

- If you develop the symptoms described above – to be effective, antiviral drugs must be taken early on.

- If you have a bruised sensation on one side of your face or body.

- If facial skin lesions spread close to your eyes.

- If an inflamed area is infected or lasts more than 10 days without real improvement.

- If you are unable to endure the pain.

REMINDER: If you have a medical condition, consult your doctor before taking supplements.

What it is

Shingles, known medically as herpes zoster, is a form of the same herpes virus infection that causes chicken pox. After a childhood attack of chicken pox the virus does not die but lies dormant in nerve cells. It can be reactivated later in life, when it produces intensely painful clumps of skin blisters. Shingles itself is not contagious, but the open sores it causes can transmit the chicken pox virus to young children, or to others who have never been infected.

What causes it

The virus responsible for shingles is thought to be revitalised when the immune system is weakened by age, stress or flu, or by certain drugs or illnesses that impair immunity. But no one knows for sure what causes the virus to resurface and produce symptoms.

How supplements can help

Therapies for shingles are designed to treat acute flare-ups (for which supplements should be taken until the lesions heal) and post-shingles pain, which can persist for months or even years. The supplements for an acute shingles attack – which should be taken together – can be further divided into two groups: topical therapies applied directly to skin lesions, and supplements ingested to boost the immune system and to help in the healing of inflamed skin and nerves.

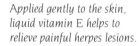

Applied gently to the skin, liquid vitamin E helps to relieve painful herpes lesions.

Aloe vera gel	**Dosage:** apply gel liberally to the skin as needed. **Advice:** use fresh aloe leaf or shop-bought gel.
Vitamin E	**Dosage:** apply topical oil for acute attacks. **Advice:** for post-shingles pain, take 250 mg orally twice a day.
Vitamin C/ flavonoids	**Dosage:** 500 mg vitamin C and 250 mg flavonoids twice a day. **Advice:** reduce vitamin C dose if diarrhoea develops.
St John's wort	**Dosage:** 300 mg extract three times a day. **Advice:** standardised to contain 0.3% hypericin.
Echinacea/ goldenseal	**Dosage:** 200 mg echinacea extract and 125 mg goldenseal extract four times a day. **Advice:** use only during acute stage; available in combination.
Lysine	**Dosage:** 1000 mg L-lysine three times a day only during the acute stage. **Advice:** take on an empty stomach; do not take with milk.
Selenium	**Dosage:** 100 mcg a day only during the acute stage. **Caution:** high doses of selenium are toxic; do not take more than 350 mcg.

Note: consider using supplements in blue first; the one in black may also be beneficial. Some dosages may be supplied by supplements you are already taking – see page 195.

Topical treatments, such as **aloe vera gel** combined with **vitamin E** oil, may provide immediate relief. They act as soothing emollients, relieve pain and itching, enhance healing, and reduce the likelihood that shingles lesions will become infected. A melissa or liquorice cream applied to the affected areas of the skin may also be effective.

For internal treatment during flare-ups, **vitamin C** and **flavonoids** are antioxidants that help to protect against cell damage. Along with the herbs **echinacea** and **goldenseal** they boost the function of the immune system, helping it to fight the herpes virus and bacterial skin infections. St John's wort also has strong antiviral properties, and has a long tradition of use as a treatment for shingles. The amino acid **lysine** and the mineral **selenium** promote healthy skin growth and speed up the healing process.

For lingering post-shingles pain, stick with the supplements that worked for you during the acute phase, adding vitamin E (250 mg twice a day) to protect against cell damage and vitamin B_{12} (1000 mcg with 400 mcg of folic acid every morning) to nourish the sheaths that cover and protect the nerves.

What else you can do

☑ Keep affected areas clean and dry. Never scratch or try to burst blisters, as this can cause a bacterial infection.

☑ Use cool, wet compresses or ice packs to soothe the area and reduce pain. You can also apply calamine lotion to the skin.

Capsaicin, the peppery liquid responsible for the hotness of chilli peppers, is available in an ointment formula for topical application. Studies in pain clinics have found that chilli ointment helps to reduce the lingering nerve pain that afflicts some people after an attack of shingles. Check with your doctor before using chilli ointment. It must not be applied to active shingles infections, as it can cause intense burning on open skin wounds. Use it only for long-term pain, after lesions have completely healed up.

DID YOU KNOW?
Shingles strikes hundreds of thousands of people every year, most of them over the age of 50, though younger people can also be afflicted by the disease.

FACTS & TIPS

■ Natural supplements can be used in combination with prescription medicines such as acyclovir which also promote healing.

■ Colloidal oatmeal, a form of finely ground oatmeal sold in pharmacies, can be added to baths to help to relieve itching. You can make your own blend by grinding oatmeal in a food processor and adding several cups to your bath water. Be careful when getting out of the bath: oatmeal makes smooth surfaces very slippery.

Sinusitis

The sinus cavities produce lubricating mucus which helps to keep the respiratory system free of debris. When the sinuses become inflamed or blocked and the flow of mucus is prevented, a number of uncomfortable and sometimes painful symptoms can result.

Symptoms

- *Pressure or headache above the eyes.*
- *A feeling of fullness in the face.*
- *Pain that worsens when the head is bent forwards.*
- *Tenderness above the sinuses.*
- *Trouble breathing through the nose.*
- *Postnasal drip (excessive mucus at the back of the throat).*
- *Yellowish-green nasal discharge.*
- *Toothache or symptoms of fever.*

SEE YOUR DOCTOR ...

- If symptoms do not clear up within a week, or if they are accompanied by a bloody discharge.
- If sinusitis recurs more than three times a year.
- If redness, pain, bulging or paralysis develops in the eyes – you may have orbital cellulitis, a condition that can damage the eye and facial nerves: get medical help immediately.

REMINDER: If you have a medical condition, consult your doctor before taking supplements.

What it is

Sinusitis is a condition caused by blocked sinuses. The sinuses are four pairs of openings in the bones at the front of the skull, located above the eyes on either side of the nose, behind the bridge of the nose and behind the cheekbones. They are lined with a thin membrane which secretes mucus. The mucus passes into the nose through small openings in the sinuses, sweeping away inhaled dust, pollen, germs and other matter, then drains into the back of the throat where it is swallowed. (Most dangerous bacteria are destroyed by stomach acid.)

Normally the work of the sinuses is so subtle that you don't even notice it, but the membrane can become irritated or inflamed, which results in the production of more (or thicker) mucus and blocks the tiny sinus openings. When this occurs the sinuses cannot drain properly; this causes headaches, a feeling of fullness in the face and postnasal drip (an excessive amount of mucus running down the back of the throat). The mucus build-up also provides a breeding ground for bacteria.

What causes it

Sinusitis can be a complication of an upper respiratory infection, such as a cold or flu. The linings of the sinuses can also be irritated by smoke, air pollution or allergies. Malformations in the nose such as a deviated septum or nasal polyps may increase the chances of developing sinusitis.

How supplements can help

Some cases of sinusitis – bacterial infections, for instance – require antibiotic treatment, but conventional medicine is beginning to question the universal use of these drugs, especially for people with chronic sinus conditions which may not originate from bacteria. Antibiotics do not prevent future sinus infections.

Supplements can help to clear up an acute infection, even if you are taking antibiotics. A lack of any of several nutrients can exacerbate

Vitamin C is a natural antihistamine that fights the inflammation caused by sinusitis.

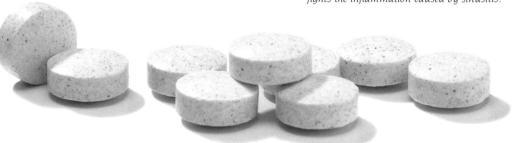

SUPPLEMENT RECOMMENDATIONS

Vitamin C/ flavonoids	**Dosage:** 500 mg vitamin C and 250 mg flavonoids twice a day. **Advice:** reduce dose if diarrhoea develops.
Fish oils	**Dosage:** 2 teaspoons to supply 2 grams omega-3 fatty acids a day. **Caution:** consult your doctor if you take anticoagulant drugs. **Advice:** vegetarians can substitute 1 tablespoon of flaxseed oil.
Echinacea	**Dosage:** 200 mg of extract four times a day. **Advice:** standardised to contain at least 3.5% echinacosides.
Astragalus	**Dosage:** 200 mg extract twice a day between meals. **Advice:** supplying 0.5% glucosides and 70% polysaccharides.
Cat's claw	**Dosage:** 250 mg of standardised extract twice a day. **Caution:** do not use during pregnancy. **Advice:** take between meals.
Reishi/ maitake mushrooms	**Dosage:** 500 mg reishi mushrooms and/or 200 mg maitake mushrooms three times a day. **Caution:** avoid reishi mushrooms if you take anticoagulant drugs.

Note: consider using supplements in blue first; those in black may also be beneficial. Some dosages may be supplied by supplements you are already taking – see page 195.

see page 195

inflammation, so a general multivitamin and multimineral formulation should always be taken by regular sufferers. The recommended vitamins and herbs are particularly valuable for those with recurring problems, and do not cause the side effects provoked by conventional prescription medicines for sinusitis (such as a dry mouth).

One of the best ways to prevent and treat sinusitis is to strengthen the body's defences against germs. Start off by taking the immune strengtheners **vitamin C** and **flavonoids**, which offer additional benefits for those whose allergy attacks develop into sinusitis. Both substances minimise the effect of histamine – an inflammatory substance produced by the cells in response to allergens. Modern diets often exacerbate inflammation because they are too high in omega-6 fats and too low in omega-3 fats: inflammation can be reduced by taking omega-3 fats as **fish oils** (or flaxseed oil) to balance the omega-6 fatty acids.

In addition, choose one of the following immune-boosting herbs: **echinacea**, **astragalus**, **cat's claw** or **reishi** or **maitake mushrooms**. For acute attacks, take just one of these herbs until the infection clears up. For chronic sinusitis, try alternating them in two-week rotations to build and maintain immunity.

What else you can do

☑ Avoid cigarette smoke and excess dust.
☑ Drink plenty of fluids to thin the mucus.
☑ Use a humidifier to keep indoor air moist.
☑ Put warm compresses on your face to help to open up the sinuses.
☑ Consider using a sinus irrigator, a device available from some health-food and chemists' shops, which uses salt water to flush out mucus.

RECENT FINDINGS

Milk has often been cited as a culprit in increased mucus production – some say that it should be avoided during a bout of sinusitis. But in a recent study healthy participants who drank half a pint of milk a day showed no significant increase in congestion or thickening of the mucus.

DID YOU KNOW?

In medical terminology, the suffix '-itis' (as in sinusitis, for example) means inflammation.

FACTS & TIPS

■ You can reduce congestion by inhaling eucalyptus-scented steam. Add a few drops of eucalyptus oil to a pan of water. Heat to boiling and remove from the stove. Place a towel over your head and the pan and breathe in the steam through both nostrils. Blow your nose frequently.

■ Some practitioners believe that spicy foods such as horseradish or garlic may help to clear out congested sinuses. No major scientific studies have been conducted to prove this theory.

Skin problems

A disorder of the skin may affect any part of the body, and its seriousness can range from irritating to life-threatening. A diet abundant in fruit and vegetables, drinking plenty of water and a judicious use of supplements can all have positive effects.

Symptoms

- Itchy, red or inflamed skin.
- Dull, dry, scaly or cracking skin; brown spots or discoloration.
- Thickening or thinning of the skin.
- Excessive bruising.

SEE YOUR DOCTOR ...

- If you suffer from a recurrent skin complaint.
- If you experience severe, persistent itching, particularly when the skin is warm – you may have scabies, which is a highly contagious disease.
- If you have a persistent rash – it could be a sign of shingles.

REMINDER: If you have a medical condition, consult your doctor before taking supplements.

What they are

The skin is the largest organ in the body, responsible for many functions and vulnerable to a wide variety of disorders, the causes of which are not always evident. For example, itching and bruising afflict everyone, occasionally, but in some cases indicate a serious underlying condition. Some skin problems result from a malfunction of the body's excretory system. The many causes of skin inflammation include eczema (or dermatitis), lupus, acne and psoriasis. Among other skin problems are verrucas, warts, cold sores, sunburn, corns and calluses, cuts and grazes, and contagious diseases such as impetigo and scabies.

What causes them

A diet high in processed foods, sugar or fat takes its toll on the skin, as do pollution, stress, smoking and ultraviolet light. Dry skin is usually genetic in origin but is made worse by exposure to the elements and poor diet. Very dry skin is often due to a simple shortage of oil or oil and moisture, although it is sometimes linked to hypothyroidism.

Drugs such as antispasmodics, antihistamines and diuretics, the sun and smoking are all drying agents. Thinning of the skin is a natural result of ageing but can also be caused by steroids. Eczema and rashes are often caused by allergies to metals, sunlight, cosmetics, plants, foods or other substances, while stress can provoke psoriasis. Poor elimination of toxins from the body as a result of kidney or liver problems can cause skin rashes. Extensive bruising may be the result of nutritional deficiencies, anaemia, anticoagulant drugs or being overweight; it is sometimes an early sign of cancer. Corns and calluses can be caused by friction, for example from badly-fitting shoes.

How supplements can help

To counteract dry skin and to treat eczema and rashes, ensure that you are obtaining the proper balance of omega-3 and omega-6 essential fatty acids by taking **fish oils** (or flaxseed oil). These oils can also relieve the

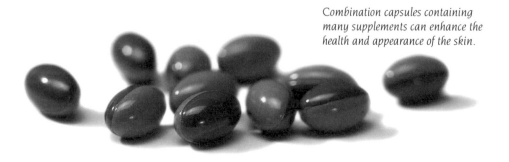

Combination capsules containing many supplements can enhance the health and appearance of the skin.

Fish oils	**Dosage:** 2 teaspoons to supply 2 grams omega-3 fatty acids a day. **Caution:** consult your doctor if you take anticoagulant drugs. **Advice:** vegetarians can substitute 1 tablespoon of flaxseed oil.
Vitamin C	**Dosage:** 500 mg a day. **Advice:** reduce dose if diarrhoea develops.
Vitamin E	**Dosage:** 250 mg a day. **Caution:** consult your doctor if you take anticoagulant drugs.
Zinc	**Dosage:** 15 mg a day. **Advice:** if you take a zinc supplement for more than a month, use one that includes 2 mg copper.
Echinacea	**Dosage:** 200 mg three or four times a day. **Advice:** in cases of acute infection take every few hours.
Evening primrose oil	**Dosage:** 1000 mg two or three times a day. **Advice:** take with meals.

Note: consider using supplements in blue first; the one in black may also be beneficial. Some dosages may be supplied by supplements you are already taking – see page 195.

itching and inflammation of many skin problems, from erysipelas to scabies. They need to be taken with antioxidants such as **vitamin C** and **vitamin E**, which help to protect the skin from external damage and from free radicals (unstable oxygen molecules) which can damage cells. These vitamins ease rashes and eczema, repair tissue damage caused by burns or cuts and grazes, inhibit inflammation and encourage healing – all of which relieves itching and dryness.

To treat dry skin, acne and psoriasis, and to promote tissue repair, **zinc** has been shown to be useful. For dry skin, eczema and rashes take an 'A-Z' multivitamin and multimineral formula which contains zinc and selenium. By boosting the immune system **echinacea** fights skin infections – it can also be applied directly to the skin to heal wounds, eczema, burns and boils. **Evening primrose oil** is useful for many skin problems, particularly inflammatory skin disorders, and can also be applied externally.

Tea tree oil and lavender oil can be applied directly to the skin to aid healing of insect bites, cuts and grazes and guard against infection. Aloe vera soothes sunburn and heals injured skin. Chamomile cream, chickweed cream and yoghurt can be applied topically to relieve itching, and calendula cream can be used to reduce inflammation.

What else you can do

☑ Drink at least six glasses of water a day: this helps to eliminate waste products that can cause skin disorders, and boosts the healing process.
☑ Reduce the amount of fatty foods in your diet and increase your intake of fresh fruit and vegetables, especially carrots (which contain the anti-oxidant beta-carotene), for general skin health and to combat acne.

FACTS & TIPS

■ Washing less often than usual, using lukewarm water and unperfumed products, and gently patting your skin dry rather than rubbing it can help to reduce dryness.

■ Food allergies, particularly to eggs, milk and peanuts, may be responsible for as many as 75% of cases of skin rashes in children. An allergy test can reveal if a particular food is to blame. Research suggests that excluding gluten from the diet as well as dairy products may bring relief to dermatitis sufferers.

■ Teas made from infusions of dandelion, nettle, red clover, sarsaparilla, yellow dock and burdock stimulate liver and kidney function, which promotes elimination of toxins and improves the appearance of the skin.

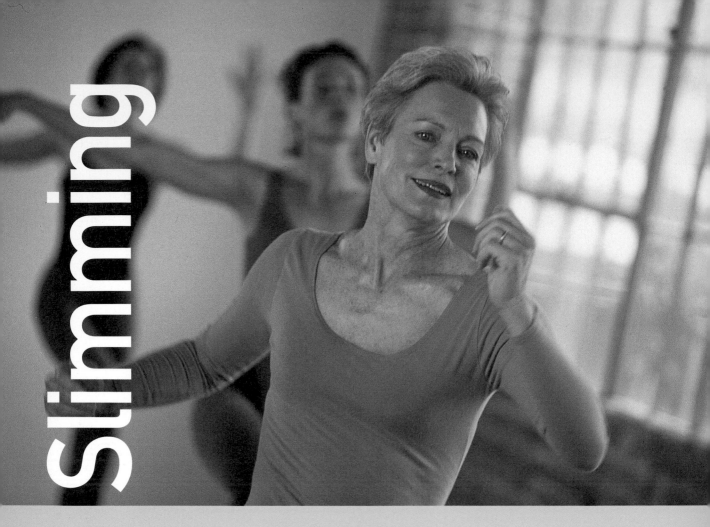

slimming

Many of us have tried to lose weight, or 'slim', at some stage in our lives, with varying degrees of success. But when is it appropriate to slim? Can you do it effectively and safely? And can supplements help?

COUNTING CALORIES: ENERGY AND DIET

■ **Energy in food is measured in Calories. Recommended daily intakes are 2500 for men and 2000 for women.**

■ **Individual needs depend on age, lifestyle and basal metabolic rate – the rate at which we use energy for our body's basic functions – which between them consume almost 90% of our energy.**

■ Maintaining a healthy weight is crucial to well-being.

■ Obesity increases the risk of health problems, such as heart disease, stroke and certain cancers – all major causes of death in the UK. It can also contribute to other ailments and significantly reduce the quality of your life.

■ Obesity is linked with an increased risk of high blood pressure, diabetes, osteo-arthritis, respiratory disorders, gallbladder disease, infertility, sweating, breathlessness and sleeping difficulties.

■ Estimates from the 1997 Health Survey for England show that 62% of men and 53% of women are overweight.

ARE YOU OVERWEIGHT?

There is a simple way to check whether your weight and shape are healthy. The Body Mass Index (BMI) assesses weight and height. To work out your BMI, divide your weight in kilograms by the square of your height in metres. The healthy range is 20-25. If your BMI is above 25 you should consider losing weight. If it is 30 or higher you are suffering from obesity and should consult your doctor.

The BMI cannot distinguish the weight of muscle from that of fat, but unless you have particularly well-developed muscles your BMI rating will be a good indication of your total body fat content.

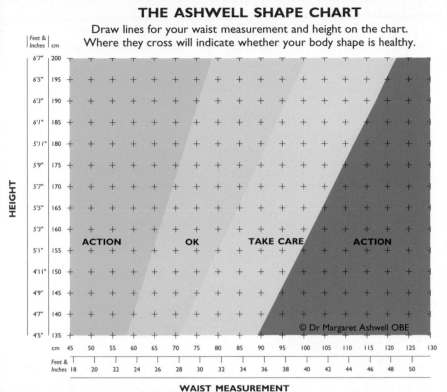

THE ASHWELL SHAPE CHART

Draw lines for your waist measurement and height on the chart.
Where they cross will indicate whether your body shape is healthy.

Feet & Inches | cm

6'7"	200
6'5"	195
6'3"	190
6'1"	185
5'11"	180
5'9"	175
5'7"	170
5'5"	165
5'3"	160
5'1"	155
4'11"	150
4'9"	145
4'7"	140
4'5"	135

HEIGHT

ACTION   OK   TAKE CARE   ACTION

© Dr Margaret Ashwell OBE

cm 45 50 55 60 65 70 75 80 85 90 95 100 105 110 115 120 125 130
Feet & Inches 18 20 22 24 26 28 30 32 34 36 38 40 42 44 46 48 50

WAIST MEASUREMENT

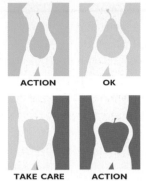

ACTION   OK

TAKE CARE   ACTION

Green *If your shape falls in this area you are underweight and should take action*

Blue *This pear region indicates a healthy shape, with any excess fat only just beneath the skin*

Yellow *In the 'pear/apple' area you are verging on an unhealthy shape and need to take care*

Red *If you are apple-shaped your excess fat lies deep down in the stomach. Your health is at risk and you need to take action*

The distribution of fat also has a bearing on health. If it is spread evenly, mainly round the hips and thighs (in a 'pear' shape), you will be less prone to heart disease, diabetes and strokes than 'apple'-shaped people, who have a 'spare tyre' or pot belly.

HOW TO LOSE WEIGHT

The key to losing weight safely and effectively is to reduce your calorie intake while following a balanced diet (*see pages 15-22*), and exercising. Remember that, weight for weight, fat supplies more than twice as many calories as carbohydrate or protein.

Aim to lose no more than 1 kg per week at a steady rate: crash diets and 'yo-yo' dieting are thought to damage health.

THE ROLE OF DIETARY SUPPLEMENTS

If you are trying to lose weight, taking an A-Z multivitamin and multimineral supplement will help to guard against the micronutrient deficiencies which might arise from having a reduced intake of energy-producing foods.

Although fat consumption should be reduced, omega-3 and omega-6 essential fatty acids are still necessary for healthy cell membranes and the effective functioning of the immune system. Eat oily fish twice a week or take a daily supplement of fish oils or flaxseed oil to maintain your intake. If you cut down on dairy products, maintain your intake

of calcium with a 'bone formula' which also contains magnesium and vitamin D.

Losing weight is all about using up more energy than you take in. Some supplements may help to boost your energy expenditure while others may help to reduce your intake by making you feel full.

SUPPLEMENTS TO BOOST ENERGY EXPENDITURE

A number of herbs can be used to raise metabolic rate and improve blood circulation, and may be helpful in weight loss.
■ Extracts of the rind of the **brindall berry** contain hydroxycitric acid (HCA), which research suggests may reduce the conversion of

carbohydrates into stored fat. The normal dose is 500 mg three times a day.

■ **Kelp** may be helpful for those who are overweight as a result of reduced thyroid activity. Although its benefits are not scientifically proven, medical herbalists use this plant to stimulate the thyroid gland and so raise the metabolic rate of those with hyperthyroidism.

HOW TO EAT LESS

■ **Use small plates and bowls and take small portions.**

■ **Eat as slowly as you can, to give your body more time to signal satisfaction to your brain and for your brain to tell you to stop eating.**

■ **Eat all food – snacks included – from a plate, using a knife, fork and spoon.**

■ **Take small mouthfuls and put down your cutlery until you have swallowed.**

■ **Eat only in one place, at a table – away from TV, radio, newspapers, books and other distractions – and concentrate on what you are eating.**

■ **Stop eating when you no longer feel hungry.**

■ **Don't feel that you must leave a clean plate.**

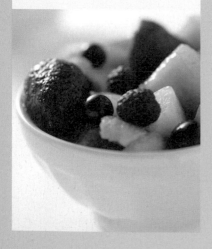

■ **Chromium** enables cells to recognise insulin, so the body needs adequate supplies of this trace element. Clinical studies have shown that chromium improves blood glucose control in diabetics, and preliminary research suggests that it may be helpful for weight loss.

A low intake of chromium is associated with high blood cholesterol levels, as well as with low insulin sensitivity, so supplements may also be helpful for general health. An A-Z multivitamin and multimineral formulation usually contains about 200 mcg, which would normally be sufficient. This can safely be increased to 400 mcg (as chromium picolinate) by taking a separate supplement.

In overweight and obese people the body's cells become increasingly insensitive to insulin. This hormone helps to regulate blood glucose levels by allowing glucose to enter cells for conversion into energy. Without insulin, glucose cannot enter cells and is converted into fat. If the insulin sensitivity of cells is improved, glucose is 'burnt' as energy rather than being stored as fat, helping weight loss. Regular exercise improves insulin sensitivity.

SUPPLEMENTS TO REDUCE HUNGER

There is increasing evidence that the brain neurotransmitter serotonin is involved in appetite control; low levels, which occur during dieting, are linked with increased appetite. The brain is thought to convert a substance

called **5-HTP** into serotonin. Studies of overweight women found that a supplement of 5-HTP promoted the sensation of satiety, and that they then consumed less food at meals.

The usual dose is 50-100 mg of 5-HTP, taken 20 minutes before meals for at least two weeks; if weight loss is less than 0.5 kg per week, the dosage may be progressively increased up to a maximum of 300 mg. Higher doses can cause nausea.

FILLING UP ON FIBRE

Eating foods high in fibre provides bulk, which produces a feeling of fullness and reduces hunger pangs. The gummy substances from plants, known as soluble fibre, are most effective; they bind much more water than insoluble fibre from woody tissues and wheat bran.

Although research has not proved that soluble fibre aids reduced calorie intake by promoting satiety, it may help to prevent cravings for food caused by low levels of blood glucose, which are common when dieting. This is because soluble fibre slows down the rate of absorption of sugars from the intestine and so helps to smooth out fluctuations in blood glucose.

Guar gum, a soluble fibre extracted from the Indian cluster bean, has exceptional water-binding properties and is widely used as a gelling agent in foods such as dairy desserts.

Guar gum granules may be helpful to slimmers because they take up water, producing a feeling of fullness in the stomach, and normalise blood glucose levels. Don't take large amounts of guar gum granules – they may cause flatulence – and don't take tablets or capsules, which can swell up in the throat and cause a blockage.

Two other types of soluble fibre with similar effects to guar gum – **psyllium husks** and **glucomannan** – are often used as supplements.

Psyllium husks come from the seeds of the Indian plantain. Herbalists have known for centuries that the seeds act as laxatives, and pharmaceutical companies use them to make laxatives that bulk out the stools. Powder made from the husks can be taken with meals, mixed with water or fruit juice.

Glucomannan is a soluble fibre prepared from the root of the oriental Konjac plant and is taken in the same way.

EATING DISORDERS

The eating disorders anorexia nervosa and bulimia nervosa are the outward expression of psychological and emotional turmoil. Most sufferers have low self-esteem and find it hard to express their emotions; they use food and eating as a means of expressing their difficulties.

A true eating disorder usually follows a period of restrictive dieting, often spurred by worry about body weight and shape. Only a tiny minority of people who diet develop disorders.

Sufferers of anorexia nervosa typically refuse to maintain a minimally healthy body weight

(an anorexic's weight is at least 15% below normal), experience dramatic weight loss, have an intense fear of gaining weight, are preoccupied with food, and have abnormal patterns of food consumption.

They may also suffer a hormonal disorder which can lead to amenorrhoea (lack of menstruation) in women and loss of sexual potency in men.

Bulimia is characterised by recurrent episodes of 'binge' eating, with a feeling of loss of control. These are followed by purges through fasting, self-induced vomiting or the use of laxatives or diuretics.

Bulimics fear being over-weight but, unlike anorexics, their body weight may be high, low or average. The condition typically starts between the ages of 15 and 20, often after problems with eating habits, childhood obesity or a lifelong fluctuation in weight.

SUPPLEMENTS AND EATING DISORDERS

Food supplements cannot pre-vent eating disorders, but can help to improve general health; extra zinc may help to stimulate appetite. Dietary supplements will protect against nutritional deficiencies in those whose food intake is extremely low.

Trace elements and vitamins can be obtained from A-Z formulations; extra calcium and magnesium should be obtained from a 'bone formula'; and separate supplements will be required to provide sufficient vitamin C and vitamin E.

HOW TO BE MORE ACTIVE

■ Develop a positive attitude to activity, taking all opportunities to be on the move.

■ Try tensing your muscles and then relaxing them at intervals throughout the day.

■ If you have a sedentary job, welcome a chance to search for something in a filing cabinet. Don't phone or e-mail someone who is only two offices away.

■ At home, resist the temptation to ask anyone to fetch and carry for you. If you want the newspaper, go and get it, as briskly as possible. If you want the television channel changed, get up and change it – don't use the remote control.

■ Walk up stairs at home and at work; this uses a lot of energy because you are moving your body against gravity.

■ Perform daily activities more quickly than usual. Walk more briskly, and try walking-cum-jogging. When weeding the garden or doing housework, use maximum body movement.

■ When possible, walk or cycle rather than going by car. Take a walk during your lunch break.

■ One of the best exercise machines you can get is a dog. The regular walks it demands are a good way of increasing your own activity.

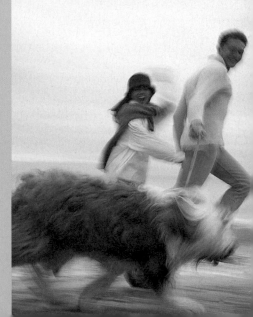

Smoking

It is never too late to stop smoking, but unfortunately a tobacco addiction is one of the most difficult habits to overcome. A number of natural supplements can boost your chances of success, helping you to cope with cravings and reducing the anxiety that often accompanies giving up.

Symptoms

Caused by smoking

- Persistent cough or recurring bouts of bronchitis or pneumonia.

- Hoarseness, sore throat, bad breath and yellowed teeth.

- Premature greying, balding and wrinkling of the skin.

- In some men, impotence.

Caused by giving up smoking

- Anxiety, depression, craving for cigarettes, compulsive eating, nervousness and irritability.

- Drowsiness, fatigue, headaches, a productive cough and constipation.

SEE YOUR DOCTOR ...

- If you develop symptoms of a serious smoking-related illness: pains in your chest or upper back; chronic wheezing or coughing; pink or blood-tinged mucus; or persistent sores or white patches on the mouth, tongue or throat.

- If you need help to give up smoking.

REMINDER: If you have a medical condition, consult your doctor before taking supplements.

What it is

Smoking is a habit with serious health consequences, though it is not considered an illness. Within minutes of lighting a cigarette, pipe or cigar, a smoker's blood pressure and pulse rate rise and oxygen levels drop. After a few months of smoking, symptoms such as a cough, fatigue, sinus congestion or shortness of breath, can appear. In the long term, smoking can lead to cancer, chronic lung disorders, heart disease and stroke.

What causes it

Despite the well-documented risks to health, millions of people continue to smoke because smoking is an extremely powerful addiction. Not only does the addictive drug in tobacco – nicotine – cause physical effects throughout the body, but it also travels almost directly to the brain, where it temporarily lifts the spirits and soothes anxiety. Social rituals associated with lighting a cigarette can also be calming. Giving up smoking causes nicotine levels to drop, which results in jittery feelings and a range of physical complaints.

How supplements can help

If you are trying to give up smoking there are various supplements that may help to soothe frayed nerves and powerful cravings. They can be used over a period of weeks or months, and all can be taken with other stop-smoking aids such as nicotine patches or gum. Under your doctor's supervision they can also be taken with antidepressant drugs.

Begin by increasing your intake of **B vitamins** and **vitamin C**, which are depleted in smokers. Vitamin B complex promotes healthy nerves and can lessen anxiety. Vitamin C has an antioxidant effect – meaning that it can mop up some of the excess unstable oxygen molecules called free radicals that are generated by tobacco smoke. It can also ease cravings and other withdrawal symptoms. The action of vitamin C is supported by **vitamin E** – together they reduce the risk of heart and arterial disease caused by free radicals. A number of additional

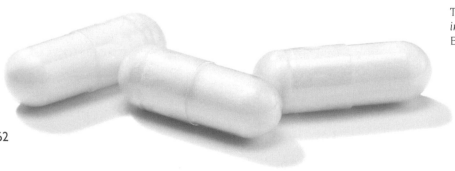

The stress of giving up smoking increases the body's need for the B vitamin pantothenic acid.

SUPPLEMENT RECOMMENDATIONS

Vitamin B complex	**Dosage:** one tablet twice a day with food. **Advice:** look for a B-50 complex with 50 mcg vitamin B_{12} and biotin, 400 mcg folic acid and 50 mg all other B vitamins.
Vitamin C	**Dosage:** 500 mg twice a day. **Advice:** reduce dose if diarrhoea develops.
Vitamin E	**Dosage:** 400 mg a day. **Caution:** consult your doctor if you take anticoagulant drugs.
Oat extract	**Dosage:** ½ teaspoon of tincture four times a day. **Advice:** this is an alcohol-based extract, also called *Avena sativa*.
Pantothenic acid	**Dosage:** 100 mg twice a day. **Advice:** use calcium pantothenate – the least expensive form.

Note: consider using supplements in blue first; the one in black may also be beneficial. Some dosages may be supplied by supplements you are already taking – see page 195.

nutrients – used singly or together – may also lessen cravings. One option is **oat extract**, which healers in India have used for centuries to treat opium addiction. In one study it significantly reduced the craving for cigarettes, even two months after people stopped taking it, possibly by affecting levels of the brain chemicals responsible for addiction. Bottled oat juice is available for those who do not wish to take an alcoholic tincture.

The anxiety caused by nicotine withdrawal usually dissipates within a month or so. People who are trying to stop smoking may benefit from the B vitamin **pantothenic acid**, which boosts the production by the adrenal glands of antistress hormones.

Liquorice root and dandelion root may also be helpful in reducing the craving for tobacco (they should be chewed when the urge is strong); mullein tea has a similar effect. Cat's claw extract can be used to stimulate the removal of toxins from the body (but should not be taken during pregnancy).

What else you can do

☑ Eat plenty of fruit, vegetables and nuts to reduce the harmful effects of tobacco smoke on the body. Choose green leafy vegetables, carrots, berried fruits (especially bilberries and blueberries) and any kind of nuts, which all help to protect against cancer and the deterioration of the eyes.
☑ Consider nicotine gums or patches, the prescription antidepressant drug bupropion, acupuncture or hypnosis, which can all reduce cravings.
☑ Exercise to cut down on stress. A brisk walk can also help to overcome an intense craving, which usually lasts only a few minutes.

RECENT FINDINGS

Researchers have long known that drinkers tend to smoke more than non-drinkers, and that drinking often serves as a social cue to smoke. A recent American study shows that, in smokers, alcohol can actually increase the craving to smoke.

The *Journal of the National Cancer Institute* reports that people who give up smoking for longer than three months are much less likely to relapse than those who give up for a shorter time – another reason to use supplements and other strategies to bridge the gap.

DID YOU KNOW?

Within three months of giving up, a former smoker's lung capacity increases. After about 15 years most of the elevated health risks return to normal.

FACTS & TIPS

■ The pepped-up feeling produced by smoking comes from compounds that mimic the effects of the brain chemical acetylcholine, which plays a vital role in mental alertness. A balanced diet and a daily high-potency multi-vitamin can boost the natural production of acetylcholine, reducing the need to smoke.

■ 'Environmental' tobacco smoke is classified as a Class A carcinogen by the US Environmental Protection Agency – along with arsenic, asbestos, benzene and radon gas.

Sore throats

Stress and tiredness, as well as colds and flu, can make us susceptible to sore throats. Fortunately this ailment responds exceptionally well to natural treatments: not only do they alleviate the pain and discomfort, but they can also reduce inflammation in the throat.

Symptoms

- *Redness, pain or burning in the throat; sometimes pain in the ears.*
- *Difficulty in swallowing.*
- *A lump-like feeling in the throat.*
- *Hoarseness.*
- *Swollen lymph glands under the jaw.*

SEE YOUR DOCTOR ...

- If a sore throat is severe and comes on suddenly – it could be a bacterial infection.
- If you have a temperature of 38°C or higher and no symptoms of a cold.
- If you have extreme difficulty in swallowing.
- If a rash develops.
- If a mild sore throat persists for more than a week.

REMINDER: If you have a medical condition, consult your doctor before taking supplements.

What they are

Sore throats are not illnesses in themselves but symptoms of illness. The feeling of rawness or burning which begins at the back of the mouth and extends to the middle of the throat is usually caused by inflammation. When the throat is infected or otherwise irritated, the body responds by sending more blood to the area. The blood carries white cells and other substances to fight the infection – these fighting substances cause redness, swelling and pain in the throat.

What causes them

Allergies, bacterial or viral infections and environmental triggers such as dust, dry air and smoke are the most common causes of sore throats. In the case of an allergy or a viral infection, a sore throat is often the result of postnasal drip – the draining of excessive mucus from the nose or sinuses down the back of the throat. The viruses that cause colds also attack throat tissue directly. A viral sore throat usually develops slowly over several days. It lasts longer but is milder than a bacterial infection, which often strikes suddenly – sometimes in a matter of hours – and induces severe throat pain, difficulty in swallowing and a temperature.

How supplements can help

The recommended remedies are intended to strengthen the immune system, help to heal inflamed throat tissue and ease pain. Unless otherwise noted, they should be used together for as long as symptoms last. These supplements can be combined with over-the-counter or prescription medications for colds or allergies, or taken with antibiotics.

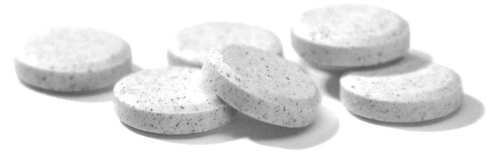

Zinc lozenges may help you to fight a cold, preventing the development of an associated sore throat.

Vitamin C	**Dosage:** 500 mg twice a day. **Advice:** reduce dose if diarrhoea develops.
Echinacea	**Dosage:** 200 mg of extract four times a day. **Advice:** standardised to contain at least 3.5% echinacosides.
Garlic	**Dosage:** 400-600 mg of dried concentrate four times a day with food. **Advice:** each tablet should provide 4000 mcg allicin potential.
Zinc	**Dosage:** one lozenge every three or four hours. **Caution:** do not continue for more than five days.
Slippery elm	**Dosage:** as a tea, 1 teaspoon per cup of hot water, as required. **Advice:** can be combined with or replaced by an infusion of marshmallow root.

Some dosages may be supplied by supplements you are already taking – see page 195.

Vitamin C helps the body to fight the upper respiratory tract infections that often cause sore throats. It is a natural antihistamine, and can also reduce the production of inflammatory compounds in the bodies of allergy sufferers. The herbs **echinacea** and **garlic** have antiviral and antibacterial properties; take them at the first sign of throat irritation.

If you have a cold, try **zinc** lozenges to help to ward off a sore throat; studies have shown that they may shorten the duration of the illness. If you dislike the taste of zinc or do not have a cold, drink **slippery elm** or marshmallow root tea. These herbs coat the throat, making swallowing easier and relieving pain. Slippery elm also contains compounds known as oligomeric proanthocyanidin complexes (OPCs), which fight infection and allergic reactions. For an extra boost to the immune system add a few drops of goldenseal tincture to your tea – this is especially effective against bacterial infections because it contains an anti-bacterial compound known as berberine. If you are congested you can add liquorice (in dried herb or tincture form), but do not take it if you suffer from high blood pressure.

What else you can do

☑ Use a humidifier to keep the throat lubricated.
☑ Do not smoke, and stay out of smoke-filled rooms.
☑ Drink eight or more cups or glasses of liquid daily. Warm liquids, such as soup or tea, can be especially helpful.

New research shows that zinc lozenges do not work as a treatment for children. A study involving 249 school-age children found that those using the lozenges took just as long to get over their colds as children taking a placebo (nine days, on average). Other studies in adults have shown that zinc lozenges can cut the duration of a cold almost in half. The reason for the different results is not known.

FACTS & TIPS

■ Gargling several times a day reduces the pain of a sore throat. Try these herbal gargles: boiling water with equal parts of goldenseal, liquorice, slippery elm and raspberry leaf, cooled to lukewarm; or ½ cup of boiling water added to 1 teaspoon of red sage, cooled and strained.

■ Your doctor should not prescribe antibiotics for a sore throat unless it has been confirmed that the soreness is related to a bacterial infection. If you do have to take antibiotics they may destroy the 'friendly' bacteria that keep your digestive system functioning well, so replenish your internal supply with probiotics.

Sprains and strains

Whether it is caused by a sudden 'twist' of the ankle, strenuous exercise or repeated wrenching, a sprain or strain can create severe discomfort and affect mobility. Whatever the cause, natural therapies can go a long way to relieving the symptoms.

Symptoms

Sprains

- *Mild to severe pain at time of injury; tenderness and swelling of the joint; bruising.*

- *Lack of, or very painful, movement in injured joint.*

Strains

- *Stiff, sore muscles, tenderness and swelling.*

- *Slight skin discoloration, which may appear after several days.*

SEE YOUR DOCTOR ...

- **If swelling is severe or gets worse, or an injured joint becomes conspicuously mis-shapen — it may be a fracture.**

- **If pain continues to be extreme despite self-treatment, or if pain spreads to other parts of the injured area.**

- **If severe bruising or skin discoloration occurs.**

- **If the injured area cannot sustain movement or bear the body's weight.**

REMINDER: If you have a medical condition, consult your doctor before taking supplements.

What they are

Strains are minor injuries to the muscles. They usually occur in the calf, thigh, groin or shoulder, and cause soreness and stiffness. Sprains are similar to strains, but are more serious and painful and take longer to heal. They can entail damage to ligaments, tendons or muscles – usually those surrounding a joint.

What causes them

Strains and sprains result from physical stress to the muscles and other tissues. Lifting a heavy object, using the muscles for long periods without resting, or overstretching before a physical workout can lead to a strain. Sprains, on the other hand, are the result of a sudden force to a muscle, tendon or ligament. Any unexpected movement, such as a fall or a twisting motion, can yank and tear these structures.

How supplements can help

In addition to self-care measures, supplements – either taken internally or applied externally – can promote tissue repair, strengthen injured areas and reduce inflammation. They can be very effective in alleviating the symptoms of sprains or strains, and most need to be used only for a week or so, or until the injury begins to improve.

Various oral supplements have been shown to speed up the healing process. They can all be taken in combination with conventional painkillers. **Bromelain**, an enzyme derived from the pineapple plant, may prevent swelling and reduce inflammation, and so relieve pain. It also promotes blood circulation and hastens healing. The antioxidants **vitamin C** and **flavonoids** aid in healing and in limiting further injury to connective tissues and muscles.

Topical therapies may also be effective. Apply ointments containing the plant extract **arnica** to sore muscles or joints to reduce pain and

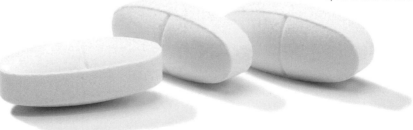

Glucosamine strengthens and protects joints, which helps sprains and strains to heal faster.

SUPPLEMENT RECOMMENDATIONS

Bromelain	**Dosage:** 500 mg three times a day on an empty stomach. **Advice:** should provide 6000 GDU or 9000 MCU daily.
Vitamin C/ flavonoids	**Dosage:** 500 mg vitamin C and 200 mg flavonoids two or three times a day. **Advice:** reduce dose of vitamin C if diarrhoea develops.
Arnica	**Dosage:** apply ointment to painful area four times a day. **Caution:** never ingest arnica and do not put it on broken skin.
Glucosamine	**Dosage:** 500 mg glucosamine sulphate three times a day. **Advice:** take with food to minimise digestive upset.
Turmeric	**Dosage:** 300 mg extract up to three times a day. **Advice:** take with meals; can also be applied externally.
Gotu kola	**Dosage:** 200 mg extract twice a day. **Advice:** can also be applied externally as a tincture.
Horse chestnut	**Dosage:** 500 mg extract each morning. **Advice:** standardised to contain 16%-21% aescin.
Sweet marjoram oil	**Dosage:** add a few drops to a basin of cold water. **Advice:** soak towel in solution, wring out and apply.
Rosemary oil	**Dosage:** add a few drops to a basin of cold water. **Advice:** soak towel in solution, wring out and apply.

Note: consider using supplements in blue first; those in black may also be beneficial. Some dosages may be supplied by supplements you are already taking – see page 195.

see page 195

A recent study of 59 people with strains and torn ligaments who were given 500 mg of bromelain three times a day for one to three weeks found that the supplement caused a marked reduction in swelling, tenderness and pain, at rest and during movement. The results were comparable to those in people taking NSAIDs (nonsteroidal anti-inflammatory drugs) such as aspirin.

DID YOU KNOW?

Sprains can weaken ligaments and lead to recurring injuries. Ensure that you warm up before exercising and adapt your exercise regime accordingly. An elastic support bandage may help to protect weakened joints.

FACTS & TIPS

■ Common treatments for sprains and strains include NSAIDs. Supplements are safer alternatives because they have very few of the potentially dangerous side effects, such as stomach bleeding, that may be associated with the drugs.

■ Although scientists have found no evidence to confirm that magnets have any benefits, some people insist that applying magnets to painful areas can speed healing. Magnet therapy is especially popular in Japan.

swelling and encourage healing. By building up cartilage, sometimes known as the 'shock absorber' of the body, **glucosamine** serves to strengthen and protect the joints and ligaments.

Turmeric is a traditional remedy used externally or internally to relieve inflammation; if it is mixed with hot water to form a paste and applied on a gauze dressing, it can help to reduce swelling and ease bruising. **Gotu kola** improves healing by building connective tissue and improving blood flow. **Horse chestnut** is also useful for controlling inflammation. Compresses soaked in a mixture of either **sweet marjoram oil** or **rosemary oil** and water can produce a soothing, pain-relieving effect and are useful in reducing swelling.

What else you can do

☑ Follow the RICE acronym: Rest the injured part; Ice the painful area; Compress the injury with an elastic support bandage; and Elevate the injured area above the level of the heart. Apply ice for 10 to 20 minutes at a time; reapply it every two or three hours for one to two days following the injury. A bag of frozen vegetables is a good substitute for ice and can be easily moulded around the injured area – peas work best.

☑ Once the swelling subsides, use a hot compress or heating pad on the area to boost blood circulation.

☑ Witch hazel water, comfrey cream and even raw cabbage juice are traditional remedies which can be applied to the skin to improve healing.

Stress

Modern life can often exhaust our natural defences, leaving the body susceptible to stress and its broad range of associated health problems. Certain nutrients can help you to cope, and herbs and other nutritional supplements can calm the mind and restore equanimity.

Symptoms

- *Fatigue, insomnia or difficulty in concentrating.*
- *Nervousness, agitation or unusual excitability.*
- *Loss of appetite, nausea, upset stomach, diarrhoea or constipation.*
- *Headaches.*
- *Loss of sexual interest.*
- *Irritability, anger, resentment, apathy or pessimism.*

SEE YOUR DOCTOR ...

- If you have prolonged or pronounced symptoms of stress. These weaken your immune system and increase your risk of medical problems – heart disease, high blood pressure, digestive disorders, ulcers, migraines and possibly cancer.

- If stress symptoms cause problems with relationships, work or everyday activities, or lead to substance abuse – you may need to be treated for depression.

REMINDER: If you have a medical or psychiatric condition, consult your doctor before taking supplements.

What it is

Stress is simply an individual's response to taxing physical, emotional or intellectual demands. The body is equipped to deal with brief episodes, but high-level stress on a regular basis can be severely detrimental to physical and mental health.

What causes it

A variety of predicaments can produce stress: family discord, financial problems, job pressures, injuries, illness, traumatic events and so on. The body's initial reaction to stress is to prepare itself for impending danger. The adrenal glands – two small glands, one on top of each kidney – release adrenaline and other so-called 'stress' hormones which provide an instant burst of energy and strength, allowing the body to confront an enemy or escape to safety.

This 'fight or flight' response is a natural and healthy reaction, but problems can arise if the stress persists. Over time, chronically high levels of stress hormones deplete both nutrient and energy reserves, creating an overall state of exhaustion. Blood pressure and cholesterol levels increase (sometimes damaging heart and blood vessels); the stomach secretes too much acid; sex hormones diminish; and the brain becomes starved of glucose (its only energy source), which impairs mental ability. These effects place additional demands on the immune system, which may become so weakened that the body can muster little resistance to infection and illness.

How supplements can help

Many nutrients are crucial to the body's natural ability to cope, so a daily multivitamin and multimineral formulation is especially important during times of stress. Take the **B complex vitamins** as well; the extra

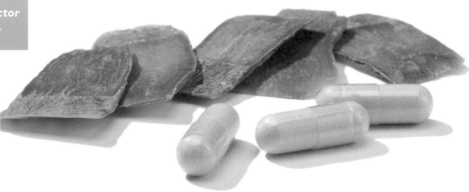

The dried root of Panax ginseng, often packaged in capsule form, helps to build up the body's defences against stress.

Vitamin B complex	**Dosage:** one tablet twice a day with food. **Advice:** choose a B-50 complex with 50 mcg vitamin B_{12} and biotin, 400 mcg folic acid and 50 mg all other B vitamins.
Calcium/ magnesium	**Dosage:** 500 mg calcium and 200 mg magnesium twice a day with food. **Advice:** sometimes sold as a single supplement.
Siberian ginseng	**Dosage:** 100-300 mg extract three times a day. **Advice:** standardised to contain at least 0.8% eleutherosides.
Panax ginseng	**Dosage:** 100-250 mg extract twice a day. **Advice:** standardised to contain at least 7% ginsenosides.
Valerian	**Dosage:** 300 mg extract twice a day. **Caution:** may cause drowsiness if you are short of sleep. **Advice:** standardised to contain 0.5% valerenic acid.
St John's wort	**Dosage:** 300 mg of extract three times a day. **Advice:** standardised to contain 0.3% hypericin.

Note: consider using supplements in blue first; those in black may also be beneficial. Some dosages may be supplied by supplements you are already taking – see page 195.

B vitamins it supplies promote the health of the nervous and immune systems and can counteract fatigue. **Calcium** and **magnesium** are worth while because they can relieve muscle tension and strengthen the heart. **Siberian ginseng** and **Panax ginseng** may also be effective because they bolster the adrenal glands. These stress-fighting herbs are sometimes called 'adaptogens' (because they help the body to 'adapt' to challenges) or 'tonics' (because they 'tone' the body, making it more resilient). These supplements can be taken in combination, with the exception of the two ginsengs, which should not be taken together.

Other herbs and nutritional supplements, used singly or together, or combined with the supplements above, may be valuable in particular circumstances. Take **valerian** if worry is keeping you awake at night, and **St John's wort** if the stress is accompanied by mild depression.

What else you can do

☑ Exercise regularly and try relaxation techniques such as breathing exercises, yoga, t'ai chi, meditation, massage or biofeedback.
☑ Eliminate or restrict your intake of caffeine and alcohol. They can contribute to anxiety and insomnia.
☑ Consider psychological counselling and therapy to increase your ability to cope with stressful situations.
☑ Maintain social ties. A close network of family and friends – or even a cherished pet – is vital to good health.

RECENT FINDINGS

An American researcher has suggested that the healing effects of poorly understood alternative therapies such as crystal therapy – in which crystals are laid on certain 'energy centres' in the patient's body – may partly arise from their ability to reduce stress. The lowering of stress levels is known to cause changes in the brain and the immune system that increase the body's ability to fight disease.

Compared with routine stress, being highly stressed for more than a month doubles your chances of catching a cold. Among life events, work-related stress, moving house and problems with personal relationships have the greatest impact on stress levels.

DID YOU KNOW?

In 1984 the Ministry of Health in the USSR reported improvements in performance among telegraph operators using Siberian ginseng. After taking the herb, workers transmitted text faster and made fewer mistakes.

FACTS & TIPS

■ Adrenal formulas sold in health-food shops may be a convenient addition to a stress-management routine. These contain B vitamins, liquorice, Siberian ginseng or other stress-fighting substances.

Sunburn

A round of golf or a seaside outing may be a warm-weather treat, but even if you protect yourself from the sun's rays your skin can sometimes burn. A number of healing supplements can relieve the pain – and will also help to prevent long-term skin damage.

Symptoms

Mild sunburn
- Pink or reddish skin that is hot to the touch.

Moderate sunburn
- Red skin with small, fluid-filled blisters that may itch or burst.

Severe sunburn
- Deep red to purplish skin, with or without blisters, accompanied by shivering, headache, nausea, dizziness or a temperature.

SEE YOUR DOCTOR ...

- If you experience shivering, headache, nausea, dizziness or a temperature.

- If large blisters form – these can become infected.

- If you experience unusually severe itching or pain.

REMINDER: *If you have a medical condition, consult your doctor before taking supplements.*

What it is

Sunburn is the reddening and inflammation of the skin's outer layers that results from overexposure to the sun. It may be mild, with some redness; moderate, with small blisters; or severe, with purple skin, shivering and a temperature. Symptoms appear gradually and may not reach a peak until 24 hours after exposure. Sunburn is best avoided – not only because it may make your skin sore but also because it speeds up the skin's ageing process and increases the risk of skin cancers later in life.

What causes it

The amount of exposure that produces sunburn varies, depending on an individual's skin pigmentation, the geographical location, the season, the time of day and the weather. Melanin, a skin pigment that absorbs the sun's ultraviolet (UV) rays, is the body's natural defence against sunburn. Fair-haired people with pale eyes have less melanin than darker-skinned people, and are more prone to sunburn. Some antibiotics and other drugs can also make the skin more sensitive to the sun.

How supplements can help

Supplements cannot prevent sunburn, but applied to the skin and taken orally they can lessen the discomfort and damage that it causes. Topical treatments provide immediate soothing relief. For mild sunburn, add 10 drops each of **chamomile oil** and **lavender oil** to a cool bath and soak for

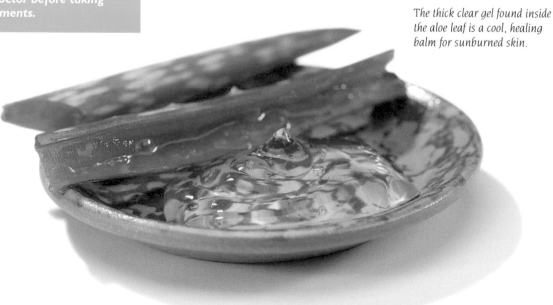

The thick clear gel found inside the aloe leaf is a cool, healing balm for sunburned skin.

SUPPLEMENT RECOMMENDATIONS

Chamomile oil	**Dosage:** add a few drops to a cool bath, or mix them with 1 tablespoon of almond oil (or another neutral oil) and apply to the skin twice a day. **Advice:** use with lavender oil; chamomile or calendula ointment applied several times a day also promotes healing.
Lavender oil	**Dosage:** add a few drops to a cool bath, or mix them with 1 tablespoon of almond oil (or another neutral oil) and apply to the skin twice a day. **Advice:** use with chamomile oil.
Aloe vera gel	**Dosage:** apply gel to affected areas of skin as required. **Advice:** use fresh aloe leaf or shop-bought gel.
Vitamin C	**Dosage:** 500 mg twice a day. **Advice:** reduce dose if diarrhoea develops.
Vitamin E	**Dosage:** 250 mg twice a day, or apply topical cream as required. **Caution:** do not use if you take anticoagulant drugs.
Fish oils	**Dosage:** 2 teaspoons to supply 2 grams omega-3 fatty acids a day. **Caution:** do not use if you take anticoagulant drugs. **Advice:** vegetarians can substitute 1 tablespoon of flaxseed oil.

Some dosages may be supplied by supplements you are already taking – see page 195.

30 minutes or more, to relieve discomfort and moisturise the skin. A lukewarm bath containing a cup of dissolved baking soda can be a good alternative. If the burn is more serious, prepare a topical remedy using a few drops of chamomile oil or lavender oil, or both, and a tablespoon of a neutral oil such as almond, and apply it gently to the affected areas twice a day. **Aloe vera gel** and chamomile or calendula cream also soothe the skin and help to speed up the healing process.

Sun exposure releases free radicals, unstable oxygen molecules that can cause damage to the skin. Antioxidants such as **vitamin C** and **vitamin E**, taken orally, render these free radicals harmless. They can be used over a long period, if necessary. For bad burns, vitamin E cream can be applied to help the skin to heal and prevent scarring. **Fish oils** (or flaxseed oil) can also be taken orally. These are a rich resource of omega-3 fatty acids, which can reduce inflammation and promote skin healing.

What else you can do

☑ Use a sunscreen with a sun protection factor (SPF) of at least 15. Keep out of the sun between 10am and 3pm, when the rays are strongest, and cover yourself up with clothing and a wide-brimmed hat.

☑ Relieve severe sunburn pain by soaking a cotton towel or shirt, or a gauze pad, in cold milk and placing it gently on the affected areas. Alternatively, place cooled used tea bags on the affected areas – the tannin in the tea can also ease the pain.

☑ Add a cup of finely ground oatmeal (sold as colloidal oatmeal in chemists) to a bath. It can help to relieve pain and itching.

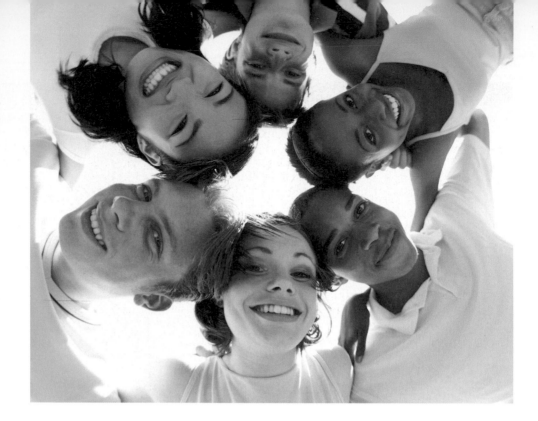

Good nutrition is vital during adolescence, a time of physical and emotion upheaval, but as a young person's independence increases food choices are distorted by fads and peer pressure. Supplements can help to make up any nutritional shortfall in the teenage diet.

■ Rapid growth occurs in girls between the ages of 10 and 12 and in boys between 12 and 15. These spurts make great nutritional demands, and can lead to deficiencies of the B group vitamins, vitamin C, calcium, iron, magnesium and zinc.

■ Teenage requirements are either similar to those of adults, or slightly higher, so it is safe to take adult supplements.

DIETING
More than 10% of UK children are considered overweight. Even so, many diet needlessly, compromising their bone strength and development, and, if girls, their pregnancy outcomes in later life. Faddy diets often mean major food groups are cut down or missed out.

Obsession with weight-loss can also lead to serious eating disorders (*see pages 358-61*). Excessive exercise in underweight girls may lead to the cessation of periods, and the associated loss of oestrogen will weaken the skeleton.

VEGETARIAN DIETS
As long as sources of iron, such as beans, dried apricots, egg yolk, green leafy vegetables and nuts are taken with foods rich in vitamin C, vegetarian diets can provide adequate nutrients. Cheese and cream should be eaten in moderation. Vegan diets can lead to low intakes of major nutrients, particularly of B_{12}, folic acid and iron.

Vegetarians and vegans should take vitamin B_{12} supplements. This vitamin is found in most foods of animal origin, but does not occur naturally in plants.

SMOKING AND DRINKING
Deficiencies can arise from smoking and excessive alcohol consumption; girls who are dieting or using oral contraceptives are particularly at risk. Smokers need extra B complex vitamins and vitamin C. Heavy drinkers should take vitamins B_1 and B_2 in a multivitamin and multimineral formula; additional B complex vitamins and vitamin C are also advisable.

NUTRIENTS REQUIRED BY GROWING TEENAGERS

NUTRIENT	EFFECTS	FOOD SOURCES	DEFICIENCY SYMPTOMS	DAILY REQUIREMENTS (BOYS/GIRLS)
Vitamin B group	**Energy metabolism** (B_1, B_2); **Protein metabolism** (B_6); **Blood formation** (B_6, B_{12}, folic acid); **Nervous system support** (B_{12})	Yeast extract, dried brewer's yeast, red meat (especially pig's liver and kidney), wheatgerm, nuts, wholegrains, brown rice, fatty fish and soya flour. Green leafy vegetables and citrus fruit are good sources of folic acid	Fatigue, muscle weakness, loss of appetite, irritability, mental confusion, poor memory, depression, sore or cracked skin, poor growth, hair loss, fluid retention, anaemia	**Vitamin B_1:** 0.9-1.1 mg/ 0.7-0.8 mg **B_2:** 1.2-1.3 mg/1.1 mg **B_6:** 1.2-1.5 mg/1-1.2 mg **B_{12}:** 1.2-1.5 mcg/ 1.2-1.5 mcg **Folic acid:** 200 mcg/200 mcg
Vitamin C	Aids wound healing and iron absorption; helps to prevent free radical damage; maintains health of immune system	Fruit and vegetables, though most teenagers' vitamin C intake mainly comes from fruit drinks and squashes	Mild deficiency: fatigue, greatly raised susceptibility to infection. Severe deficiency: scurvy	35-40 mg/35-40 mg
Calcium	Bone formation. During adolescence, 45% of the adult skeleton is laid down	Milk, yoghurt and other dairy products, canned sardines. Less rich sources include white bread, tofu, pulses, dried figs, almonds, wholemeal bread and green vegetables	Demineralisation of bones, leading to osteoporosis in later life	1000mg/800mg *ADVICE: encourage consumption of milk shakes, yoghurts and cheese before considering supplements*
Iron	Oxygen transportation in the blood; builds resistance to infection	Red meat, especially liver, some oily fish and eggs. Iron from vegetable sources (e.g. fortified breakfast cereals, green vegetables, bread) is less well absorbed. Vitamin C enhances absorption	Anaemia, especially common in girls who have started menstruation and also have low iron intakes	11.3mg/14.8mg. *CAUTION: self-prescription of iron-only supplements can be dangerous – they should be taken only under a doctor's supervision; anaemia requires accurate diagnosis and tailored treatment. A multivitamin and multimineral supplement is the safest way to take extra iron*
Magnesium	Bone formation; transmission of nerve impulses; muscle contraction; co-factor in many key enzymes	Wholegrain products such as wholemeal bread, bran-rich cereals, nuts and seeds	Muscle cramps, nausea, palpitations, fatigue, weakness, premenstrual syndrome, kidney stones, insomnia	280-300mg/280-300mg *CAUTION: Do not take magnesium if you have kidney disease* *ADVICE: take a magnesium-only supplement (150mg) or a 'bone-building' calcium plus magnesium supplement (250mg). Too much magnesium can cause diarrhoea*
Zinc	Protein, carbohydrate and fat metabolism; sexual maturation, especially in males. Zinc is a component of more than 200 enzymes	Protein foods such as beef, pork, liver, dark poultry meat and eggs. Vegetarian sources, including cheese, beans and wheatgerm, are less well absorbed	Poor growth, poor wound healing, frequent infections, skin problems, poor hair and nail growth, loss of senses of taste and smell, sleep disturbances	9-9.5mg/9mg *CAUTION: zinc lozenges should be taken for no longer than five days* *ADVICE: usually included in multivitamin and multimineral formulas*

Thrush

The unpleasant burning and itching sensation of thrush can be provoked by many factors, from an unbalanced diet to hormonal changes – even by wearing synthetic underwear. Supplements can strengthen the body's overall defences against an excessive growth of yeast in the vagina.

Symptoms

- *Intense genital itching.*

- *Inflammation and redness in the external genital area.*

- *White, curd-like or thick vaginal discharge that may be odourless or smell 'yeasty' (similar to bread).*

SEE YOUR DOCTOR ...

- **If you experience any of above symptoms for the first time.**

- **If vaginal discharge has a strong, foul-smelling odour, or is tinged with blood.**

- **If symptoms do not disappear in five days, despite treatment.**

- **If the yeast infection returns within two months.**

REMINDER: If you have a medical condition, consult your doctor before taking supplements.

What it is

Thrush is an infection caused by *Candida albicans*, an organism which is normally present in the body in small, harmless amounts. Under certain conditions yeast multiplies rapidly and causes soreness and discharge. *Candida albicans*, like most fungi, thrives in warm moist areas such as the vagina. Other species of *Candida* can also contribute to yeast infections.

What causes it

Anything that disturbs the normal balance of yeast and bacteria or the pH (acid/alkaline) level in the vagina can create ideal conditions for the uncontrolled growth of yeast. The normal vaginal environment can be upset by something as simple as wearing tight jeans or nylon underwear. The risk of yeast infections is also increased by hormonal changes during pregnancy, by the use of birth control pills or spermicides, or by diabetes.

A yeast infection is also likely to develop when the immune system is weakened by illness, stress or lack of sleep, or if it is severely compromised by HIV infection or chemotherapy. Taking antibiotics such as ampicillin or tetracycline commonly leads to yeast infections, because these drugs destroy not only the bacteria causing the illness but also the 'friendly' bacteria that keep yeast levels in check.

How supplements can help

Thrush can be an indication of a general nutritional deficiency, so it is advisable to take a multivitamin and multimineral formulation in addition to the other supplements listed in the chart.

Begin taking the recommended supplements from the time when you first notice symptoms until the infection disappears. With the exception of the pessaries, all of them can be used alongside prescription or over-the-counter yeast treatments. Strengthening your immune system with **vitamin C** and **echinacea** helps your body to

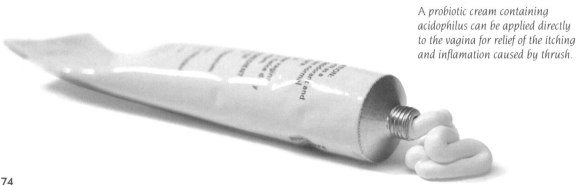

A probiotic cream containing acidophilus can be applied directly to the vagina for relief of the itching and inflamation caused by thrush.

Vitamin C	**Dosage:** 500 mg twice a day. **Advice:** reduce dose if diarrhoea develops.
Echinacea	**Dosage:** 200 mg extract three times a day. **Advice:** for recurrent infections, use in a cycle of three weeks on, one week off; standardised to contain at least 3.5% echinacosides.
Probiotics	**Dosage:** two capsules three times a day on an empty stomach, or two or three small pots of bioyoghurt a day. **Advice:** buy acidophilus or bifidus cultures, or a mixture of the two; also available as a cream for twice daily application to the vagina.
FOS	**Dosage:** 2000 mg twice a day. **Advice:** use in combination with probiotics.
Tea tree oil	**Dosage:** insert pessary into vagina every 12 hours for five days. **Advice:** available in health-food shops.
Calendula	**Dosage:** insert pessary into vagina every 12 hours for five days. **Advice:** available in health-food shops.

Note: consider using supplements in blue first; those in black may also be beneficial. Some dosages may be supplied by supplements you are already taking – see page 195.

fight an acute yeast infection. The herb echinacea seems to stimulate white blood cells to destroy the yeast, and vitamin C may inhibit yeast growth. If you are susceptible to yeast infections take echinacea for three weeks, stop using it for a week, then resume use.

Continue taking echinacea for six months, along with vitamin C and **probiotics**, which boost your body's supply of 'friendly' bacteria. Available as bioyoghurts as well as in the form of oral supplements and a topically applied cream, probiotics are especially important if your infection is linked to the use of antibiotics. Add **FOS** (fructo-oligosaccharides) – indigestible carbohydrates which feed the helpful bacteria and promote their growth.

If you would rather not use standard antithrush creams, try ready-made pessaries of **tea tree oil** or **calendula**. Clinical studies have proved that tea tree oil and anti-inflammatory calendula (marigold) are effective antifungal agents.

What else you can do

☑ Wear cotton underwear; stop wearing tights.
☑ Avoid deodorant tampons, feminine sprays and commercial douches.
☑ Use mild, unperfumed soap to wash the vaginal area.

FACTS & TIPS

■ Men can get genital yeast infections too, especially if they are uncircumcised. The only symptom may be an inflammation of the head of the penis, but often there are no symptoms. A man with a yeast infection may infect his partner, and needs treatment.

■ In place of pessaries or capsules, lukewarm tea made with pau d'arco or goldenseal can be used as a douche twice a day for up to seven days. Use two cups of liquid per application.

■ Contrary to popular belief, a diet high in carbohydrates or sugar does not increase your risk of a yeast infection. There is no benefit to be had from a 'yeast-free' diet. The yeast used to leaven bread is not the same as the type that causes yeast infections.

Thyroid disease

Many more women than men are affected by thyroid disease – a condition which is often left undiagnosed. Fortunately, once identified, thyroid disease is treatable. Under the supervision of a doctor, supplements can complement conventional medical care.

Symptoms

Hyperthyroidism

- *Mood changes, restlessness, anxiety, difficulty in sleeping.*

- *Weight loss, despite increased appetite; diarrhoea; rapid heartbeat; increased sweating; intolerance of heat.*

- *Goitre (painless swelling in the throat); bulging, irritated eyes; muscle weakness; lightness or absence of menstruation.*

Hypothyroidism

- *Fatigue, lethargy or slowed movement; depression; memory problems.*

- *Weight gain; constipation; intolerance of cold.*

- *Dry hair and skin; goitre; puffiness around the eyes; heavy menstruation.*

SEE YOUR DOCTOR ...

- **If you have any of the above symptoms – a blood test will confirm the diagnosis.**

REMINDER: If you have a medical condition, consult your doctor before taking supplements.

What it is

The thyroid gland, consisting of two large lobes situated at the base of the throat, produces hormones essential for the proper functioning and maintenance of all the cells in the body. If the gland releases too much thyroid hormone – a condition known as hyperthyroidism – the body runs too fast, like an overheated engine. Conversely, if it secretes too little – a disorder called hypothyroidism – the body's metabolism can become sluggish. Symptoms of either condition can appear very quickly, or may develop gradually, often mimicking long-term mild depression.

What causes it

Most cases of thyroid disease result from an autoimmune disorder in which the body's immune system attacks the thyroid gland. Genetic factors, hormonal disturbances elsewhere in the body, surgery, radiation or medication are other possible causes. Insufficient amounts of iodine in the diet can also lead to hypothyroidism.

How supplements can help

The supplements listed here may benefit people with thyroid disorders, including those already taking conventional drugs, but always consult your doctor before using them, because some nutrients may alter your response to your prescription drug dose. It may be a month or so before any benefits are noticed.

Many nutrients are important for maintaining the health of the thyroid gland. **Vitamin C**, **vitamin E** and the **B complex vitamins** may help in the treatment of hyperthyroidism and hypothyroidism because

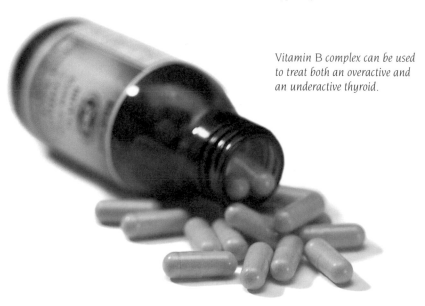

Vitamin B complex can be used to treat both an overactive and an underactive thyroid.

Vitamin C	**Dosage:** 500 mg twice a day. **Advice:** useful for both hyperthyroidism and hypothyroidism; reduce dose if diarrhoea develops.
Vitamin E	**Dosage:** 250 mg a day. **Caution:** consult your doctor if you take anticoagulant drugs.
Vitamin B complex	**Dosage:** one tablet each morning for hyperthyroidism or hypothyroidism. **Advice:** look for a B-50 complex with 50 mcg vitamin B_{12} and biotin, 400 mcg folic acid and 50 mg all other B vitamins.
Zinc	**Dosage:** 25 mg a day. **Advice:** if you take a zinc supplement for more than a month, use one that includes 2 mg copper.
Selenium	**Dosage:** 200 mcg a day. **Caution:** high doses of selenium are toxic; do not exceed the recommended dose.
Kelp	**Dosage:** 400-600 mg of powdered kelp a day. **Advice:** should supply 200-300 mcg iodine.

Note: consider using supplements in blue first; those in black may also be beneficial. Some dosages may be supplied by supplements you are already taking – see page 195.

they play key roles in improving the overall healthy function of the thyroid gland and the immune system.

If you have a sluggish thyroid you may need to take prescribed supplements under a doctor's supervision. Extra **zinc** (take with copper when using long term, because zinc inhibits copper absorption) may also be necessary to help to boost thyroid function. People with hypothyroidism need to make sure that they obtain sufficient **selenium** from their diet, since a low selenium intake (which seems common in Britain) is associated with impaired thyroid function.

If the condition is the result of an iodine deficiency, **kelp** (which contains good quantities of iodine) can be used to complement the conventional treatment.

What else you can do

☑ Regularly check the area of your neck just below the Adam's apple for any bulging, which may be a sign of thyroid problems.
☑ If you have an overactive thyroid, eat plenty of raw cruciferous vegetables such as broccoli, Brussels sprouts, cabbage, cauliflower, kale and collard greens, which contain a natural thyroid blocker. Avoid iodised salt and iodine-containing foods, including saltwater fish and shellfish.
☑ If you have an underactive thyroid, avoid eating cruciferous vegetables, use iodised salt and eat iodine-rich foods.

Tinnitus

A persistent buzzing, humming, whistling or ringing in the ears afflicts about one in six adults at some point in their lives. Though there is no outright cure, vitamins, minerals and herbs can help by improving the circulation and nerve function in the head and the ears.

Symptoms

- Persistent ringing, buzzing or humming in one or both ears.
- Sleep disturbances, distress or anxiety.
- In some cases, hearing loss.

SEE YOUR DOCTOR ...

- If you experience unusual or unrelenting noise in one or both ears that persists and interferes with daily tasks or sleep.
- If ringing is accompanied by facial numbness, dizziness, nausea or loss of balance.
- If ringing affects only one ear for an extended period.

REMINDER: If you have a medical condition, consult your doctor before taking supplements.

What it is

The medical name for persistent noise in the ears – *tinnitus* – is a Latin word meaning 'ringing'. In 99% of cases the condition does not interfere with day-to-day life, and only a third of tinnitus sufferers seek medical help for it. In certain people (usually those over 60) the ringing may become so intrusive that it interferes with sleep or leads to depression and anxiety. Many sufferers experience some degree of hearing loss.

What causes it

Most cases of tinnitus probably stem from repeated exposure to loud noise (rock music, gunshots or machinery, for example), which damages the nerves and tiny hairs in the inner ear that detect sound. Other causes include excess earwax, ear infections, excess alcohol consumption, poor circulation and the side effects of some medications such as antibiotics or aspirin. Recent research indicates that tinnitus probably involves a nerve malfunction in the brain, rather than just damage to the ear.

How supplements can help

For the many chronic cases with no treatable cause, supplements may be effective. The supplements listed can safely be used together, and will usually have to be taken long term, though benefits may be noticed within a month.

Because poor blood circulation to certain parts of the brain may affect the inner ears and cause ringing, the herb **ginkgo biloba** may relieve some cases, though its benefits may take weeks or months to be felt. Blood circulation can also be improved by concentrated **garlic** (taken with, or instead of, ginkgo). Other supplements may help by improving the health of the nerves – including those that lead to the

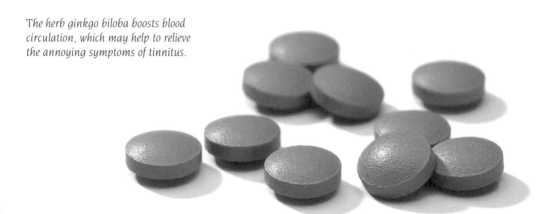

The herb ginkgo biloba boosts blood circulation, which may help to relieve the annoying symptoms of tinnitus.

SUPPLEMENT RECOMMENDATIONS	
Ginkgo biloba	**Dosage:** 40 mg extract 3 times a day. **Advice:** standardised to contain at least 24% flavone glycosides.
Garlic	**Dosage:** 400-600 mg dried concentrate four times a day with food. **Advice:** each tablet should provide 4000 mcg allicin potential.
Vitamin B$_6$	**Dosage:** 50 mg once a day. **Advice:** not necessary if taking a vitamin B complex supplement.
Vitamin B$_{12}$/ Folic acid	**Dosage:** 1000 mcg vitamin B$_{12}$ and 400 mcg folic acid a day. **Advice:** take sublingual form for best absorption.
Magnesium	**Dosage:** 200 mg twice a day. **Advice:** take with food; reduce dose if diarrhoea develops.
Zinc	**Dosage:** 25 mg a day. **Advice:** if you take a zinc supplement for more than one month, use one that includes 2 mg copper.

Some dosages may be supplied by supplements you are already taking – see page 195.

inner ear. **Vitamin B$_6$** has beneficial effects on nerve function, as does **vitamin B$_{12}$**, which the body uses to make myelin, a fatty substance that covers and protects the nerves and enables them to function efficiently. (Vitamin B$_{12}$ should be taken with **folic acid** to prevent deficiencies of either B vitamin.) If your symptoms do not improve after three months, discontinue the regimen of B$_6$, B$_{12}$ and folic acid.

Magnesium also plays an important role in maintaining good nerve function and hearing. Low magnesium levels can cause blood vessels to constrict, inhibiting circulation in the brain. Insufficient zinc might contribute to tinnitus, because the inner ear has a higher concentration of **zinc** than most other parts of the body. Even a slight deficiency can worsen the hearing loss associated with ageing. Zinc interferes with copper absorption, so take a formulation that includes copper.

Several plants are used by herbalists to treat tinnitus, although their efficacy has not been proved by clinical trials. Depending upon its cause, one or more of the following may be prescribed: black cohosh, cayenne (chilli), echinacea, feverfew or hawthorn (for good circulation and nerve function), white willow or goldenseal (anti-inflammatories).

What else you can do

☑ Cut back on caffeine, alcohol, nicotine and aspirin: they can exacerbate ringing in the ears.

☑ Ask your doctor for information about ear devices that cover up, or mask, tinnitus. Low-volume white noise, such as television or radio static, may also help.

☑ Exercise to improve circulation and so, possibly, to ease symptoms.

☑ Consider acupuncture to relieve the buzzing.

Travel ailments

Motion sickness, the effects of jet lag and the occasional stomach upset are common travellers' complaints. Luckily they are usually short-lived. Dizziness and vertigo can be more persistent problems, but in most circumstances natural remedies bring relief.

Symptoms

- *Nausea and vomiting.*
- *Dizziness, weakness, unsteadiness or faintness.*
- *Cold sweats.*
- *Yawning, fatigue and sleepiness.*

SEE YOUR DOCTOR ...

- **If you experience persistent nausea, which may indicate a liver disorder.**
- **If dizziness is accompanied by numbness, rapid heartbeat, fainting or blurred vision, or if your speech is affected.**
- **If dizziness starts suddenly, especially if it is accompanied by nausea or vomiting.**
- **If dizzy spells increase in frequency or persist.**

REMINDER: If you have a medical condition, consult your doctor before taking supplements.

What they are

Most of us have experienced dizziness or nausea when travelling by road, air or sea. Anyone who has taken a long-distance flight will be familiar with the fatigue and disrupted sleep patterns caused by jet lag. The loose or watery stools associated with diarrhoea are the body's way of flushing out harmful toxins and usually last only for a few days. Continued sensations of unsteadiness or faintness, or vertigo, when you feel as if the world is spinning around you, may be due to other factors.

What causes them

Travel sickness occurs when the eyes try to focus on constantly moving scenery while the inner ear, which helps to orientate the body to movement, sends conflicting signals to the brain. Jet lag is experienced when the body's natural rhythms do not synchronise with actual time. The pineal gland secretes melatonin to regulate our cycle of sleep and wakefulness according to light cues. This becomes disrupted by travel to different time zones. Diarrhoea is usually the result of a viral or bacterial infection caused by consuming contaminated food or water.

How supplements can help

Fresh or preserved **ginger** is very effective at preventing and treating the nausea associated with travel sickness and mild vertigo. It takes effect almost instantly and has none of the side effects of conventional drugs, such as drowsiness or blurred vision. **Magnesium** is a good general tonic for calming the nerves, which can ease travel sickness, and **vitamin B$_6$** can help to relieve feelings of nausea. Peppermint in all its forms is a

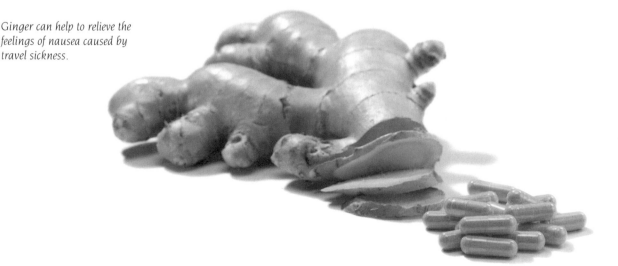

Ginger can help to relieve the feelings of nausea caused by travel sickness.

SUPPLEMENT RECOMMENDATIONS

Ginger	**Dosage for travel sickness:** 100 to 200 mg of standardised extract in capsule form three or four hours before departure and then every four hours as needed. **Advice:** take capsules with fluid.
Magnesium	**Dosage for travel sickness:** 500 mg one hour before travelling. **Advice:** take with food.
Vitamin B$_6$	**Dosage for travel sickness:** 100 mg one hour before travelling; 100 mg two hours later; **for dizziness:** 50 mg three times a day. **Caution:** do not take more than 100 mg at any one time. Taking 200 mg daily long term can cause nerve damage.
Ginkgo biloba	**Dosage for dizziness:** 80 mg extract three times a day. **Advice:** standardised to contain 24% ginkgo flavone glycosides.

Some dosages may be supplied by supplements you are already taking – see page 195.

Some dosages may be supplied by supplements you are already taking – see page 195.

helpful antidote to travel sickness and nausea. Try drinking peppermint tea, taking a drop of oil on the tongue or inhaling the oil from a tissue.

To combat the fatigue of jet lag, Chinese ginseng is a good general tonic which can be taken alongside other remedies and also relieves stress. If you have persistent dizziness or vertigo, seek medical advice to rule out serious underlying causes. You may be prescribed drugs, but other supplements may also be beneficial. One study has shown that **ginkgo biloba**, which boosts blood flow to the brain, helped almost half the patients with chronic vertigo, although it may take between 8 and 12 weeks for the effects to be noticed. Magnesium may help to prevent dizziness. Vitamin B$_6$, essential for normal brain and nervous system function, may be useful for some cases of chronic dizziness.

What else you can do

For travel sickness:

☑ Keep your head as still as possible and limit visual stimulation. Deep breathing and fresh air can also help.

☑ Eat light, non-fatty food. Avoid anything that may upset your stomach.

☑ Drink chamomile tea to calm an upset stomach.

For jet lag:

☑ Inhaling rosemary oil may ease symptoms.

☑ Soon after take off adjust your watch and other routines such as eating and sleeping to local arrival time.

☑ Avoid drinking alcohol and increase the amount of water and other liquids you drink. Try to avoid caffeine.

For dizziness or vertigo:

☑ Avoid sudden changes in body position, particularly moving from lying down to standing up, and extreme movements of the head.

☑ Desensitisation techniques may help. Move your head in a way that makes you feel dizzy and repeat this several times a day for a few weeks.

☑ Cut down on caffeine, nicotine and salt, all of which can reduce blood flow to the brain.

DID YOU KNOW?
Dizziness and travel sickness can be made worse by anxiety or stress. One solution is to practise yoga or meditation techniques in addition to taking supplements.

FACTS & TIPS

■ Although travel sickness can be prevented, it is hard to cure, so take any remedy before symptoms appear.

■ Sitting in a plane for more than four hours dramatically increases the risk of blood clotting in the legs, because of reduced blood flow and the dehydrating atmosphere. Regular consumption of fish oils reduces the risk. Walking around during the flight and drinking plenty of fluids are good preventative measures. If you feel pain or swelling in the legs, seek medical advice.

■ Taking naps when you are very tired can help to relieve jet lag, but sleeping for over four hours makes it hard to adjust to a new time zone. If you are staying in a new time zone for a short period only, adjustment is unnecessary.

Ulcers

Erosions in the lining of the stomach or intestine are painful and occasionally life-threatening. They can often be quickly and effectively treated with conventional drugs, and a number of useful natural remedies speed up the healing process through their effects on the digestive tract.

Symptoms

Typical symptoms

■ *A gnawing or aching pain in the stomach, either just before or several hours after a meal. The pain may feel like heartburn, or may be accompanied by indigestion, nausea, vomiting or weight loss. It may be relieved by antacids, bland foods or milk.*

Emergency symptoms

■ *Passing black or bloody stools, or vomiting blood or particles that look like coffee grounds, may indicate internal bleeding. Sudden, severe abdominal pain could indicate a perforated intestinal wall. These are life-threatening emergencies.*

SEE YOUR DOCTOR ...

■ If you have ulcer symptoms.

■ If you experience any signs of internal bleeding or perforation (blood in the vomit, black and tar-like stools or severe pain in the abdomen) – these require immediate medical attention.

REMINDER: If you have a medical condition, consult your doctor before taking supplements.

What they are

An ulcer is a crater-like erosion in the protective lining of the stomach or the duodenum (the first section of the small intestine). Normally glands in the stomach secrete substances that aid digestion, including acids and the enzyme pepsin, and at the same time the stomach and duodenum secrete mucus, which protects the lining from damage by these gastric juices. An ulcer is formed when this balance breaks down, causing the juices to begin digesting away the stomach or intestinal lining.

What causes them

Until recently, conventional wisdom held that a stressful lifestyle and a diet rich in fats and spicy foods lead to an ulcer, but researchers have now discovered that most ulcers are caused by a bacterium known as *Helicobacter pylori*. Once the digestive tract is infected the protective mucous membrane is weakened, and even small amounts of digestive juices can eat into the intestinal wall. Once an ulcer has appeared, secondary influences such as stress, diet, alcohol, caffeine and smoking can aggravate it. Other contributing factors include heredity – ulcers often run in families – and the long-term use of aspirin, ibuprofen or other nonsteroidal anti-inflammatory drugs (NSAIDs).

How supplements can help

If you have a suspected ulcer your doctor is likely to arrange a blood test for H. *pylori*, and will prescribe antibiotics and other drugs if the result is positive. Whether or not bacteria are present, the natural remedies listed (all of which are safe to use in

Aloe vera juice contains the astringent ulcer-healing gel found inside the leaf of the aloe vera plant.

Carotenoids	**Dosage:** 15 mg twice a day. **Caution:** take natural beta-carotene, not the synthetic form.
Vitamin C	**Dosage:** 500 mg twice a day. **Advice:** dose may be increased to 1000 mg for up to seven days; reduce dose if diarrhoea develops.
Zinc	**Dosage:** 25 mg a day. **Advice:** if you take a zinc supplement for more than a month, use one that includes 2 mg copper.
Liquorice (DGL)	**Dosage:** chew one or two 380 mg deglycyrrhizinated liquorice (DGL) tablets three times a day. **Advice:** take 30 minutes before meals.
Glutamine	**Dosage:** 500 mg L-glutamine three times a day for one month. **Advice:** take on an empty stomach.
Gamma-oryzanol	**Dosage:** 150 mg twice a day for one month. **Advice:** also known as rice bran oil; take on an empty stomach.
Aloe vera juice	**Dosage:** 300 ml juice three times a day for one month. **Advice:** should contain 98% aloe vera and no aloin or aloe-emodin.

Some dosages may be supplied by supplements you are already taking – see page 195.

DID YOU KNOW?

Folk healers have long recommended cabbage juice as a treament for ulcers. It is good advice – cabbage is rich in the healing amino acid glutamine.

FACTS & TIPS

■ Antibiotics are probably the best way to eliminate *H. pylori*, but supplements offer a safer alternative to most conventional ulcer drugs – most have few, if any, known adverse effects.

combination with each other and conventional drugs) can speed up the healing process. Pain will usually diminish in a week, but the ulcer may take up to eight weeks to heal. The body converts the beta-carotene in mixed **carotenoids** into vitamin A, which helps to protect the lining of the stomach and small intestine, allowing ulcers to heal. **Vitamin C** may directly inhibit the growth of the H. *pylori* bacterium.

Other substances that encourage healing include **zinc** (taken with copper) and deglycyrrhizinated **liquorice (DGL)** tablets. The tablets, which, unlike ordinary liquorice root, do not raise blood pressure, should be used for three months to maximise healing. **Glutamine**, an amino acid, helps the healing process by nourishing the cells that line the digestive tract; **gamma-oryzanol**, an extract of rice bran oil which promotes healthy levels of digestive juices, also seems to be beneficial.

Practitioners often treat ulcers with juice from the **aloe vera** plant, which may reduce stomach acid secretions and relieve symptoms in some people. This popular herb, currently being investigated in clinical trials, also contains astringent compounds that may help to prevent internal bleeding. It may also be worth trying herbal teas made from chamomile, marshmallow, slippery elm, meadowsweet or calendula, which soothe irritated mucous linings.

What else you can do

☑ Eat a sensible diet rich in fibre and avoid foods that cause discomfort.
☑ Avoid alcohol, coffee, cola drinks and acidic fruit juices, which irritate the lining of the digestive tract.
☑ Do not smoke. Smoking can delay healing.

Urinary tract infections

Modern science has now proved a long-held belief of folk healers: that the uncomfortable and potentially serious symptoms of urinary tract infections, a common problem for women, can be relieved by herbs and other natural remedies.

Symptoms

- *Frequent urge to urinate.*
- *Voiding a small amount of urine, despite frequent urges.*
- *Burning sensation or searing pain when urinating.*
- *Foul-smelling, cloudy or unusually dark urine.*
- *Cramps or a heavy feeling in the lower abdomen.*

SEE YOUR DOCTOR ...

- If a burning sensation, pain or other symptoms persist after 24 to 36 hours of self-treatment.
- If a burning sensation is accompanied by a vaginal or penile discharge.
- If the symptoms described above are accompanied by back pain, shivering or a temperature.
- If there is blood in your urine.

REMINDER: If you have a medical condition, consult your doctor before taking supplements.

What it is

A urinary tract infection (UTI), also referred to as cystitis, is an infection that causes inflammation in the bladder or urethra (the tube that transports urine out of the bladder). The problem most frequently affects females – one in five women suffers from a UTI at least once a year – but men can also contract such an infection. Treatment should be prompt and antibiotics may be necessary, because recurring UTIs can lead to potentially serious kidney infections.

What causes it

A UTI results from a bacterial infection. Normally urine is sterile (free of bacteria) when it is excreted by the kidneys and stored in the bladder; it washes out the small amount of bacteria in the urethra as it passes to the outside. Sometimes bacteria in the urinary tract overwhelm the body's immune defences and multiply, causing an infection. Ignoring the urge to urinate may increase the likelihood of UTIs. Lack of personal hygiene can be a contributory factor, as can pregnancy, when the bladder is compressed by the foetus and is unable to empty completely.

How supplements can help

Take the recommended supplements at the first hint of burning during urination. Start with **vitamin C** and **cranberry**. Vitamin C helps to acidify urine, making the bladder a less inviting environment for harmful bacteria to colonise; it also strengthens the body's immune defences. Cranberry also acidifies the urine, but more importantly it prevents infectious bacteria from clinging to the lining of the urinary tract. The supplements can be used alongside the herb **echinacea**, which boosts the immune

Cranberry extract helps to keep the urinary tract free of harmful bacteria, and can be used to treat or prevent infections.

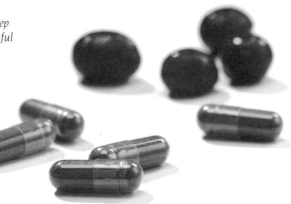

Vitamin C	**Dosage:** 250 mg every other hour, as tolerated. **Advice:** reduce dose if diarrhoea develops.
Cranberry	**Dosage:** 400 mg extract twice a day. **Advice:** alternatively, drink 300 ml a day of pure, unsweetened cranberry juice.
Echinacea	**Dosage:** one cup of echinacea tea several times a day. **Advice:** echinacea can be blended with goldenseal or nettle.
Probiotics	**Dosage:** two capsules three times a day on an empty stomach, or two or three small pots of bioyoghurt a day. **Advice:** buy acidophilus or bifidus cultures, or a mixture of the two.

Some dosages may be supplied by supplements you are already taking – see page 195.

system. Drink plenty of fluids to wash the bacteria and toxins away. Herbalists use many plants (either singly or in mixtures) in the treatment of urinary tract infections, although the workings of these herbs are not always understood. They include buchu, wild carrot, corn silk, couch grass, elder flowers and horsetail, which can be taken as tinctures or teas. When the urine is alkaline (as happens in strict vegetarians) another herb, uva ursi, is recommended.

Some UTIs can progress to more serious kidney infections, so it is important that these natural therapies be tried for only 24 to 36 hours before you seek professional advice. If an infection is confirmed your doctor is likely to prescribe antibiotics, but unfortunately they kill the healthy bacteria which help to protect the digestive and urinary tracts as well as the harmful bacteria. **Probiotics** (cultures of 'friendly' bacteria) are helpful specifically for those taking antibiotics because they reintroduce healthy bacteria. The other recommended supplements can also be continued while taking antibiotics.

What else you can do

☑ Drink at least one glass of water every hour. This will increase urine flow, which helps to flush harmful substances out of your system. Always urinate as soon as you feel the urge.

☑ Keep genital and anal areas clean and dry. Wash before and after intercourse. Always wipe the anal area from the front to the back to avoid the transmission of bacteria to the urinary tract

☑ Wear cotton (breathable) underwear, and change into dry clothing quickly after exercising or swimming.

FACTS & TIPS

■ To make a UTI-fighting herbal tea, pour a cup of very hot water over 2 teaspoons of buchu, corn silk or wild carrot (or a combination of these herbs). Steep for 15 minutes and strain. Sweeten to taste with honey.

■ In addition to their use in teas, buchu and echinacea can be used as cleansers to help to prevent recurrences in women who are prone to bladder infections. Prepare a cup of tea using either one herb or a blend and let it cool. Swab the genital area with the cooled solution.

■ Avoid using scented douches and feminine hygiene sprays. These products can irritate the urinary tract.

Varicose veins

Bulging blue varicose veins – often an inherited condition – can be unsightly and painful. You may avoid invasive surgery by eating the right food, making a few lifestyle changes and using vitamins and herbs that strengthen the blood vessels and inhibit swelling.

Symptoms

- *Swollen, snaking blue veins, usually on the calf, behind the knee or inside the thigh.*

- *Painful, aching legs, especially after long periods of standing.*

- *In severe cases, swollen ankles.*

SEE YOUR DOCTOR ...

- If the area around the varicose veins turns red – this may indicate vein inflammation, which can be serious.

- If pain makes it hard to walk.

- If skin around the vein is discoloured or peeling.

- If a small, persistent sore develops over a varicose vein.

- If your ankles are swollen – a possible sign that you are retaining water.

REMINDER: If you have a medical condition, consult your doctor before taking supplements.

What they are

Normal veins – the vessels that carry blood to the heart – contain valves that open and close to permit blood flow in only one direction. If these valves become weak and do not close completely, blood flows backwards and collects, and the result is the bulging veins commonly referred to as varicose veins. The condition almost always occurs in the legs (although haemorrhoids are actually varicose veins in the anus).

In most people varicose veins produce only mild discomfort. In severe cases, however, blood and other fluids leak out of the veins into the surrounding tissue; this causes scaly, itchy skin or swelling in the ankles from fluid that has pooled in the legs. Sometimes the legs ache or feel heavy, particularly after long periods of standing. Without treatment, varicose veins tend to worsen over time.

What causes them

Genetic and hormonal factors play key roles in the development of varicose veins. The condition tends to run in families, and is four times more common in women than men.

Other possible causes of the disorder include obesity, pregnancy and frequent heavy lifting – all of which put excessive pressure on the veins. Pregnancy also stimulates hormonal changes that are believed to weaken the veins in the legs. The condition tends to affect people who spend a lot of time on their feet or habitually cross their legs, or those who take too little exercise. The risk is also increased by liver disease or a failure of the blood circulation system.

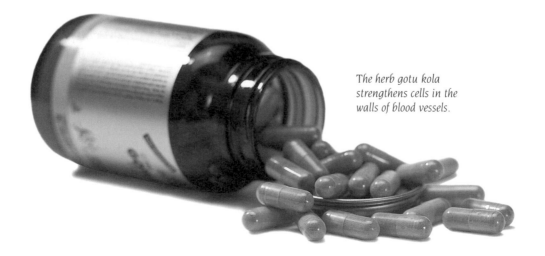

The herb gotu kola strengthens cells in the walls of blood vessels.

SUPPLEMENT RECOMMENDATIONS

Vitamin C/ flavonoids	**Dosage:** 500 mg vitamin C and 250 mg flavonoids twice a day. **Advice:** reduce vitamin C dose if diarrhoea develops.
Vitamin E	**Dosage:** 250 mg twice a day. **Caution:** consult your doctor if you take anticoagulant drugs.
Gotu kola	**Dosage:** 200 mg extract or 400-500 mg crude herb three times a day. **Caution:** do not use during pregnancy. **Advice:** extract standardised to contain 10% asiaticosides.
Bilberry	**Dosage:** 80 mg extract three times a day. **Advice:** standardised to contain 25% anthocyanosides.
Horse chestnut	**Dosage:** 500 mg extract each morning. **Advice:** standardised to contain 16%–21% escin.
Butcher's broom	**Dosage:** 150 mg extract 3 times a day. **Advice:** standardised to contain 9%–11% ruscogenin.

Note: consider using supplements in blue first; those in black may also be beneficial. Some dosages may be supplied by supplements you are already taking – see page 195.

How supplements can help

If you have varicose veins, taking **vitamin C** with **flavonoids** (which help the body to use vitamin C) and **vitamin E** can improve blood circulation and strengthen the walls of the veins and capillaries.

Gotu kola can be added to these vitamins – a very valuable herb for this condition because it enhances blood flow, increases the tone of the connective tissue surrounding the veins and keeps the veins themselves supple. **Bilberry** complements gotu kola; the two herbs are often sold as a single supplement. **Horse chestnut** can be used in place of gotu kola and bilberry; it appears to control inflammation and swelling and reduce the accumulation of fluid. If you cannot find the standardised extract of horse chestnut, substitute **butcher's broom**.

You can take the supplements and herbs that work best for you indefinitely. It may take up to three months to see results.

What else you can do

☑ Exercise, but avoid high-impact activities. Walk, cycle or swim rather than jog. If you lift weights, do not use very heavy ones.
☑ Elevate your legs whenever possible; this helps to prevent the blood from pooling in the veins.
☑ Avoid prolonged standing or sitting, and do not cross your legs.
☑ Don't wear tight clothing, including shoes, tights or belts. These items constrict veins in and around the legs, and can make it hard for blood to move upwards as it should.

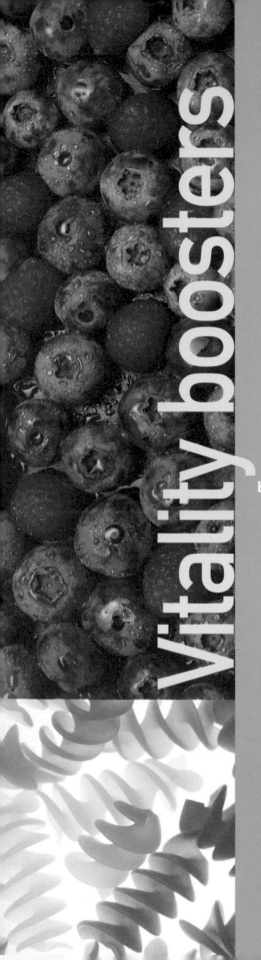

The keys to vitality are readily available energy and a healthy immune system. If you suffer from frequent colds and continuing fatigue, this may indicate that you are suffering from impaired immunity. To achieve and maintain optimum health your diet must provide all the vitamins and minerals you need in adequate amounts, and may need boosting with supplements.

DIET AND ENERGY

■ The nutrients required for the release of energy from foods and the body's reserves include the B complex vitamins and magnesium.

■ Iron is also required because it forms haemoglobin in the blood, which carries the oxygen necessary for energy utilisation.

■ These nutrients, together with antioxidants, omega-3 fatty acids and phytochemicals, are necessary for the health of the immune system.

AN EFFICIENT IMMUNE SYSTEM

■ Eating plenty of fruit and vegetables is the best way to support the body's defences against infection and also degenerative disease.

■ Immunity can be enhanced by taking fish oils or flaxseed oil, which provide the omega-3 fatty acids important for the structure of cell membranes. A daily multivitamin and multi-mineral supplement will also be of benefit.

■ Ageing weakens the immune response, so older people should maintain a good diet. Several studies have shown that the age-related decline in immune function can be reduced by the use of extra antioxidant nutrients and B complex vitamins.

■ Chronic stress can also weaken the immune system by increasing blood levels of adrenalin and corticosterone, hormones produced by the adrenal glands. Since vitamin B_6, vitamin C, magnesium and pantothenic acid (vitamin B$_5$) are needed to manufacture these hormones, requirements for these nutrients can double during periods of prolonged stress. If this demand is not met, immune function can suffer. A multivitamin and multimineral supplement, and practising relaxation techniques, can help to reduce adverse effects.

HERBS TO BOOST IMMUNITY
■ Panax ginseng has been used in China for thousands of years to fight the physical symptoms of stress. It has been shown to improve the functions of the immune and the nervous systems, although it should be avoided by anyone with high blood pressure.
■ St John's wort is used by medical herbalists to increase vitality. Its antiviral properties make it especially helpful for alleviating the fatigue that often follows viral infections.

REMEDIES FOR EXTREME TIREDNESS
When the liver is 'sluggish', toxic end products of metabolism may accumulate in the body, causing fatigue and headaches. Liver function can be improved by taking dandelion root, while milk thistle seed can be taken to help to neutralise the uncontrolled free radicals that can cause liver damage.

Another common reason for persistent fatigue is anaemia, which results in the tissues of the body failing to get enough oxygen. The problem is usually caused by a shortage of iron,

which may occur in heavily menstruating women through excessive blood loss, and among vegetarians and vegans, who usually have a low dietary intake of iron.

Consult a doctor if you suspect that you have anaemia. It is best to obtain extra iron through a multivitamin and multimineral supplement. Iron-only supplements should be taken only under the direction of a doctor.

If you experience fatigue unrelated to a lack of sleep for a period of more than six months, you could be suffering from

chronic fatigue syndrome (CFS) and should consult a doctor. Common symptoms include loss of concentration and memory, low fever and aching muscles.

CFS sufferers are likely to benefit from a good diet and a multivitamin and multimineral supplement, and extra vitamins C and E. Immunity-enhancing herbs, especially St John's wort, echinacea and pau d'arco, can be used to support this regime. If there is no improvement after about two months, a consultation with a medical herbalist may be beneficial.

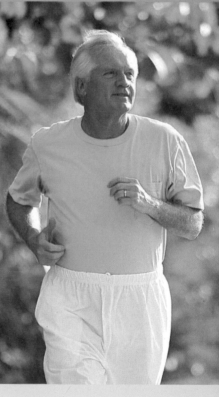

THE RELATIONSHIP BETWEEN VITALITY AND EXERCISE
Regular physical exertion, practised long term, has a tonic effect on all the body's systems, including the immune system. Exercise also produces a feeling of well-being by stimulating the release of beta endorphins and serotonin in the brain.

Their high energy expenditure means that athletes and people who take plenty of strenuous exercise need a greater calorie intake than those with a sedentary lifestyle.

For the body to perform at its best, insulin and other hormones must be secreted to supply glucose for the muscles to convert into energy – a chain of events that is put under great pressure at times of strenuous exercise. Minerals, including chromium, magnesium and zinc, are needed for these processes – together with B complex vitamins for the utilisation of energy.

During strenuous exercise we take in more oxygen than usual; this stimulates the production of free radicals, the unstable molecules that can damage cells. An excess of these may cause muscle ache which can be counteracted by anti-oxidants. Novices, older people or those who train particularly vigorously may benefit from supplements of vitamins C and E.

Warts and verrucas

About 10% of people in the UK suffer from warts or verrucas at some time in their lives. Although many warts and verrucas disappear on their own, supplements can hasten healing for the millions who suffer from these sometimes unsightly blemishes.

Symptoms

Warts may grow on their own or in clusters; some may also itch or cause discomfort, though most are painless.

- *Common wart: a flat or raised growth, usually just a little darker than the skin, generally on the hands or fingers.*

- *Verruca: a flat or slightly raised bump on the bottom of the foot that can resemble a callus.*

- *Genital wart: usually a reddish-pink growth, with a small 'flowery' head, in the genital or anal area.*

SEE YOUR DOCTOR ...

- If you have any unusual or worrying skin growths, or if a growth changes size or colour.

- If a wart develops after you reach the age of 45.

- If a wart is larger than the size of a pencil rubber; bleeds, hurts or interferes with daily tasks; or if it is located in the genital area.

- If a wart does not respond to self-care within 12 weeks.

REMINDER: If you have a medical condition, consult your doctor before taking supplements.

What they are

Although warts and verrucas may look unpleasant they are normally harmless. These small growths are areas of skin which have grown more quickly than the rest of the skin and become toughened as the result of a virus. There are many different kinds, including common warts, which are usually found on the fingers or hands, and verrucas, which appear on the feet. Genital warts are considered to be more serious than the other types because they may be linked to an increased risk of skin, cervical or penile cancers.

What causes them

Warts and verrucas are formed when a human papilloma virus, of which there are dozens of different types, invades the top layer of skin. Normally the virus is transmitted by direct contact and enters through a small cut or abrasion. Genital warts are the most common form of sexually transmitted disease. Once infection has taken place, it may take months, or sometimes several years, for a wart to appear. This means that a person does not need to have warts to transmit the virus. Low immunity may play a role in activating the wart virus and causing the growths to emerge.

How supplements can help

Warts often develop in response to a depressed immune system, so take a multivitamin and multimineral formula alongside immune-boosting **mixed carotenoids** and **vitamin C**, which may help to eliminate the growths and, taken long term, may prevent recurrences. In addition, try a

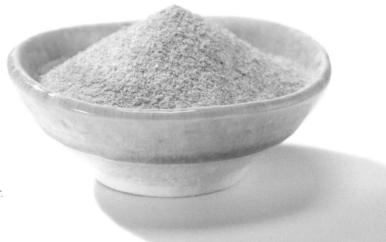

Mixed with a little water and applied to a compress, vitamin C in powder form may help warts to disappear.

Mixed carotenoids	**Dosage:** 15 mg twice a day. **Caution:** use only the natural form of beta-carotene.
Vitamin C	**Dosage:** 500 mg twice a day. **Advice:** reduce dose if diarrhoea develops; you can also mix ½ teaspoon of powdered vitamin C with a little water and apply as a skin compress twice a day.
Vitamin E	**Dosage:** break open a capsule; add contents to a skin compress. **Advice:** apply at bedtime and take off in morning until wart heals.
Garlic oil	**Dosage:** moisten a skin compress with the oil. **Advice:** apply at bedtime and take off in morning until wart heals.
Tea tree oil	**Dosage:** put several drops on a skin compress. **Advice:** apply at bedtime and take off in morning until wart heals.
Goldenseal	**Dosage:** soak a skin compress with tincture. **Advice:** apply at bedtime and take off in morning until wart heals; can also be applied directly to the wart several times a day.
Pau d'arco	**Dosage:** soak a skin compress with tincture. **Advice:** apply at bedtime and take off in morning until wart heals.
Aloe vera gel	**Dosage:** put dab of gel on skin compress. **Advice:** use fresh aloe leaf or shop-bought gel.

Note: consider using supplements in blue first; those in black may also be beneficial. Some dosages may be supplied by supplements you are already taking – see page 195.

topical treatment such as: **vitamin E**, **garlic oil** or **tea tree oil**, **goldenseal** or **pau d'arco** tincture or **aloe vera gel**. Powdered vitamin C mixed with water can also be used topically. Apply these treatments with a skin compress of cotton wool or gauze. The herbs contain virus-fighting ingredients, and vitamins C and E promote healing. If skin irritation develops, dilute the preparation with water or vegetable oil and protect the surrounding skin with petroleum jelly. Always dilute preparations if you are applying them to the genital area. Change the compresses daily. Benefits should occur in three or four days; continue treatment until the wart heals. Other supplements that can be applied as compresses are castor oil (mix with a little bicarbonate of soda) and oil of cloves. Consult your doctor before trying these, especially in the case of genital warts.

What else you can do

☑ Wear flip-flops or sandals if you visit a gym or swimming pool. Some verruca viruses can be picked up from communal changing-room floors.
☑ Persistent warts or verrucas may need prescription wart removers, or freezing, burning or laser treatment conducted by a doctor or chiropodist.
☑ Echinacea is effective in building up the immune system, which may be weakened, especially if you have several warts. Apply directly to the affected area or take 200 mg three or four times a day.
☑ For stubborn warts, soak the affected area in very warm water for about 20 minutes before applying a topical treatment. Soaking may help the remedy to penetrate the skin.

Can alcohol make you more susceptible to genital warts? Researchers in Seattle, USA – after taking into account diet, sexual behaviour and other possible contributory factors – found that those who drank two to four alcoholic beverages a week doubled their risk of genital warts. Five or more drinks a week further increased risks.

Another recent study points to smoking as a possible risk factor for genital warts. Women who smoked were five times more likely to develop genital warts than nonsmokers.

FACTS & TIPS

■ Over-the-counter wart remedies are sometimes effective, but be careful – and never use them on the sensitive genital area. They can contain harsh chemicals that are much more likely than natural supplements to irritate the skin.

■ If warts are on the face, legs or other areas that may be shaved, avoid straight razors, which can cause them to spread. Try an electric shaver or a depilatory. Cutting or scratching a wart can result in bleeding, infection and scarring.

■ Cutting a wart will not cause it to disappear because the virus will still be present in the skin.

Drug interactions

Vitamins, minerals and other supplements are not safe to use in all circumstances. Some may interact adversely with prescription or over-the-counter (OTC) drugs, intensifying the action of the medications or even producing dangerous side effects.

This section lists most of the popular classes of drug and highlights reactions that may occur when specific supplements interact with them. Few studies have been done to determine the risks involved in taking supplements and medications together. Further research is needed, and caution is always advisable when combining any supplements with drugs.

To find out more about specific supplements listed here, refer to the individual entries in the A-Z of supplements on pages 38–193 of this book.

CHECKING FOR POSSIBLE INTERACTIONS

If you are taking a drug for a particular condition, scan the general categories listed alphabetically on the right to see if your drug presents a potential problem if used together with a particular supplement.

The most popular members of each drug class are listed by generic name, but not every drug in the group is included. (If you have any questions, consult your doctor or pharmacist.) Remember that all drugs within a category are likely to have similar interactions. Even if you don't see the name of your particular medication listed, the interaction may nevertheless apply to all the drugs in that class.

CONSULTING YOUR DOCTOR

Unless your doctor recommends it, avoid taking drugs and supplements with similar effects. For example, if you are using a herb such as kava or valerian to treat insomnia, it may induce excessive sleepiness when combined with a conventional sleeping aid or with any drug that can cause drowsiness – a narcotic pain reliever, an OTC antihistamine, or even alcohol.

Similarly, if you are already taking a prescription antidepressant, a nutritional supplement that affects brain chemicals and enhances mood, such as 5-HTP, is best tried only under the supervision of a doctor.

If you are taking any type of prescription drug you should not stop taking it without your doctor's advice or consent. If you have a medical or psychiatric condition, or are taking any prescription or OTC medication, always consult your doctor or pharmacist before trying any herb or supplement.

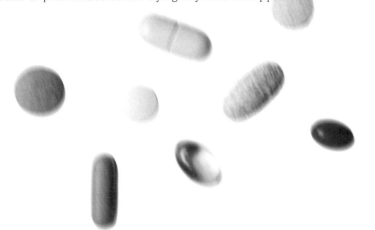

GENERAL CAUTIONS

Listed below are supplements that require special caution if you are taking particular conventional drugs.

■ **BETAINE HCl** increases levels of digestive acids in the stomach. It is essential that people taking aspirin or other anti-inflammatory medicines (NSAIDs) avoid this supplement, because in combination they increase the risk of stomach bleeding.

■ **GYMNEMA SYLVESTRE** may alter required dosages for insulin or oral diabetes drugs; consult your doctor before taking this herb with any medication for diabetes.

■ **LIQUORICE** can increase blood pressure and should be avoided by people taking drugs to counteract high blood pressure or any medication that alters blood pressure; take deglycyrrhised liquorice (DGL) instead.

■ **PSYLLIUM** should not be used within two hours of taking any drug because it may delay absorption of that medication.

■ **ST JOHN'S WORT** interacts with several medicines, and can increase or decrease their effectiveness. Consult your doctor before taking this herb with any other medication or supplement.

■ **VALERIAN** may cause excessive drowsiness in those people who are also using sedatives or drugs with sedative effects.

ACNE DRUGS

Isotretinoin and other acne drugs

Supplement interactions:

■ **VITAMIN A** if taken together with acne drugs, may cause high blood levels of vitamin A, increasing the chance of side effects.

ANTACIDS

All antacids

Supplement interactions:

■ **FOLIC ACID** absorption is decreased by antacids; take folic acid supplements either two hours before or two hours after an antacid.

ANTIBIOTICS

All oral antibiotics

Supplement interactions:

■ **IRON** may make the antibiotic less effective; take iron supplements either two hours before or two hours after the drug.

Doxycycline, Minocycline and Tetracycline

Supplement interactions:

■ **BROMELAIN** may enhance absorption of amoxicillin, which is not necessarily a negative effect.

■ **CALCIUM** may decrease absorption of the drug; avoid taking calcium within one to three hours of taking any of these antibiotics.

■ **IRON** may make the antibiotic less effective; take iron supplements either two hours before or two hours after the drug.

■ **MAGNESIUM** may make the antibiotic less effective; take magnesium supplements one to three hours before or after the drug.

■ **PSYLLIUM** may make the antibiotic less effective; consult your doctor.

■ **VITAMIN C** may enhance absorption of tetracycline, which is not necessarily a negative effect.

■ **ZINC** may make the antibiotic less effective; take zinc supplements at least two hours after the drug.

ANTICOAGULANTS

Enoxaparin, Warfarin and other anti-coagulants (*blood thinners*)

Supplement interactions:

■ **BROMELAIN** use with caution; intensifies the blood-thinning effect of the medication; may lead to excessive bleeding.

■ **FEVERFEW** use with caution; intensifies the blood-thinning effect of the medication; may lead to excessive bleeding.

■ **FISH OILS** use with caution; intensifies the blood-thinning effect of the medication; may eventually lead to internal or excessive bleeding.

■ **GARLIC** may intensify the blood-thinning effect of the medication; consult your doctor before taking the two together.

■ **MEDICINAL MUSHROOMS** reishi mushrooms may intensify the blood-thinning effect of the medication; consult your doctor.

■ **PAU D'ARCO** use with caution; intensifies the blood-thinning effect of the medication; may lead to excessive bleeding.

■ **ST JOHN'S WORT** may enhance liver function, and could also reduce the effectiveness of anticoagulants; consult your doctor before taking this herb.

■ **VITAMIN E** may intensify the blood-thinning effect of the medication; consult your doctor before taking together.

■ **VITAMIN K** may counteract the effects of the medication.

ANTIDEPRESSANTS

Prozac and other antidepressants

Supplement interactions:

■ **5-HTP** avoid taking within four weeks of using a monoamine-oxidase (MAO) inhibitor; may cause anxiety, confusion and other potentially serious side effects; consult your doctor before combining with conventional antidepressants.

■ **GINSENG (PANAX)** consult your doctor if you are taking an MAO inhibitor.

■ **ST JOHN'S WORT** taking this herb with conventional antidepressants may lead to adverse reactions; consult your doctor.

ANTIHISTAMINES

Supplement interactions:

■ **5-HTP, VALERIAN** any of these may cause excessive drowsiness when taken with sedative anti-histamines.

CHOLESTEROL DRUGS

Atorvastatin, Lovastatin, Simvastatin and other 'statin' drugs

Supplement interactions:

■ **SOLUBLE FIBRE** may reduce absorption of these drugs; avoid excessive consumption.

COLD REMEDIES

OTC Prescription remedies containing ephedrine or pseudephedrine

Supplement interactions:

■ **5-HTP** may cause anxiety, confusion or other serious side effects if taken with these cold remedies; use with caution.

DIABETES DRUGS

Insulin and oral diabetes drugs

Supplement interactions:

■ **ALPHA-LIPOIC ACID** long-term use of supplements may require a change in dosage of insulin or diabetes medication.

■ **CAT'S CLAW** do not take with glipizide; adverse effects have been reported.

■ **CHROMIUM** may alter required dosages of insulin or other drugs; consult your doctor.

■ **DANDELION** use with caution; may intensify the blood-sugar-lowering effect of glipizide.

■ **GINSENG (PANAX)** long-term use of supplements may require a change in the dosage of insulin or other diabetes medications; check with your doctor.

■ **GINSENG (SIBERIAN)** use with caution; may intensify the blood-sugar-lowering effect of glipizide.

■ **GYMNEMA SYLVESTRE** may require a change in the dosage of insulin or other diabetes medications; consult your doctor.

DIURETICS

Amiloride, Spironolactone and Triamterene (*potassium-sparing diuretics*)

Supplement interactions:

■ **PHOSPHORUS** when used with phosphates containing potassium, phosphorus may increase the risk of hyperkalaemia (too much potassium in the blood), possibly leading to serious side effects; consult your doctor before taking together.

■ **POTASSIUM** do not take with diuretics; may increase the risk of hyperkalaemia (too much potassium in the blood), possibly leading to serious side effects.

Bumetanide, Ethacrynic acid, Furosemide and Torsemide (*loop diuretics*)
Supplement interactions:

■ **DANDELION** may boost the diuretic effects of these drugs when taken in high doses.

■ **GINSENG (PANAX)** if you are taking furosemide, may intensify the blood-pressure-lowering effects of the drug.

■ **GLUCOSAMINE** higher doses of the diuretic may be necessary.

Chlorothiazide, Hydrochlorothiazide and Indapamide (*thiazide diuretics*)
Supplement interactions:

■ **CALCIUM** may cause build-up of excessive, possibly toxic, calcium levels in the body, leading to kidney failure, if taken with a thiazide diuretic; consult your doctor.

■ **DANDELION** may boost the diuretic effects of these drugs when taken in high doses.

■ **GLUCOSAMINE** higher doses of the drug may be necessary.

■ **LIQUORICE** may lead to dangerously low levels of potassium in the body; deglycyrrhised liquorice (DGL) should be taken instead.

■ **POTASSIUM** if taking together with thiazide diuretic, do not suddenly discontinue the use of the diuretic; it may cause hyperkalaemia (too much potassium in the blood), possibly resulting in serious side effects.

■ **VITAMIN D** may cause build-up of excessive – possibly toxic – levels of calcium in the body, resulting in kidney failure; consult your doctor.

HEART/BLOOD PRESSURE DRUGS
All antihypertensives
Supplement interactions:

■ **BLACK COHOSH** may intensify the drug's effect of lowering blood pressure.

■ **CALCIUM SUPPLEMENTS** may reduce blood pressure; consult your doctor.

■ **GARLIC** may increase the potency of blood pressure medication; consult your doctor.

■ **GINSENG (PANAX OR SIBERIAN)** consult your doctor if you are taking blood pressure medications.

■ **HAWTHORN** may intensify the drug's effect of lowering blood pressure. A lower dose of the medication may be advisable; consult your doctor.

■ **VITAMIN D** may reduce blood pressure; consult your doctor.

Amlodipine, Diltiazem, Verapamil and other calcium channel blockers
Supplement interactions:

■ **FLAVONOIDS** when using a calcium channel blocker do not take a citrus bioflavonoid preparation containing naringin (a flavonoid that is present in grapefruit but not in oranges).

Benazepril, Enalapril, Fosinopril and other ACE inhibitors
Supplement interactions:

■ **PHOSPHORUS** do not take together; when used with phosphates containing potassium, may increase

the risk of hyperkalaemia (too much potassium in the blood) and lead to serious side effects.

■ **POTASSIUM** do not take together; may increase the risk of hyperkalaemia (too much potassium in the blood) and lead to serious side effects.

Digitoxin and Digoxin (*digitalis drugs, cardiac glycosides*)
Supplement interactions:

■ **GINSENG (SIBERIAN)** increases medication levels needed; consult your doctor before using them together.

■ **HAWTHORN** may intensify the drug's effect of lowering blood pressure, so a lower dose of the medication may be advisable; consult your doctor.

■ **PHOSPHORUS** using digitalis with phosphates containing potassium may increase the risk of hyperkalaemia (too much potassium in the blood), possibly leading to serious side effects; consult your doctor.

■ **POTASSIUM** when taken together, may increase the risk of hyperkalaemia (too much potassium in the blood), possibly leading to serious side effects; consult your doctor before taking together.

Amyl nitrite, Isosorbide mononitrate or dinitrate and Nitroglycerin (*Nitrates*)
Supplement interactions:

■ **NAC (N-ACETYLCYSTEINE)** do not take with nitrates; this may cause severe headaches.

MUSCLE RELAXANTS
Carisoprodol, Cyclobenzaprine and other muscle relaxants
Supplement interactions:

■ **5-HTP, VALERIAN** either of these may cause excessive drowsiness when taken with muscle relaxants.

NARCOTIC PAIN RELIEVERS
Codeine, Hydrocodone/ Acetaminophen and other narcotic analgesics
Supplement interactions:

■ **5-HTP, VALERIAN** either of these may cause excessive drowsiness when taken with narcotic pain relievers.

NEUROLOGY DRUGS
Methylphenidate (*Ritalin*) and other nervous system stimulants
Supplement interactions:

■ **FLAVONOIDS** use with caution when taking a citrus bioflavonoid preparation containing naringin (a flavonoid present in grapefruit but not in oranges) with methylphenidate.

■ **GINSENG (PANAX)** increases the risk of over-stimulation of the nervous system and stomach upset.

NONSTEROIDAL ANTI-INFLAMMATORY DRUGS (NSAIDs)
Etodolac, Ibuprofen, Ketoprofen, Naproxen and other NSAIDs
Supplement interactions:

■ **BETAINE HCl** do not take together; increases the risk of potentially serious stomach bleeding.

■ **PHOSPHORUS** when used with phosphates containing potassium, may increase the risk of hyperkalaemia (too much potassium in the blood), possibly leading to serious side effects; consult your doctor before taking with NSAIDs.

■ **POTASSIUM** when taken together, may increase the risk of hyperkalaemia (too much potassium in the blood), possibly leading to serious side effects; consult your doctor.

Aspirin
Supplement interactions:

■ **BETAINE HCI** do not take together; increases the risk of potentially serious stomach bleeding.

■ **FEVERFEW** intensifies the blood-thinning effect of long-term aspirin use; may lead to excessive bleeding.

■ **FISH OILS** intensify the blood-thinning effect of long-term aspirin use; may lead to internal or excessive bleeding.

■ **GARLIC** may increase the blood-thinning effect of long-term aspirin use; consult your doctor.

■ **GINKGO BILOBA** intensifies the blood-thinning effect of long-term aspirin use; may lead to excessive bleeding.

■ **MEDICINAL MUSHROOMS** reishi mushrooms may intensify the blood-thinning effect of long-term aspirin use; consult your doctor.

■ **VITAMIN E** intensifies the blood-thinning effect caused by long-term aspirin use, and may lead to excessive bleeding.

■ **VITAMIN K** may counteract the blood-thinning effect of long-term aspirin use.

OBSTETRIC AND GYNAECOLOGICAL DRUGS
Conjugated oestrogens, Oestrogen-progestogen products and other female hormones
Supplement interactions:

■ **BLACK COHOSH** may interact adversely when taken together; consult your doctor.

■ **CAT'S CLAW** use with caution; may affect levels of female sex hormones.

■ **FLAVONOIDS** use with caution when taking a citrus bioflavonoid preparation containing naringin (a flavonoid which is present in grapefruit but not in oranges) together with oestrogens.

■ **ST JOHN'S WORT** may enhance liver function, resulting in decreased levels of oestrogen in the blood; consult your doctor before taking this herb.

Oral contraceptives (*combination oestrogen-progestogen products*)
Supplement interactions:

■ **BLACK COHOSH** may interact adversely; consult your doctor.

■ **CAT'S CLAW** use with caution; may affect levels of female sex hormones.

■ **ST JOHN'S WORT** may enhance liver function, resulting in decreased levels of oestrogen in the blood; consult your doctor before taking this herb.

PARKINSON'S DISEASE DRUGS
Levodopa
Supplement interactions:

■ **5-HTP** may cause anxiety, confusion and other serious side effects when taken together; consult your doctor.

■ **VITAMIN B6** may prevent the medication from working properly.

PSYCHIATRIC DRUGS
Antipsychotics
Supplement interactions:

■ **GINSENG (PANAX)** consult your doctor if you are taking antipsychotics.

Buspirone (*anti-anxiety*)
Supplement interactions:

■ **5-HTP** may cause anxiety, confusion and other serious side effects when taken together; consult your doctor.

Lithium (*antimanic agent*)
Supplement interactions:

■ **5-HTP** may cause anxiety, confusion and other serious side effects when taken together; consult your doctor.

SEDATIVES AND TRANQUILLISERS
Sleeping aids and other sedatives
Supplement interactions:

■ **BLACK COHOSH, 5-HTP, VALERIAN** any of these may cause excessive drowsiness when taken with sedatives.

SEIZURE /EPILEPSY DRUGS
Carbamazepine, Gabapentin, Phenytoin and other anticonvulsants
Supplement interactions:

■ **FOLIC ACID** has been shown to interfere with some anticonvulsants when consumed in amounts exceeding a total daily dose of 1 mg; let your doctor know if you are taking folic acid and never exceed recommended dosages.

STEROIDS
Beclomethasone, Methylprednisolone, Prednisone and other oral corticosteroids
Supplement interactions:

■ **BETAINE HCI** do not take together.

■ **GINSENG (PANAX)** use with caution; may interact when taken together.

THYROID DRUGS
Methimazol and Propylthiouracil
Supplement interactions:

■ **IODINE** may decrease effectiveness of these and other antithyroid agents.

■ **KELP** taking high doses could provide too much iodine and interfere with the actions of these medications.

TRANSPLANT DRUGS
Cyclosporine and other immunosuppressants
Supplement interactions:

■ **FLAVONOIDS** do not take a citrus bioflavonoid preparation containing naringin (a flavonoid present in grapefruit but not in oranges) when using an immunosuppressant.

■ **ST JOHN'S WORT** may enhance liver function, and could reduce levels of immunosuppressive drugs; consult your doctor before taking this herb.

Useful addresses

The following organisations can provide information about nutritional and herbal therapies and practitioners.

BRITISH NUTRITION FOUNDATION
High Holborn House
52-54 High Holborn
London WC1V 6RQ
020 7404 6504
www.nutrition.org.uk
Provides fact sheets on various aspects of nutrition, but does not give nutritional advice to individuals.

BRITISH SOCIETY FOR ECOLOGICAL MEDICINE
PO Box 7
Knighton LD7 1WT
01547 550378
www.bsaenm.org
Society of doctors who emphasise the importance of nutritional therapy.

COMPLEMENTARY MEDICAL ASSOCIATION
67 Eagle Heights
The Falcons
Bramlands Close
London SW11 2LJ
0845 129 8434
www.the-cma.org.uk
Runs a free referral scheme for registered practitioners. Send two loose first-class stamps for details of qualified and insured practitioners in your area.

GENERAL COUNCIL AND REGISTER OF NATUROPATHS
Goswell House Clinic
2 Goswell Road
Street, Somerset BA16 OJG
0870 7456 984
www.naturopathy.org.uk
Provides a register of naturopaths, downloadable from the web site or by post from the secretary.

INSTITUTE FOR COMPLEMENTARY MEDICINE
PO Box 194
London SE16 7QZ
020 7237 5165
www.i-c-m.org.uk
Provides information and has a searchable online database of accredited practitioners in a variety of disciplines.

INSTITUTE FOR OPTIMUM NUTRITION
Avalon House
72 Mortlake Road
Richmond, Surrey TW9 2JY
0870 979 1122
www.ion.ac.uk
Educational trust offering an information service and a membership scheme.

INTERNATIONAL REGISTER OF CONSULTANT HERBALISTS AND HOMEOPATHS
32 King Edward Road
Swansea SA1 4LL
01792 655886
www.irch.org
Can provide a list of qualified practitioners.

NATIONAL INSTITUTE FOR MEDICAL HERBALISTS
Elm House
54 Mary Arches Street
Exeter EX4 3BA
01392 426022
www.nimh.org.uk
Can provide a list of qualified practitioners.

NUTRITION SOCIETY
10 Cambridge Court
210 Shepherds Bush Road
London W6 7NJ
020 7602 0228
www.nutritionsociety.org
Academic society which publishes scientific journals including the British Journal of Nutrition, which is also available on its web site.

The organisations listed below can give information, advice and support in relation to specific ailments.

ALLERGY UK
3 White Oak Square
London Road
Swanley, Kent BR8 7AG
01322 619898
www.allergyuk.org
Runs a helpline offering support, details of your nearest allergy clinic, self-help and fact sheets.

ALZHEIMER'S SOCIETY
Gordon House
10 Greencoat Place
London SW1P 1PH
0207 306 0606
www.alzheimers.org.uk
Book ordering and library service, leaflets, information and advice.

ARTHRITIC ASSOCIATION
One Upperton Gardens
Eastbourne BN21 2AA
01323 416550
0800 652 3188: freefone
www.arthriticassociation.org.uk
Offers membership and support, and gives advice on a home treatment plan using natural methods.

BRITISH ASSOCIATION OF DERMATOLOGISTS
4 Fitzroy Square
London W1T 5HQ
020 7383 0266
www.bad.org.uk
Provides a list of registered dermatologists; telephone callers only.

DIABETES UK
Macleod House
10 Parkway
London NW1 7AA
www.diabetes.org.uk
020 7424 1000: enquiries
0845 1202 960: careline

FORESIGHT
Association for the Promotion of Preconceptual Care
178 Hawthorn Road
West Bognor
West Sussex PO21 2UY
01243 868001
www.foresight-preconception.org.uk
Advice on all aspects of preparing for pregnancy.

IBS (IRRITABLE BOWEL SYNDROME) NETWORK
Unit 5, 53 Mowbray Street
Sheffield S3 8EN
0114 272 3253: helpline
www.ibsnetwork.org.uk
An independent self-help group offering membership, advice, support and useful publications.

ME (MYALGIC ENCEPHALOMYELITIS) ASSOCIATION
4 Top Angel
Buckingham Industrial Park
Buckingham
Bucks MK18 1TH
0870 444 8233: info line
www.meassociation.org.uk
'Listening Ear' programme for people who need some- one to talk to (afternoons, evenings and weekends).

NATIONAL ASSOCIATION FOR COLITIS AND CROHN'S DISEASE
4 Beaumont House
St Albans, Herts AL1 5HH
0845 130 2233
www.nacc.org.uk
National charity supplying information and support.

NATIONAL ECZEMA SOCIETY
www.eczema.org.uk
email: info@eczema.org.uk
Online information and advice.

NATIONAL MULTIPLE SCLEROSIS SOCIETY
MS National Centre
372 Edgware Road
London NW2 6ND
0208 438 0700
0808 800 8000: helpline
www.mssociety.org.uk
Information and support for
people with MS and their
families.

PARKINSON'S DISEASE SOCIETY
United Scientific House
215 Vauxhall Bridge Road
London SW1V 1EJ
020 7931 8080
0808 800 0303: helpline
www.parkinsons.org.uk
Support group and
information service.

RAYNAUD'S AND SCLERODERMA ASSOCIATION
112 Crewe Road
Alsager
Cheshire ST7 2JA
01270 872776
www.raynauds.org.uk
Information pack, details of
heating aids, research and
treatment programme.

Suppliers of supplements and other products
HEALTH PLUS
Dolphin House
27 Cradle Hill Ind. Estate
Seaford
East Sussex BN25 3JE
01323 872277
www.healthplus.co.uk
Mail order service.

HIGHER NATURE
Burwash Common
East Sussex TN19 7LX
01435 883484
www.highernature.co.uk
Supplies supplements and
some books by mail order.

NATURE'S BEST
Century Place
Tunbridge Wells TN2 3BE
01892 552118

01892 552175: nutrition advice
www.naturesbest.co.uk
Vitamins and minerals by
mail order.

THE NUTRI CENTRE
7 Park Crescent
London W1B 1PF
020 7436 5122
www.nutricentre.com
Supplies supplements,
including DGL chewable
liquorice tablets and
homeopathic remedies.

SOLGAR
Beggars Lane
Aldbury
Tring
Herts HP23 5PT
01442 890355
www.solgar.com
Contact for information on
local stockists (does not
supply direct).

Other useful organisations
THE SOIL ASSOCIATION
Bristol House
40-56 Victoria Street
Bristol BS1 6BY
0117 314 5000
www.soilassociation.org
Provides list of organic
suppliers.

BREAKSPEAR HOSPITAL
Hertfordshire House
Wood Lane
Hemel Hempstead
Herts HP2 4FD
01442 262333
www.breakspearmedical.com
Private hospital offering
treatment for allergies and
environmentally induced
conditions with emphasis on
nutrition and supplements.

WEB SITES
*It can be dangerous to follow
medical advice given on the
internet without first
consulting your doctor. Sites
run by well established
organisations are likely to be
more reliable than those*

*hosted by individuals. Many
of the web sites listed have
searchable databases, links
to other relevant sites and
up-to-date information on
specific ailments or nutritional and herbal medicine in
general.*

www.bmj.com
Current and archived issues
of the *British Medical Journal*
with searchable topics and
links to related sites.

www.healthcentre.org.uk
Medical information site with
some 4000 links to mostly UK
sites covering a wide range of
medical topics. Maintained
by a GP in North Yorkshire.

www.healthfinder.gov
User-friendly US site with
information on particular
ailments and family health.

www.healthnotes.com
US complementary and
integrative medicine site,
with information on drug and
nutrient interactions and
details of research on herbal
medicine and nutrition.

www.hebs.scot.nhs.uk
Information from the Health
Education Board in Scotland,
with a virtual health centre,
searchable database of
health information and
advice about diet and drugs.

www.hsis.org
Health suppliers' information
service for consumers and
the media, with details
of specific supplements,
information about
supplement myths and
facts, and useful links.
Coordinated by the
Proprietary Association of
Great Britain.

www.immunesupport.com
US site for sufferers from

chronic fatigue syndrome
and fibromyalgia; includes
directory of support groups

www.inciid.org
Site for the International
Council on Infertility, based
in the USA, offering fact
sheets and a global directory
of professionals in the field.

www.mca.gov.uk
A government site belonging
to the Medicines and Healthcare products Regulatory
Agency (MHRA) dedicated to
safety issues associated with
herbal medicines. Gives
general advice on the use
of herbal remedies and also
covers specific safety issues.

www.nhsdirect.nhs.uk
National Health Service site,
covering the latest health
stories and practical advice
for healthy living and treating
minor ailments at home,
with a 24 hour nurse-led
telephone advice service and
online support.

www.nlm.nih.gov
US National Library of
Medicine site, offering a
searchable library of medical
information with details of
research programmes.
Includes Medline
(registration required), which
has references from more
than 4000 medical journals.

www.patient.co.uk
Site edited by two GPs which
aims to give non-medically
trained individuals
information about health
issues. Includes a section
devoted to vitamins.

www.thinknatural.com
Comprehensive, searchable
UK site with sections on
vitamins, minerals and herbs,
health features and an
online shop.

Glossary

ABSORPTION The uptake by the body of a supplement, drug or other substance through the digestive tract, skin or mucous membranes.

ACUTE Short, severe, not chronic; designates an illness or condition typically lasting no more than a week or two.

AMINO ACIDS Chemical substances from which proteins are built. They are produced in the body and found in foods.

ANTIBIOTIC A drug that kills or inhibits infection-causing bacteria.

ANTICOAGULANT A drug, such as warfarin or aspirin, that deters blood clotting; often used by those at risk of heart attacks. Also known as a blood thinner.

ANTICONVULSANT A drug that prevents seizures; used to treat epilepsy.

ANTIFUNGAL A drug that combats athlete's foot or other infections caused by a fungus.

ANTI-INFLAMMATORY A drug or supplement that fights inflammation, a bodily response to injury or irritation, characterised by redness, heat, swelling and pain.

ANTIOXIDANT A substance that protects cells from the damaging effects of highly reactive molecules called free radicals. Some anti-oxidants are made by the body; others, such as vitamins C and E, are obtained through diet or nutritional supplements.

ANTISEPTIC An infection-fighting herb, drug or other substance.

ANTISPASMODIC A drug or supplement that prevents spasms or cramps in the digestive tract or elsewhere.

ATHEROSCLEROSIS The build-up of cholesterol and other substances in the artery walls ('hardening of the arteries'), leading to heart disease, angina, heart attack, stroke and other ailments.

AUTOIMMUNE DISORDER An ailment, such as lupus or rheumatoid arthritis, in which the immune system mistakenly attacks the body's own healthy tissues.

BETA-BLOCKER A type of drug that affects the heart, blood vessels and other body parts; often prescribed to treat high blood pressure or angina.

BILE A fat-digesting substance produced in the liver, stored in the gallbladder, and released into the intestine when needed.

BOTANICAL A herb or plant with healing properties.

CAPILLARIES Tiny blood vessels that link veins and arteries. In the capillaries oxygen and nutrients are transferred from the blood to the cells, and waste products are removed.

CARTILAGE A dense yet flexible tissue in the joints, spine, throat, ears, nose and other areas. It is not as hard as bone, but it does provide protection and support.

CHOLESTEROL A fat-like substance that circulates in the blood and helps to build cell membranes; high levels can increase the risk of heart attack. *See also* HDL *and* LDL.

CHRONIC Persistent or long term; describes an illness or condition that often requires months or years of treatment.

COENZYME A substance that acts in concert with enzymes to speed up chemical reactions in the body.

COLLAGEN A tough, fibrous protein that provides support throughout the body and helps to form bones, cartilage, skin, joints and other tissues.

COMPLEX A combination of vitamins, minerals, herbs or other nutritional supplements. Examples include vitamin B complex, liver (lipotropic) complex and amino acid complex.

COMPRESS A soft cotton or flannel cloth or piece of gauze that has been soaked in a herbal tea or other healing substance, then folded and placed on the skin to help to reduce inflammation and pain.

DEMENTIA Loss of mental faculties as a result of Alzheimer's disease or other brain impairment.

DIURETIC A substance that draws water from the body tissues and increases the total output of urine.

DOUCHE A herbal tea, acidophilus and water mixture, for example, that can be used to flush the vagina; may be recommended for infections.

ENDORPHINS Natural pain-reducing substances released by the pituitary gland, producing an effect similar to that of narcotic pain relievers.

ENTERIC COATING A protective covering that enables a pill to pass intact through the stomach into the small intestine, where the coating dissolves and the contents are absorbed.

ENZYME A protein that speeds up specific chemical reactions and processes in the body, such as digestion and energy production.

ESSENTIAL FATTY ACIDS (EFAs) The building blocks that the body uses to make fats. To ensure good health the body must obtain various kinds of EFAs through diet or supplements (such as fish oils and flaxseed oil).

ESSENTIAL OIL A concentrated oil extracted from herbs or other plants.

EXPECTORANT A substance that makes it easier to cough up mucus.

EXTRACT A pill, powder, tincture or other form of a herb that contains a concentrated, and usually standard, amount of therapeutic ingredients.

FLAVONOIDS A large group of phytochemicals found in plants. Most are colourless, but some are pigments responsible for the colours of many fruits and vegetables.

FREE RADICALS Highly reactive and unstable molecules, generated in the body, that can damage cells, leading potentially to heart disease, cancer and other ailments. Antioxidants help to minimise the damage they cause.

GDU (GELATIN DIGESTING UNIT) A dosage measure for bromelain, a supplement that can help to reduce pain and inflammation. Potencies of bromelain are based on GDUs or MCUs (milk clotting units – *see below*). One GDU equals 1.5 MCU.

HAEMOGLOBIN The oxygen-carrying component of red blood cells. Made of iron and protein, it transports oxygen from the lungs to the cells.

HDL (HIGH DENSITY LIPOPROTEIN) One of two types of lipoprotein in the blood that transport cholesterol around the body. High levels of HDL – which carries much less fat than LDLs, or low density lipoproteins – signal a lower than average risk of heart disease. HDL cholesterol is also known as 'good' cholesterol. *See also* cholesterol *and* LDL.

HERB A plant or plant part – the leaves, stem, roots, bark, buds or flowers – which can be used for medicinal or other purposes (such as flavouring foods).

HOMOCYSTEINE An amino acid-like substance; high levels in the blood have been linked to heart disease.

HORMONE Any of various chemical messengers (produced by the ovaries, testes, adrenal, pituitary, thyroid and other glands) that have far-reaching effects throughout the body. Hormones regulate everything from growth and tissue repair to metabolism, reproduction and blood pressure, as well as the body's response to stress.

HORMONE REPLACEMENT THERAPY (HRT) The use of supplemental oestrogen and progesterone (in the form of progestogen) – female sex hormones – to relieve the adverse effects of the menopause. The therapy may also help to prevent osteoporosis.

IMMUNE RESPONSE The body's natural defence system against infectious microbes – including disease-causing bacteria and viruses – as well as cancer cells within the body itself.

INSULIN RESISTANCE A condition in which the body's cells do not respond adequately to the hormone insulin. It can lead to higher blood sugar (glucose) levels, increased insulin production by the pancreas and, possibly, diabetes.

INTERFERONS Virus-fighting proteins that are produced by the immune system.

INTERNATIONAL UNIT (IU) A dose of a vitamin that produces a standard physiological response,

irrespective of the chemical form that is administered. (Most commonly used for vitamin E, which has several different chemical forms.)

JAUNDICE A symptom of hepatitis and other liver disorders, marked by a yellow hue to the skin and eyes.

LDL (LOW DENSITY LIPOPROTEIN) One of two types of lipoprotein in the blood that transport cholesterol around the body. LDLs carry about three-quarters of the cholesterol in the blood. High LDL levels usually reflect high cholesterol levels and imply a higher risk of heart disease. LDL cholesterol is also known as 'bad' cholesterol. *See also* cholesterol *and* HDL.

LIPOTROPIC COMBINATION A 'fat-digesting' blend of choline, inositol, methionine, milk thistle and other nutrients used to promote the health of the liver. Also called liver complex.

MACROPHAGE A type of white blood cell that can surround and digest disease-causing bacteria and other foreign microbes.

MCU (MILK CLOTTING UNIT) A dosage measure for bromelain, a supplement that can help to reduce pain and inflammation. *See also* GDU.

METABOLISM The sum of all the chemical changes that occur within the living body. (There are two directions: anabolism is the formation of more complex molecules; catabolism is the formation of less complex molecules.)

MICROGRAM (MCG) A metric measure of weight used in dosages; sometimes denoted by the symbol μ. There are 1000 mcg in 1 milligram (mg).

MINERAL An inorganic substance, such as calcium, found in the earth's crust that plays a crucial role in the human body for enzyme creation, regulation of heart rhythm, bone formation, digestion and other meta-bolic processes.

MIXED AMINO ACIDS A balanced blend (complex) of amino acids, often taken in conjunction with individual amino acid supplements.

MONOAMINE-OXIDASE (MAO) INHIBITOR A specific class of drug used to treat depression, frequently interacting with foods, drugs and supplements.

MUCOUS MEMBRANES The pink, moist, skinlike layers that line the lips, mouth, vagina, eyelids and other body cavities and passages.

NEURALGIA Sharp, some-times severe pain resulting from damage to a nerve and often affecting a specific area of the body, such as the face.

NEUROTRANSMITTER Any of various chemicals found in the brain and throughout the body that transmit signals among nerve cells.

NONSTEROIDAL ANTI-INFLAMMATORY DRUG (NSAID) A drug such as aspirin or ibuprofen that reduces inflammation and pain by blocking the pro-duction of prostaglandins. *See also* prostaglandins.

NUTRITIONAL SUPPLEMENT A nutrient that has been synthesised in the laboratory or extracted from plants or animals for medicinal use.

OESTROGEN A female sex hormone, produced mainly in the ovaries, that helps to regulate menstruation, reproduction and other processes.

OLIGOMERIC PROANTHO-CYANIDIN COMPLEXES (OPCS) A group of anti-oxidant compounds, also called proanthocyanidins – found in pine bark, grape seed extract, green tea, red wine and other substances – that may help to protect against heart and vascular disease.

OVER-THE-COUNTER (OTC) A drug that can be sold without a doctor's prescription.

PHYTOCHEMICALS Substances found in fruits, vegetables, grains, herbs and other plants that may help to protect against cancer, heart disease and other ailments.

PHYTOESTROGENS Compounds present in soya and other plants that have mild oestrogenic properties. They can help to alleviate the symptoms of hormonal imbalance in women, and may reduce the risk of certain cancers.

PLACEBO A substance that contains no medicinal ingredients. Often used in scientific studies as a control so that the effects of the drug or supplement under study can be compared with the untreated body.

POULTICE A soft, moist substance spread between layers of cloth or gauze and applied, usually heated, to the skin. Poultices can be used to reduce pain and inflammation, to treat bruises and to promote the healing of wounds and the extraction of pus.

PROBIOTICS Cultures of 'friendly' bacteria normally found in the intestine. Pro-biotics such as acidophilus and bifidus are consumed to improve digestion by multiplying and restoring the balance of the normal bacterial population of the intestine.

PROGESTERONE A female sex hormone, made by the ovaries, that helps to regulate menstruation. Progesterone belongs to the group of hormones known as progestogens, which are syn-thesised for therapeutic use.

PROLACTIN A hormone secreted by the pituitary gland whose level is raised by stress; prolactin is also involved in promoting lactation.

PROSTAGLANDINS Hormone-like chemicals produced naturally in the body in response to a stimulus. Their wide range of effects include inducing inflammation, stimulating uterine contractions during labour and protecting the lining of the stomach.

RECOMMENDED DAILY ALLOWANCE (RDA) An average of a key nutrient that people should obtain from their diets, established according to European Union regulations. RDAs apply to 'average adults' and take no account of individual nutritional requirements. They are used on labels only; Reference Nutrient Intakes (RNIs) are used for all other purposes.

REFERENCE NUTRIENT INTAKE (RNI) The daily amount of a vitamin or mineral needed by healthy individuals to meet the body's requirements and prevent a deficiency. These guidelines are set by the Department of Health.

STANDARDISED EXTRACT A concentrated form of a herb that contains a set (standardised) level of active ingredients. Standardisation helps to guarantee a consistent dosage strength, or potency, from one batch of herb to the next. Standardised extracts are available only for certain herbs, either as pills or tinctures, or in other forms.

STEROIDS A common name for corticosteroids, inflammation-fighting drugs that are sometimes prescribed to treat allergic reactions, asthma, skin rashes, multiple sclerosis, lupus and other ailments.

SUBLINGUAL Beneath the tongue. Some supplements, such as vitamin B_{12}, are formulated to dissolve in the mouth, allowing swift absorption into the blood-stream. This means that the supplement avoids metabo-lism in the liver, which can reduce circulating levels.

TANNIN An astringent substance derived from plants that can contract blood vessels and body tissues.

TESTOSTERONE The principal male sex hormone, produced in the testes, that induces changes at puberty and helps to build strong muscles and bones. Women also make a small amount of testosterone in their ovaries.

THERAPEUTIC DOSE The amount of a vitamin, mineral, herb, nutritional supplement or drug needed to produce a desired healing effect (as opposed to the minimum amount needed to prevent a deficiency – such as the RNI, for example).

TINCTURE A liquid usually made by soaking a whole herb or its parts in a mixture of water and ethyl alcohol (such as vodka). The alcohol helps to extract the herb's active components, concen-trating and preserving them.

TONIC A herb (such as ginseng) or herbal blend that is used to 'tone' the body or a specific organ, imparting added strength or vitality.

TRICLYCERIDE The chemical term for fat. People who have high triclyceride levels in their blood increase the likelihood of developing heart disease.

VITAMIN An organic substance that plays an essential role in regulating cell functions throughout the body. Most vitamins must be ingested in food or supple-ments because the body cannot produce them.

Index

H

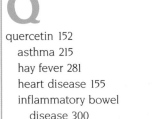

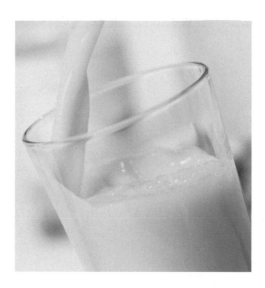

The publishers would like to thank the following for providing the illustrations in Vitamins, Minerals and Supplements. All images are Reader's Digest © except for those from GettyOne Stone, GettyOne Photodisc and Digital Vision

Ian Atkinson:359

Martin Norris:27BC, 28B, 30, 31, 34, 35, 48, 57, 60, 68, 69, 71, 72, 76, 78BR, 82, 91, 104TL, 104BL, 105, 108, 114, 128, 148, 152TL, 156, 162 (pills), 164, 170, 174, 178, 180, 192, 193, 196, 208, 2102, 212, 214, 220, 222, 224, 234, 242, 244, 246, 252, 254, 264, 266, 274, 276, 278, 282, 288, 302, 306, 308, 312, 314, 320, 328, 332, 334, 341, 356, 364, 374, 376, 378, 382, 386, 414

Paul Williams:16

Xavier Young: front cover

Digital Vision: 10, 15, 273, 310BL, 372, 389

GettyOne Photodisc: 13, 19, 20, 21, 22, 23, 24, 27C, 37, 46, 152, 153, 154, 155, 228L, 228BR, 229, 272, 273TR, 310CR, 310BR, 3113, 338, 340, 360, 388BL, 388TL

GettyOne Stone/Augusta Butera 12, **GettyOne Stone/Dale Durfee** 78, **GettyOne Stone/Chris Thomaidis** 341, **GettyOne Stone/David Madison** 358, **GettyOne Stone/Michelangelo Gratton** 361.

All other photographs are by Lisa Koenig

**READER'S DIGEST GUIDE TO
VITAMINS, MINERALS AND SUPPLEMENTS**
was published by
The Reader's Digest Association Limited, London

First edition Copyright © 2000
Paperback edition 2004
Reprinted with amendments 2007

The Reader's Digest Association Limited,
11 Westferry Circus, Canary Wharf, London E14 4HE
www.readersdigest.co.uk

We are committed to both the quality of our
products and the service we provide to our
customers. We value your comments, so please feel
free to contact us on 08705 113366,
or via our web site at www.readersdigest.co.uk
If you have any comments about the content of our
books, you can contact us at
gbeditorial@readersdigest.co.uk

Reader's Digest Association Far East Limited.
Philippines Copyright © 2000
Reader's Digest Association Far East Limited.

PRINTING AND BINDING Mateu Cromo, Madrid

**READER'S DIGEST GUIDE TO
VITAMINS, MINERALS AND SUPPLEMENTS**
was adapted from
The Healing Power of Vitamins, Minerals, and Herbs,
published by Reader's Digest Association Inc.,
Pleasantville, New York. Created by Rebus, Inc.
First edition copyright © 1999

EDITOR Henrietta Heald

ART EDITOR Louise Turpin

EDITORIAL ASSISTANTS Caroline Boucher,
Jenny Rathbone

ADDITIONAL CONSULTANTS Jane McClenaghan,
Fiona Jenkins

WRITERS Margaret Ashwell, Gaynor Bussell
Liz Clasen, Jane Egginton, Sigrid Gibson,
Azmina Govindji, Jane McClenaghan,
Fiona Wilcock

ASSISTANT EDITORS Alison Bravington,
Marion Moisy

DESIGNER Celia Rumley

PHOTOGRAPHERS Lisa Koenig,
Martin Norris

INDEXER AND PROOFREADER Laura Hicks

PROOFREADER Barry Gage

READER'S DIGEST GENERAL BOOKS, LONDON
EDITORIAL DIRECTOR Julian Browne
ART DIRECTOR Nick Clark
MANAGING EDITOR Alastair Holmes
PICTURE RESEARCH EDITOR Sarah Stewart-Richardson

The publishers would like to express their gratitude to
Pamela Mason BSc, MSc, PhD, MRPharmS for her help
in updating the information in the 2004 edition, with
editorial assistance from Jill Steed.

Concept code SA0205/IC
Book Code 400-210 UP0000-2
ISBN (10) 0 276 42930 3
ISBN (13) 978 0 276 42930 9
Oracle Code 250090174S.00.24